Soft Tissue Augmentation

Procedures in Cosmetic Dermatology

Series Editor: Jeffrey S. Dover MD FRCPC
Associate Editor: Murad Alam MD

Botulinum Toxin
Alastair Carruthers MABM BCh FRCPC FRCP(Lon) and Jean Carruthers MD FRCS(C) FRC(OPHTH)
ISBN 1 4160 2470 0

Soft Tissue Augmentation
Jean Carruthers MD FRCS(C) FRC(OPHTH) and Alastair Carruthers MABM BCh FRCPC FRCP(Lon)
ISBN 1 4160 2469 7

Cosmeceuticals
Zoe Diana Draelos MD
ISBN 1 4160 0244 8

Laser and Lights: Volume 1
Vascular • Pigmentation • Scars • Medical Applications
David J. Goldberg MD JD
ISBN 1 4160 2386 0

Laser and Lights: Volume 2
Rejuvenation • Resurfacing • Hair Removal • Treatment of Ethnic Skin
David J. Goldberg MD JD
ISBN 1 4160 2387 9

Photodynamic Therapy
Mitchel P. Goldman MD
ISBN 1 4160 2360 7

Liposuction
C. William Hanke MD MPH FACP and Gerhard Sattler MD
ISBN 1 4160 2208 2

Treatment of Scars
Kenneth A. Arndt MD

Chemical Peels
Mark Rubin MD

Hair Restoration
Dowling B. Stough MD and Robert S. Haber MD

Leg Veins
Tri H. Nguyen MD

Blepharoplasty
Ronald L. Moy MD

Face Lifting
Ronald L. Moy MD

PROCEDURES IN COSMETIC DERMATOLOGY

Series Editor: Jeffrey S. Dover MD FRCPC

Associate Editor: Murad Alam MD

Soft Tissue Augmentation

Edited by

Jean Carruthers MD FRCS(C) FRC(OPHTH)

Clinical Professor, Department of Ophthalmology, University of British Columbia, Vancouver, BC, Canada

Alastair Carruthers MABM BCh FRCPC FRCP(Lon)

Clinical Professor, Division of Dermatology, University of British Columbia, Vancouver, BC, Canada

Series Editor

Jeffrey S. Dover MD FRCPC

Associate Professor of Clinical Dermatology, Yale University School of Medicine, Adjunct Professor of Medicine (Dermatology), Dartmouth Medical School, Director, SkinCare Physicians of Chestnut Hill, Chestnut Hill, MA, USA

Associate Editor

Murad Alam MD

Chief, Section of Cutaneous and Aesthetic Surgery, Department of Dermatology, Northwestern University, Chicago, IL, USA

ELSEVIER
SAUNDERS

ELSEVIER
SAUNDERS
An Imprint of Elsevier Inc.

First published 2005

ISBN-13: 978–1–4160–2469–9
ISBN-10: 1–4160–2469–7

British Library Cataloguing in Publication Data
A catalogue record for this book is available from the British Library

Library of Congress Cataloging-in-Publication Data
A catalog record for this book is available from the Library of Congress

Printed in China

Last digit is the print number: 9 8 7 6 5 4 3

Commissioning Editors: **Sue Hodgson, Shuet-Kei Cheung**
Project Development Managers: **Martin Mellor Publishing Services Ltd, Louise Cook**
Project Managers: **Naughton Project Management, Cheryl Brant**
Illustration Manager: **Mick Ruddy**
Design Manager: **Andy Chapman**
Illustrators: **Richard Prime, Tim Loughhead**

Contents

Series Foreword
Procedures in Cosmetic Dermatology

While dermatologists have been procedurally inclined since the beginning of the specialty, particularly rapid change has occurred in the past quarter century. The advent of frozen section technique and the golden age of Mohs skin cancer surgery has led to the formal incorporation of surgery within the dermatology curriculum. More recently technological breakthroughs in minimally invasive procedural dermatology have offered an aging population new options for improving the appearance of damaged skin.

Procedures for rejuvenating the skin and adjacent regions are actively sought by our patients. Significantly, dermatologists have pioneered devices, technologies and medications, which have continued to evolve at a startling pace. Numerous major advances, including virtually all cutaneous lasers and light-source based procedures, botulinum exotoxin, soft-tissue augmentation, dilute anesthesia liposuction, leg vein treatments, chemical peels, and hair transplants, have been invented, or developed and enhanced by dermatologists. Dermatologists understand procedures, and we have special insight into the structure, function, and working of skin. Cosmetic dermatologists have made rejuvenation accessible to risk-averse patients by emphasizing safety and reducing operative trauma. No specialty is better positioned than dermatology to lead the field of cutaneous surgery while meeting patient needs.

As dermatology grows as a specialty, an ever-increasing proportion of dermatologists will become proficient in the delivery of different procedures. Not all dermatologists will perform all procedures, and some will perform very few, but even the less procedurally directed amongst us must be well-versed in the details to be able to guide and educate our patients. Whether you are a skilled dermatologic surgeon interested in further expanding your surgical repertoire, a complete surgical novice wishing to learn a few simple procedures, or somewhere in between, this book and this series is for you.

The volume you are holding is one of a series entitled "Procedures in Cosmetic Dermatology." The purpose of each book is to serve as a practical primer on a major topic area in procedural dermatology.

If you want make sure you find the right book for your needs, you may wish to know what this book is and what it is not. It is not a comprehensive text grounded in theoretical underpinnings. It is not exhaustively referenced. It is not designed to be a completely unbiased review of the world's literature on the subject. At the same time, it is not an overview of cosmetic procedures that describes these in generalities without providing enough specific information to actually permit someone to perform the procedures. And importantly, it is not so heavy that it can serve as a doorstop or a shelf filler.

What this book and this series offer is a step-by-step, practical guide to performing cutaneous surgical procedures. Each volume in the series has been edited by a known authority in that subfield. Each editor has recruited other equally practical-minded, technically skilled, hands-on clinicians to write the constituent chapters. Most chapters have two authors to ensure that different approaches and a broad range of opinions are incorporated. On the other hand, the two authors and the editors also collectively provide a consistency of tone. A uniform template has been used within each chapter so that the reader will be easily able to navigate all the books in the series. Within every chapter, the authors succinctly tell it like they do it. The emphasis is on therapeutic technique; treatment methods are discussed with an eye to appropriate indications, adverse events, and unusual cases. Finally, this book is short and can be read in its entirety on a long plane ride. We believe that brevity paradoxically results in greater information transfer because cover-to-cover mastery is practicable.

Most of the books in the series are accompanied by a high-quality DVD, demonstrating the procedures discussed in that text. Some of you will turn immediately to the DVD and use the text as a backup to clarify complex points, while others will prefer to read first and then view the DVD to see the steps in action. Choose what suits you best.

We hope you enjoy this book and the rest of the books in the series and that you benefit from the many hours of clinical wisdom that have been distilled to produce it. Please keep it nearby, where you can reach for it when you need it.

Jeffrey S. Dover MD FRCPC and Murad Alam MD

To the women in my life

My grandmothers, Bertha and Lillian
My mother, Nina
My daughters, Sophie and Isabel
And especially to my wife, Tania

For their never-ending encouragement, patience, support, love, and friendship

To my father, Mark
A great teacher and role model

To my mentor, Kenneth A. Arndt for his generosity, kindness, sense of humor, joie de vivre, and above all else curiosity and enthusiasm

At Elsevier, Sue Hodgson who conceptualized the series and brought it to reality

and

Martin Mellor for polite, persistent, and dogged determination.

Jeffrey S. Dover

The professionalism of the dedicated editorial staff at Elsevier has made this ambitious project possible. Guided by the creative vision of Sue Hodgson, Martin Mellor and Shuet-Kei Cheung have attended to the myriad tasks required to produce a state-of-the-art resource. In this, they have been ably supported by the graphics team, which has maintained production quality while ensuring portability. We are also deeply grateful to the volume editors, who have generously found time in their schedules, cheerfully accepted our guidelines, and recruited the most knowledgeable chapter authors. Finally, we thank the chapter contributors, without whose work there would be no books at all. Whatever successes are herein are due to the efforts of the above, and of my teachers, Kenneth Arndt, Jeffrey Dover, Michael Kaminer, Leonard Goldberg, and David Bickers, and of my parents, Rahat and Rehana Alam.

Murad Alam

Preface

A noted non-cosmetic physician, Sigmund Freud, famously said: "Anatomy is Destiny." His point of view was predicated on the difficulty in his day of changing personal anatomical features and patients were sent for psychotherapy. At last now in the twenty-first century, we have the means to expand, support and sculpt faces in safety and with negligible down time for our patients. The panoply of new information on both biodegradable and non-biodegradable fillers is presented in this volume. The esthetic physician can enjoy reading about the concepts of facial esthetics and the tips and tricks that make treatments art rather than just another procedure. We are so very grateful for the expertise and energy of our contributors who have made this excellent volume come to life.

Jean Carruthers and Alastair Carruthers

List of Contributors

Kenneth R. Beer MD FAAD
Voluntary Associate Professor, University of Miami; Director, Palm Beach Esthetic Center, FL, USA

Paul H. Bowman MD
Director, The Bowman Institute for Dermatologic Surgery, Tampa, FL, USA

Alastair Carruthers MABM BCh FRCPC FRCP(Lon)
Clinical Professor, Division of Dermatology, University of British Columbia, Vancouver, BC, Canada

Jean Carruthers MD FRCS(C) FRC(OPHTH)
Clinical Professor, Department of Ophthalmology, University of British Columbia, Vancouver, BC, Canada

Lisa M. Donofrio MD
Associate Clinical Professor, Department of Dermatology, Yale University School of Medicine, New Haven, CT, USA

Hayes B. Gladstone MD
Director, Division of Dermatologic Surgery, Department of Dermatology, Stanford University School of Medicine, Stanford, CA, USA

Richard G. Glogau MD
Clinical Professor of Dermatology, University of California Medical Center, San Francisco, CA, USA

Betty A. Hinderks Davis MD
Fellow in Dermatologic Surgery, Total Skin and Beauty Dermatology Center and Department of Dermatology, University of Alabama at Birmingham, Birmingham, AL, USA

Derek H. Jones MD
Clinical Professor of Medicine, Department of Dermatology, David Geffen School of Medicine, University of California, Los Angeles, CA, USA

Nicholas J. Lowe MD FRCP
Clinical Professor, University of California School of Medicine, Los Angeles, CA, USA; Consultant Dermatologist, Cranley Clinic, London, UK; Clinical Research Specialist, Santa Monica, CA, USA and London, UK

Seth L. Matarasso MD
Clinical Professor of Dermatology, University of California School of Medicine, San Francisco, CA, USA

Gary D. Monheit MD
Associate Professor, Department of Dermatology and Ophthalmology, University of Alabama at Birmingham, Birmingham, AL, USA

Rhoda S. Narins MD PC
Director, Dermatology Surgery and Laser Center, Manhattan and White Plains; Clinical Professor of Dermatology, New York University Medical Center, NY, USA

Vic A. Narurkar MD
Founder and Director, Bay Area Laser Institute, San Francisco; Assistant Clinical Professor of Dermatology, UC Davis Medical School, Sacramento, CA, USA

Joseph Niamtu III DMD
Private Practice, Oral/Maxillofacial & Cosmetic Facial Surgery, Richmond, VA, USA

David S. Orentreich MD
Dermatologist; Academic Appointment Assistant; Clinical Professor of Dermatology, Mount Sinai School of Medicine, New York, NY, USA

Stephen R. Tan MD FRCPC
Director of Dermatologic Surgery, HealthPartners Medical Group and Clinics, Minneapolis, MN, USA

Peggy Wu BS
Research Fellow, Department of Dermatologic Surgery, Stanford University, CA, USA

1 Background Information on the Use of Esthetic Fillers

Hayes B. Gladstone, Peggy Wu, Jean Carruthers

History

Human beings have used personal cosmetic enhancements for thousands of years. Initially, these applications consisted of topical inks derived from plants and animal sources. The advent of surgical procedures became possible in the second half of the 19th century due to the development of local and general anesthesia; esthetic procedures were able to become much more invasive. Initially, fat was grafted to fill volume after trauma. In the 20th century, autologous fat became the most common filler. However, cutting out fat and transplanting it still represented a major procedure, and in most cases, it did not have lasting effects.

With the slowly increasing demand for cosmetic procedures beginning in the 1970s, research into collagen production produced a bovine formulation that could be placed in a syringe and injected. Dermatologists and plastic surgeons helped develop this product, though perhaps because of its more minimally invasive nature, dermatologists such as Sam Stegman and Arnold Klein took the lead in its clinical use.

The temporary nature of bovine collagen and the requirement for double skin testing led to the development and testing of other fillers in Europe and Asia in the 1990s. Public demand was fueled by aging baby boomers demanding procedures with no down time; media hype surrounding 'lunchtime' cosmetic procedures placed fillers on center stage along with botulinum toxin (Botox). Fillers could be used as sculpting agents to dramatically change a person's appearance in a mere 15 minutes. Today, there are a number of fillers to choose from, each with its own strengths, drawbacks and indications. The development of these substances continues, often at a dizzying pace, so it is important for the esthetic specialist physician to understand the indications and uses of these fillers so that he or she can best serve the patient's needs.

Patient Esthetic Evaluation

Though there are different cultural/ethnic norms of beauty, there are certain qualities which seem globally to transcend these differences in determining what is perceptually pleasing. Esthetically pleasing features include symmetry, smooth convex contours, and even, homogeneous skin tone and texture. These features may become disrupted by natural disease such as acne or by environmental agents such as sun exposure or trauma, or merely by the inevitable and natural process of aging. Scars caused by acne or trauma leave depressions of varying depth. Depressions of an entire cosmetic unit may be caused by morphea or that of lipodystrophy secondary to infection with the human immunodeficiency virus (HIV) (Fig. 1.1). Fine rhytides, particularly in the perioral region can be caused by excessive actinic damage. Loss of maxillary and mandibular bone, subcutaneous fat and dermal collagen result in wider lower facial depressions and perioral grooves such as the melolabial and melomental folds. Any line of facial expression becomes accentuated with age, muscular hyperactivity and volume loss. The previous generations of esthetic physicians have depended on the algorithm of surgical skin redraping and tightening. *In the modern esthetic world, restoration of facial volume and contour has become the first line of treatment before surgical correction is entertained.*

Restoration of facial symmetry and volume, as well as a smooth contour and homogeneous skin tone are the newer goals of the cosmetic surgeon. Leonardo da Vinci divided the face into thirds from the hairline to the chin. Horizontally, the face is

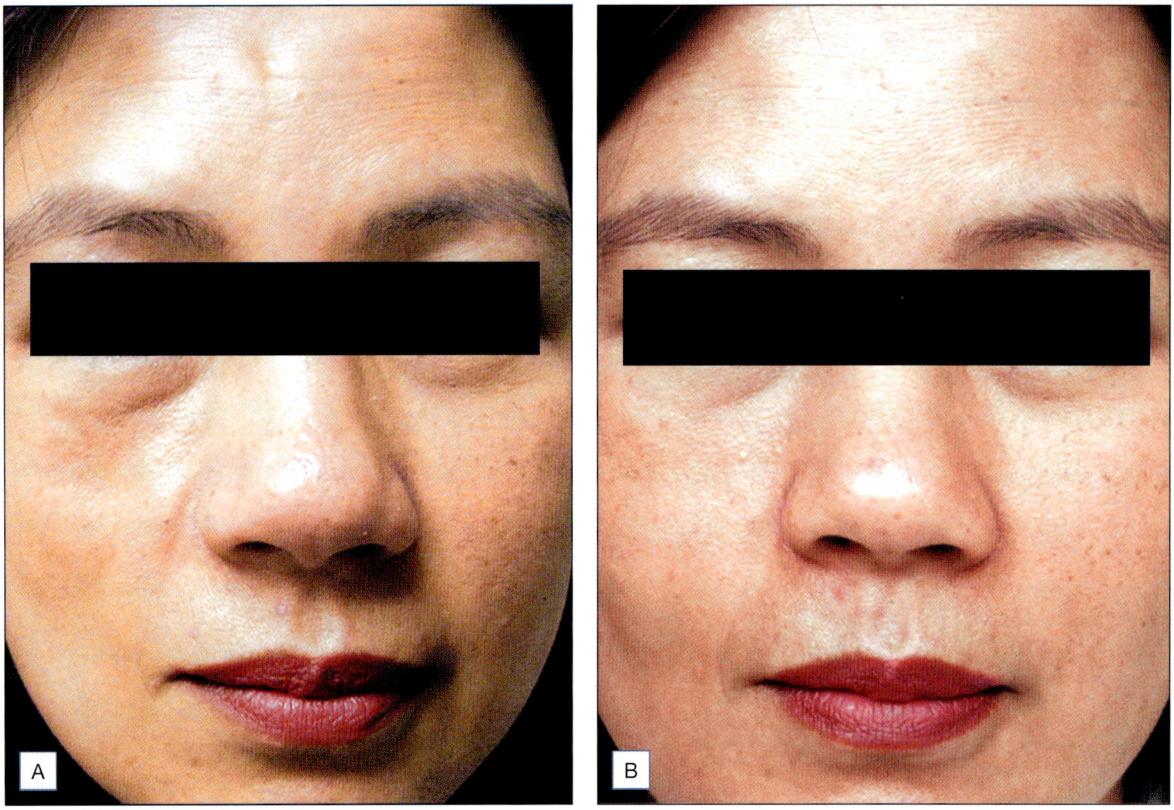

Fig. 1.1 (**A**) Patient with right-sided stable morphea. (**B**) Six months following fat transfer to the right cheek

approximately the width of five eyes. All of these esthetic divisions must be taken into consideration in making an esthetic treatment plan.

The upper, mid and lower face must be in harmony. This is particularly true of the transitions between the different facial zones. In order to achieve these objectives, a comprehensive approach must be taken, and multiple modalities utilized. Fillers play a major role in this process. The appropriate filler can restore symmetry, volume and recreate a smooth skin surface. In combination with other treatments such as chemodenervation with Botox, they may lead to more enhanced esthetic and longer lasting results.

Indications

Fillers have multiple uses, either filling pre-existing facial defects or augmenting existing facial structures. Beginning with the upper third of the face, fillers can be used to fill in depressions in the forehead from acne scars and synergistically, with Botox, to treat deep resting glabellar folds. Injection under the lateral third of the brow will elevate the previously ptotic lateral brow segment. Temporal depression below the temporal fusion line, often associated with age or acquired lipodystrophy, may also be augmented. Esthetic physicians should be aware that glabellar augmentation with deep dermal hyaluronans such as Restylane appear to be safe, unlike injections of autologous fat and bovine collagen, which have caused cases of iatrogenic blindness. In the periorbital region, low viscosity fillers may be used for 'etched-in' crow's feet, particularly those that extend inferior to the inferior orbital margin, past the origin of zygomaticus major on the zygoma.

Some practitioners advocate using filler in the upper eyelid as a substitute for blepharoplasty. In the lower eyelid, restoring this subunit's volume and contour rather than ritually removing fat has become a guiding principle in restoration of the upper third of the face. The appropriate use of a filler can remove the 'double bubble' between the lower eyelid and

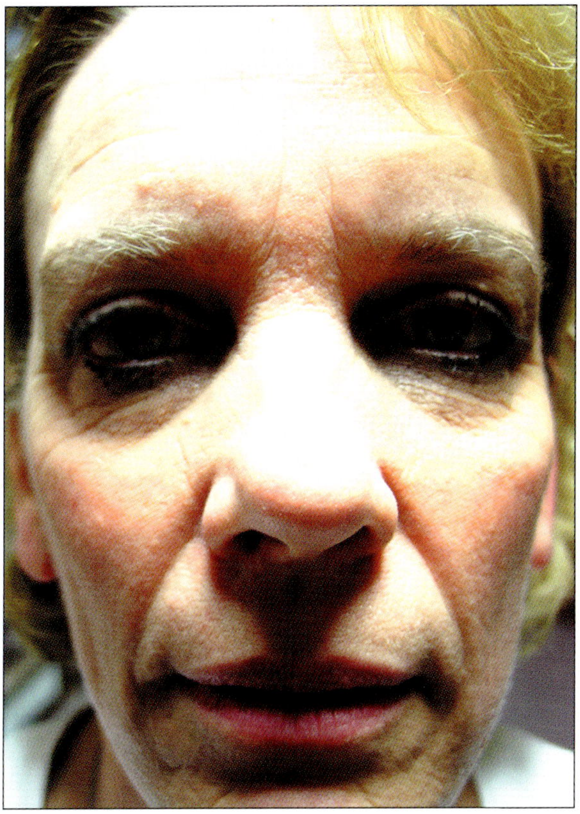

Fig. 1.2 Prominent nasolabial lines that create a sense of age, and are amenable to a filler

the upper cheek as well as filling the lateral and inferior nasojugal groove as it extends into the orbitomalar groove bisecting the malar fat pad. Fillers create a more uniform smoothness in the transition between the upper and midface by effacing the tear trough deformity; the subject promptly loses the tired appearance caused by the dark circles and is provided with a more rested, energized appearance.

In the midface, fillers can be used to fill scars from pre-existing asymmetry, and scars resulting from trauma or acne. Two common features of the aging midface are the sinking and effacing of the malar eminence and hollowing and descent of the cheeks. Fillers can be used to augment this area. The malar region can be directly built up, often by merely adding volume to the cheeks; this will increase the malar prominence and enhance the youthful convex appearance. Similarly, cheek hollowing is often seen in subjects suffering HIV-related facial lipoatrophy. While the thinness of nasal skin may lead to a higher rate of complications or unsatisfactory results, with experience, scars, particularly on the dorsum, can be effectively filled. Occasionally, subscision of the nasal tip to relax skin adhesion to the underlying cartilage is necessary before tip contour can be improved with injected filler.

The most popular anatomic area, and the one with the most prolonged results, is the nasolabial folds (NLFs) also known as 'smile' lines. The NLFs cross the transition zone between the midface and lower face. Though initially, these lines don't truly reflect the aging process, their deepening over time creates an abnormal demarcation between these two major facial regions (Fig. 1.2). The desire of even young patients to fill these lines, which initially are only a function of expression rather than senescence, reflects the esthetic aspiration for a smooth facial contour and the softening of the vertical depth of these lines, which cause a severe and angry facial expression. A variety of fillers can be used to effectively blunt these lines. A secondary effect of filling these lines will be to increase the profile of the medial cheeks, which is also esthetically desirable.

The lower face is dominated by the vermilion lips, both in contour and profile. As time passes, the vertical dimension of the vermilion lip may decrease as the vermilion display turns inside the oral cavity. Fine rhytides in the upper lip allow lipstick to 'bleed' up into the cutaneous lip, thus giving an obvious and 'smudged' appearance to the lip borders. Many types of fillers can be used in the lips to enhance and achieve a natural fullness.

Marionette or 'drool' lines are a combination of expression, aging gravity and genetics. In many individuals, these can be not only quite pronounced, but there may be multiple perioral curvilinear depressions lateral and inferior to the oral commissures. Biomechanically, marionette lines are caused by a loss of volume and support combined with a loss of dermal elasticity. While a variety of fillers can be used to reduce them, in older individuals or those with advanced actinic damage and sagging, filling them may create ripples lateral to the injection area. The concurrent use of neurotoxin relaxation (Botox) of the depressor anguli oris, the mentalis and the orbicularis oris will not only improve the esthetic result but also prolong the longevity of the filler in the highly mobile perioral region.

A sign of aging in the lower face is unevenness of the jawline. This is not only caused by loss of skin elasticity and gravity causing enhancement of the jowl contour, but also because of resorption of the bony mandible and subcutaneous fat. Selective injection of the appropriate filler, particularly in combination with the injection of a supporting strut of filler in the melomental fold and pre-joint sulcus, can create a smooth and robust mandibular line. Though permanent implants are the surgical procedure of choice for increasing chin projection, using injectable filler can create a more prominent chin albeit a temporary one. It may also be useful in allowing the patient to determine if he/she desires a permanent implant.

Pre-Procedure Planning

All patients desiring cosmetic procedures should have a comprehensive medical and social evaluation. This cosmetic evaluation should first address the patient's concerns, discuss the treatment options and devise an overall treatment plan. Subjects may be helped by prioritizing their concerns and their interest in the various treatments to optimize their appearance. During this discussion, subjects can understand the components of facial aging including lines of dynamic expression, static wrinkles and folds caused by photodamage and elastosis of the skin, and loss of posterior tissue support from bone remodeling and fat atrophy. Treatments appropriate for each component should be explained and outlined. This discussion is particularly important because subjects are more accepting of treatments that they understand and have chosen themselves. Many individuals are well informed because of the Media and the Internet. Some patients may be focused on wanting only one treatment even though it may not be appropriate for their concerns. When it is determined that fillers are the appropriate therapy, several alternatives should be discussed and a choice made as to the most appropriate choice. Outlining normal postoperative sequelae such as bruising, lumpiness and swelling is important as well as the pretreatment discussion of possible adverse events. If the filler is being used in an off-label manner, then this fact should also be discussed with the patient.

A complete medical history including medications and allergies should be taken. As with any other elective surgical procedure, the patient should not take aspirin for at least 8 days, or vitamin E, or nonsteroid anti-inflammatory drugs (NSAIDs) for at least 5 days prior to treatment. If the patient is on Coumadin, the prothrombin time (PT) should be checked. Generally if the PT is under 2.0, then the risk of hematoma or excessive bruising from injection is low. It should also be ascertained whether the patient takes herbal medications such as Gingko Biloba since these can cause bleeding. Some homeopathic medications such as Arnica Montana taken preoperatively are believed to reduce consistently bruising, but this has not been demonstrated in clinical studies.

There are very few absolute contraindications to fillers. A patient with a known allergy to a specific filler would obviously not be a candidate for the procedure. Finally, preoperative photos from the frontal, oblique and profile angles are not only important from a medico-legal standpoint, but are also an extremely important part of subsequent patient satisfaction follow-up.

Choosing the appropriate filler

The choice of filling substance to be used is perhaps the most important one after the choice that soft tissue augmentation is to be performed. A confusing array of biodegradable, nonpermanent and nonbiodegradable, permanent substances is available

Biodegradable and nonbiodegradable fillers	
Biodegradable fillers	**Nonbiodegradable fillers**
AcHyal	Aquamid
Alloderm	Artecoll (Artefill in USA)
Autologen	Arteplast
Biocell ultravital	Bioplastique
Cymetra	Evolution
Dermal grafting	Goretex
Dermologen (withdrawn)	Meta-Crill
Dermaplant	Silicone (Adatosil & Silikone 1000)
Endoplast-50	Softform
Fascian	
Fat	
Human placental collagen	
Hyal-system	
Hyalform SP Hylaformgel	**Slowly biodegradable fillers**
Isologen	Radiance
New-Fill (Sculptra)	Sculptra
Perlane	
Permacol	
Plasmagel	
Resoplast	
Restylane	
Restylane-fine/touch	
Reviderm intra	
Surgisis	
Cosmoderm & Cosmoplast	

Table 1.1 Biodegradable and nonbiodegradable fillers

(Table 1.1). Traditional fillers have been biodegradable, i.e. absorbed and ultimately excreted. Though these substances can result in hypersensitivity reactions, they have a proven safety record. The disadvantage to these fillers has been their relatively short duration, in some cases necessitating injections every 3 months. Over the past decade semipermanent fillers have been used in Europe, South America and Asia. Several of these fillers are in the final stages of FDA approval. While they do have a longer effect, they may have an increased incidence of granulomas; in many cases the granulomas are of late onset (more than 1 year after treatment). These fillers tend to have microspheres which are nonbiodegradable. Finally, there are the truly nonbiodegradable, permanent fillers. These substances may play a substantial role in patients with HIV lipoatrophy or stable morphea. Traditionally, they have resulted in a high incidence of granulomas and extrusion, but new formulations may decrease granulomas from these fillers. Ultimately, patient safety is the paramount consideration.

While autologous fat is historically the oldest available filler, bovine collagen in the form of Zyderm I, Zyderm II and Zyplast have been the most frequently used substances until 2003. They can provide excellent results for depressed acne scars, nasolabial folds and lips. The well-known disadvantages of these fillers are the potential for allergic reaction, which necessitates two separate skin tests. Depending on the site, it is rare for collagen to have a significant effect after 6 months. In areas with increased mobility such as the lips, it is unlikely that collagen will remain for more than 3 months. Recently, human collagen has been introduced. It has the advantage of not requiring skin testing, but its duration is similar to its bovine predecessor. There have been other types of collagen derived from cadavers or from the patient. While they also don't require skin testing, their efficacy is similar to that of human collagen. Though, as mentioned earlier, these fillers can be used in a variety of sites, because of their ease of injection and malleability, they offer superior results for lip augmentation.

Fat has been used since the late 19th century, though it has dramatically evolved in its technique, and has enjoyed a revival in its use. Fat has the advantage of volume, and the ease of using large amounts, which makes it very cost effective (Fig. 1.3). It provides excellent volume replacement. It can be used for pan-facial volume restoration. Specifically, it is an excellent substance for the nasolabial folds, cheeks and marionette lines. Because of its volume and viscosity, fine lines and small acne scars would not be appropriate for this filler. Generally, fat is more difficult to use in the lips, though in the hands of an experienced practitioner, it can provide outstanding results. The disadvantages of using fat are that the patient must have areas of fat deposits, and fat graft augmentation requires extraction and injection.

The hyaluronic acid group of fillers represents a recent breakthrough for augmentation technology (Fig. 1.4). Because this substance is generated by both bacteria fermentation, and from chicken combs there is no need for allergy testing. It is a very versatile filler and appears to have a longer effect than collagen. Initially, in Europe, there were reports that at 8 months, 80% of the filler remained. However, in a multi-center double-blind, randomized study comparing hyaluronic acid to collagen in the nasal labial folds, its effect appeared to begin to diminish at 6 months. Approved by the FDA in late 2003, it

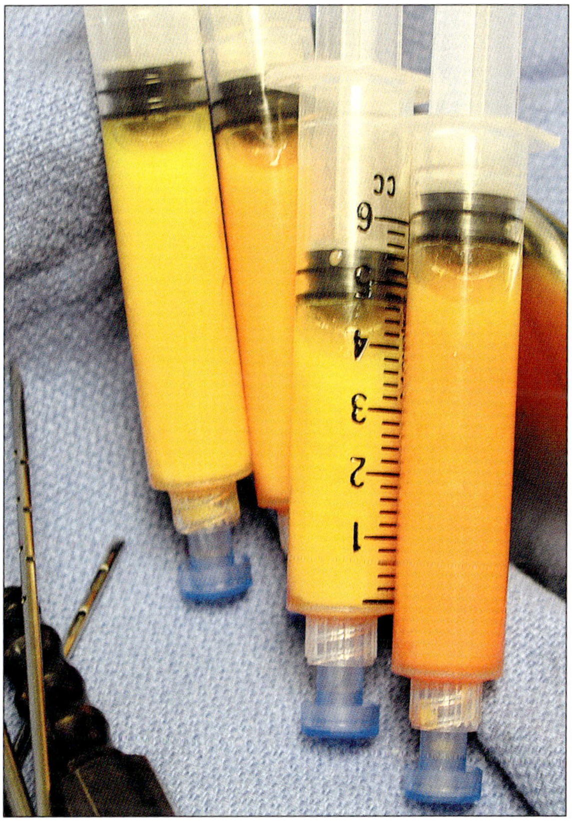

Fig. 1.3 Fat harvested by syringe for fat transfer

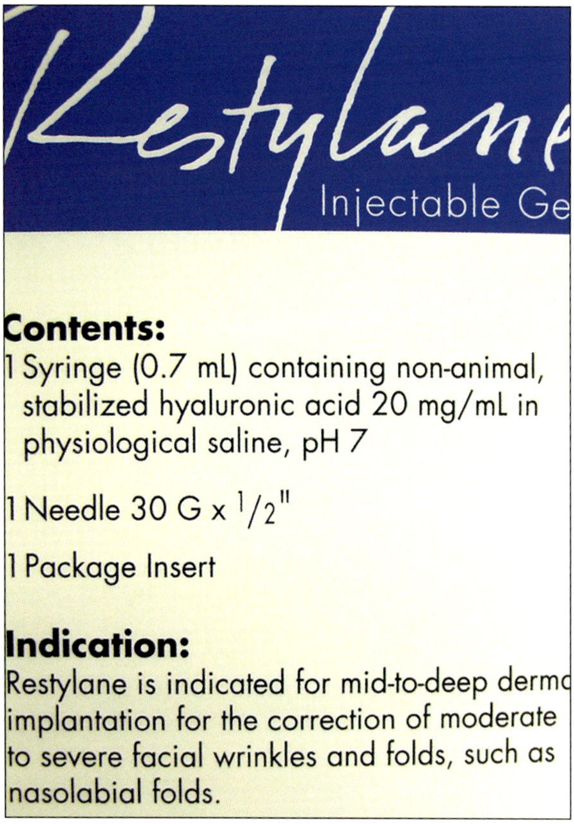

Fig. 1.4 Hyaluronic acid is a versatile filler for facial augmentation

is too early to judge the exact duration of this filler. While hyaluronic acid does not quite have the ease of use of injectable collagen, it still provides excellent long lasting results for the lips, NLFs, marionette lines and acne scars. Compared to collagen, it appears that not as much hyaluronic acid is required to fill a specific defect.

Another recent addition to fillers has been polymethylmethacrylate microspheres. This substance has the advantage of not only remaining in the skin for an extended period of time, but also causing fibrosis around the beads leading to a longer lasting effect. It has been used successfully for the deeper lines such as NLFs and marionette lines. Because of its consistency, it can lead to lumpiness and unevenness in the lips. While it can potentially last for several years; each injection sequence is not as full as one of the biodegradable fillers. Significant granulomas have been reported with Artecoll as with other permanent fillers. Calcium hydroxylapatite, another semipermanent substance which has been used as a radiologic marker and for vocal cord stabilization, has been used off-label for filling facial lines (Fig. 1.5). Based on its longevity in these other areas, it was felt that as a facial filler, it may last up to several years. That has not been the case. According to one study, it retains significant effects in NLFs for 6–9 months. Much less of this substance is needed to fill a particular defect compared to collagen. It is not difficult to inject but it should be injected in the subdermal plane. It is particularly efficacious for NLFs and marionette lines. Because of its viscosity, it is also reasonable to use for hollowing of the cheeks or substantial acne scars. Investigations are under way for use in HIV patients for lipoatrophy as well as possible chin augmentation. Similar to Artecoll, calcium hydroxyapatite can lead to lumpiness when used in the lips.

Silicone has historically been used as a facial filler. Previously, there had been reports of granulomas, foreign-body reactions and extrusion. These adverse reactions may have been secondary to impurities. Recently, the micro-droplet technique has been advocated with excellent results in selected patients using Silicone 1000. This filler is permanent, and with repeated injections can augment large defects or augment significant areas. It is currently undergoing FDA testing for cheek augmentation in subjects suffering HIV facial lipoatrophy. According to reports, it is facile to use, and has had excellent cosmetic results with a minimal side-effect profile as long as the microdroplet technique is used.

Technique

While specific techniques will be covered in the following chapters, there are several guidelines. Technique is partially dependent on the choice of filler. Having the patient positioned sitting up will enable an accurate assessment of the defects or lines. Applying a topical anesthetic at least 10–30 minutes prior to procedure will dull the pain of injection. Nerve blocks, the most common being infraorbital and submental are often indicated. Direct injection of lidocaine with epinephrine, particularly in NLFs and marionette lines, will not only make this a much more pleasant procedure, but will reduce bleeding. Generally, waiting 15 minutes will not only allow the anesthesia to take effect, but will reduce any distortion of the target site. Massaging the site will provide a more uniform distribution of lidocaine with potentially fewer needle sticks as well as reducing transient swelling.

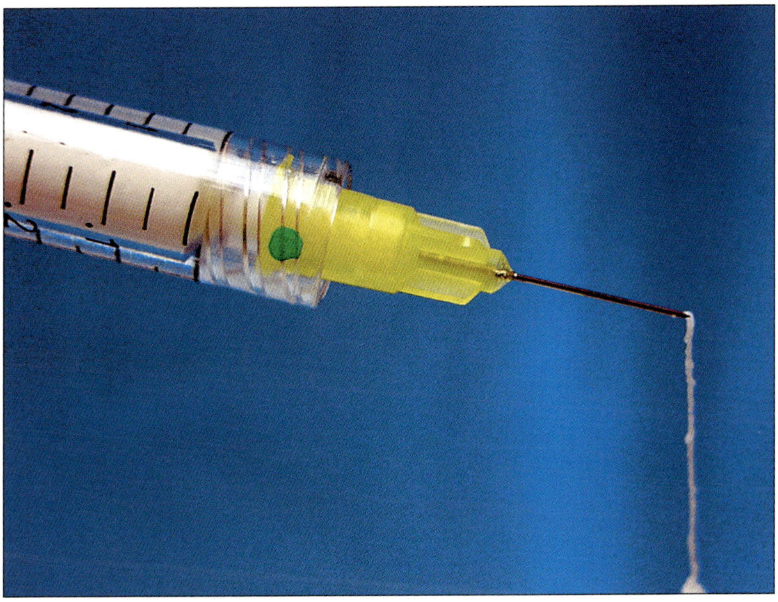

Fig. 1.5 Calcium hydroxylpatite, a semi-permanent substance, is being used off label for facial augmentation

In terms of injecting fillers such as collagen or hyaluronic acid, there are two techniques, both of which have advantages and disadvantages. For these two substances a 30 gauge needle will suffice. For thicker substances such as Artecoll or calcium hydroxylapatite, a 27 gauge needle is necessary. RJ Maxflo needles, which are also 30 gauge on the outside but 27 gauge on the inside, but permit a higher flow rate, may also be appropriate as they retain their sharpness. Fat injection requires larger gauge needles or specialized Coleman injection cannulas. Many practitioners prefer the threading technique, which injects the filler along either most or the entire length of the defect. These 'threads' are injected in toto so that they lie on top of each other. The advantage of this technique is that there are fewer needle punctures, and potentially a smoother result is obtained since it is easier to produce contiguous layering. In contrast, the multiple puncture technique requires several needle sticks. Beads of filler are injected. The advantage of this technique is more control and precise placement. With both methods, the filler is injected as the needle is retracted, thus reducing the risk of vascular injection.

The depth of injection depends on the type of filler. For Zyderm or Cosmoderm, the superficial dermis is appropriate. For Zyplast or Cosmoplast, or hyaluronic acid, the deep dermis (maintaining the needle at a 45° angle) provides the best results (Figs 1.6 and 1.7). Often, using Cosmoplast or hylauronic acid in the deep dermis and then Cosmoderm more superficially will achieve very satisfying results. The dermal-subcutaneous border or subdermal plane, is appropriate for both Artecoll and calcium hydroxylapatite. Fat is layered into the subcutaneous space. For these fillers, it is important not to inject too superficially as this will result in lumpiness and possibly in an increased incidence of granulomas. Of course, too deep an injection technique will result in a less than desirable augmentation. Injecting into the lips requires a great degree of finesse and judgment. While there are a number of different techniques, it is important to inject smoothly along the vermilion border and within the vermilion lip in order to avoid lumpiness (Fig. 1.8).

Post-Procedure Management

It may be wise to allow the patient to rest for a few minutes following the procedure, given the needle-causing anxiety of many patients. Cold compresses or ice following the procedure will reduce some of the swelling and reduce some soreness from the multiple injections after the anesthetic wears off. Dressings are generally not needed for injectables, though the donor site for fat transfer will need to be bandaged. Though the patient may not be compliant, it is worth reminding the patient to try to reduce facial expressions for the first 48 hours. For some fillers such as calcium hydroxylapatite, having the patient gently pat the area injected—without a

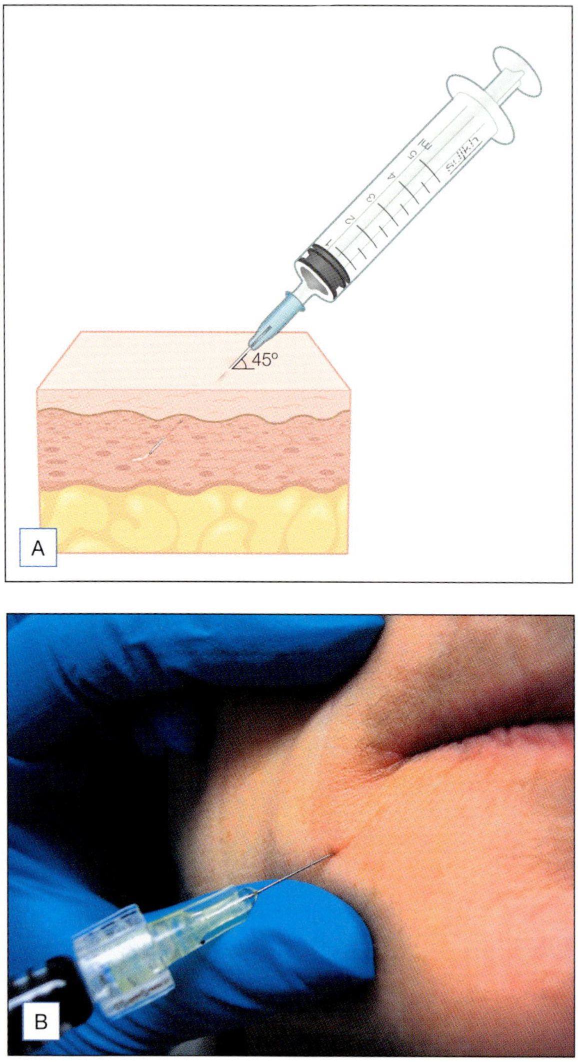

Fig. 1.6 (**A**) Diagram and (**B**) photograph showing correct angle for placement of filler into the deep dermis

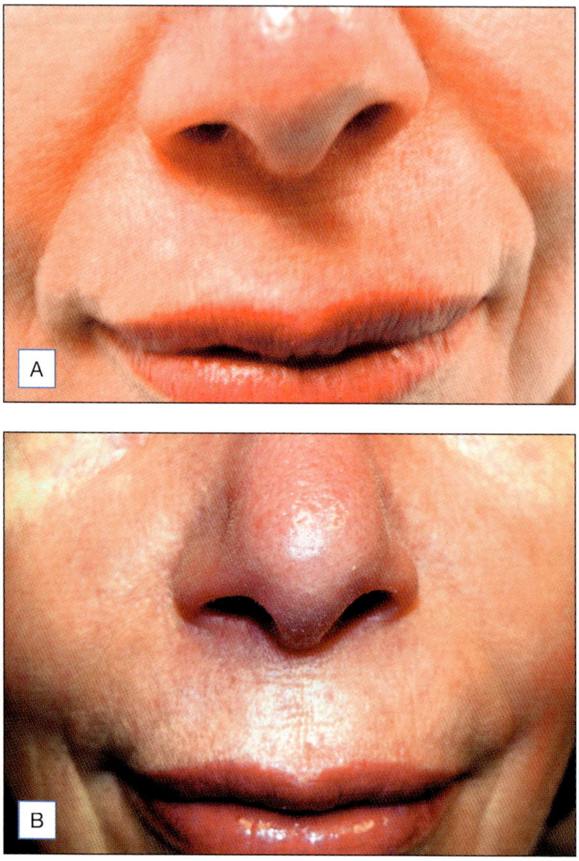

Fig. 1.7 (**A**) Prominent nasolabial or 'smile' lines. (**B**) Three months following injection of hyaluronic acid

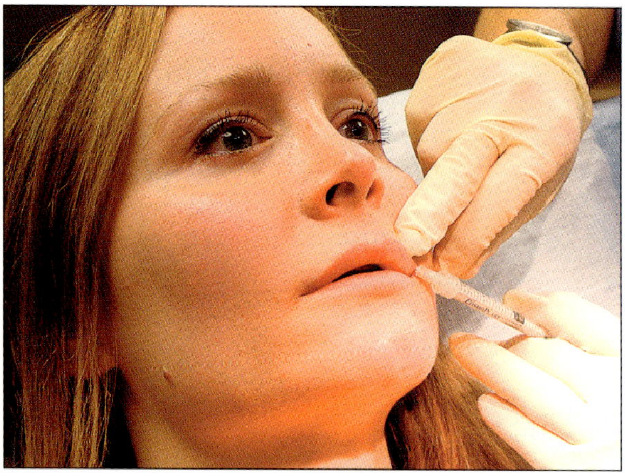

Fig. 1.8 Injecting human collagen into the upper lip. Placement of this material is at vermilion border

shearing motion—may help set the material. Pre- and post-procedure photographs are a necessity.

Complications

In addition to allergic reactions, infection and hematomas, which are rare, other adverse events may include asymmetry, granulomas, migration and extrusion. More common than the last three complications is lumpiness and dimpling, which is usually the result of placing the material in too superficial a plane. This 'bumpiness' will usually resolve over a week or two without therapy. Massage may expedite resolution of this problem. True granulomas are rare and can be treated initially with a low-dose steroid injection. Larger or persistent granulomas may need to be excised if treatment with intralesional steroid, topical tacrolimus or oral allopurinol is not successful.

Limitations: Value of Combination Therapy

It cannot be overemphasized that the approach to facial esthetics should be a comprehensive one. No one type of procedure will achieve facial harmony in all esthetic subjects. Fillers are merely one instrument to achieve this goal. Combining fillers with other modalities will often optimize results. It has been shown for instance that the combination of hyaluronans such as Restylane and Botox will provide a superior result than either alone for the upper face. Similarly the combination of a rhytidectomy and fat transfer to the cheeks, or filler injection to the peroral region, will not only provide smoother lower facial contours, but will replace the volume that a facelift alone cannot achieve. This is particularly crucial in an individual with a thin, elongated face. A facelift may also reduce the amount of filler needed in the NLFs and marionette lines. The major limitation of today's fillers, and a concern of patients is that they are very temporary in the hands of most practitioners. While this is true, permanency can present unforeseen problems when an individual's face ages, when there is deepening and subtle repositioning of lines. Perhaps in the future we will have a filler that is easy to inject, inexpensive and remains effective for 2–3 years. Until that time, appropriate education of the patient and combination therapies will result in the highest patient satisfaction.

Further Reading

Alcalay J, Alkalay R, Gat A, Yorav S 2003 Late onset granulomatous reaction to Artecol. Dermatologic Surgery 29:859–862

Alonso D, Lazarus MC, Baumann L 2002 Effects of topical arnica gel on post laser treatment bruises. Dermatologic Surgery 28:686–688

Berman M 2000 Rejuvenation of the upper eyelid complex with autologous fat transplantation. Dermatologic Surgery 26:1113–1116

Billings E, May JW 1989 Historical review and present status of free fat graft autotransplantation in plastic and reconstructive surgery. Plastic and Reconstructive Surgery 83:368–381

Carruthers J, Carruthers A 2003 A prospective randomized parallel group study analyzing the effect of BTX-A and nonanimal sourced hyaluronic acid in combination compared with NASHA alone in severe glabellar rhytides in adult female subjects: treatment of severe glabellar rhytides with a hyaluronic acid derivative compared with the derivative and BTX-A. Dermatologic Surgery 29:802–809

Carruthers J, Carruthers A 2003 Aesthetic botulinum A toxin in the mid and lower face and neck. Dermatologic Surgery 29:468–476

Conroy BF 1983 The history of facial prostheses. Clinics in Plastic Surgery 10:689–708

Danesh-Mayer HV, Savino PJ, Sergott RC 2001 Case reports and small case series: ocular and cerebral ischemia following facial injection of autologous fat. Archives of Ophthalmology 119:777–778

Donofrio L 2000 Technique of periorbital lipoaugmentation. Dermatologic Surgery 26:1129–1134

Donofrio LM 2000 Structural autologous lipoaugmentation: a panfacial technique. Dermatological Surgery 26:1129–1134

Duffy DM 1990 Silicone: a critical review. Advances in Dermatology 5:93–107

Duranti F, Salti G, Bovani B et al 1998 Injectable hyaluronic acid gel for soft tissue augmentation. A clinical and histologic study. Dermatologic Surgery 24:1317–1325

Dzubow L 1997 The Aging Face. In: Coleman WP, Hanke CW, Alt TH (eds) Cosmetic Surgery of the Skin. Mosby, St Louis, pp 7–17

Ficarra G, Mosqueda-Taylor A, Carlos R 2002 Silicone granuloma of the facial tissues: a report of seven cases. Oral Surgery, Oral Medicine, Oral Pathology, Oral Radiology and Endodontics 94:65–73

Frodel JL, Sykes JM 1996 Chin augmentation/genioplasty: chin deformities in the aging patient. Facial Plastic Surgery 12:279–283

Fulton JE, Suarez M, Silverton K, Barnes T 1998 Small volume fat transfer. Dermatological Surgery 24:857–865

Gladstone HB, Morganroth GS 2003 Evaluating calcium hydroxylapatite for facial augmentation. Presented at the Annual American Society for Dermatologic Surgery Meeting, New Orleans, LA

Goldberg RA, Edelstein C, Shorr N 1999 Fat repositioning in lower blepharoplasty to maintain infraorbital rim contour. Facial Plastic Surgery 15:225–229

Gonzalez-Ulloa M, Costillo A, Stevens E et al 1954 Preliminary study of the total restoration of the facial skin. Plastic and Reconstructive Surgery 13:151–161

Ho TT, Chan KC, Wong KH, Lee SS 1999 Indinavir-associated facial lipodystrophy in HIV infected patients. AIDS Patient Care STDS. 13:11–16

Jones DH 2003 Liquid Silicone for HIV Facial Lipostrophy: 1 Year Data of 126 Treated Patients. Presented at the Annual American Society for Dermatologic Surgery Meeting, New Orleans, LA

Jordan DR 2003 Soft tissue fillers for wrinkles, folds and volume augmentation. Canadian Journal of Ophthalmology 2:250–253

Klein AW 2001 Collagen substances. Facial Plastic Surgery Clinics of North America 9:205–218

Larrabee WF, Makielski KH 1993 Surgical Anatomy of the Face. Raven Press, New York, pp 3–12

Lemperle G, Romano JJ, Busso M 2003 Soft tissue augmentation with Artecoll: 10 year history, indications, techniques and complications. Dermatologic Surgery 29:573–587

Lombardi T, Samson J, Plantier F, Husson C, Kuffer R 2004 Orofacial granulomas after injection of cosmetic fillers: Histopathologic and clinical study of 11 cases. Journal of Oral Pathological Medicine 33:115–120

Matti BA, Nicolle FV 1990 Clinical use of Zyplast in correction of age and disease-related deficiencies of the face. Aesthetic Plastic Surgery 14:227–234

Narins RS 2002 The use of tumescent anesthetic solution for fat transfer donor and recipient sites. Journal of Drugs in Dermatology 3:279–282.

Narins RS, Brandt F, Leyden J, Lorenc ZP, Rubin M, Smith S 2003 A randomized, double blind, multicenter comparison of the efficacy and tolerability of Restylane versus Zyplast for the correction of nasolabial folds. Dermatologic Surgery 29:588–595

Orentreich D, Leone AS 2004 A case of HIV-associated facial lipoatrophy treated with 1000-cs liquid injectable silicone. Dermatologic Surgery 30:548–551

Peck H, Peck S 1970 A concept of facial esthetics. Angle Orthodontist 40:284-317

Reisberger EM, Landthaler M, West L et al 2003 Foreign body granulomas caused by polymethylmethacrylate microspheres: successful treatment with allopurinol. Archives of Dermatology 139:17–20

Sklar JA, White SM 2004 Radiance FN: a new soft tissue filler. Dermatologic Surgery 30:764–768

Watson W, Kaye RL, Klein A et al 1983 Injectable collagen: a clinical overview. Cutis 31;543–546

2 Fillers Esthetics

Stephen R. Tan, Richard G. Glogau

Wrinkles should merely indicate where smiles have been.

Mark Twain, 1897

Introduction

Over recent decades, there have been major advances in the physician's ability to improve upon the signs of aging. Filler substances have abounded, and currently available products have effects that may last from a few months to many years. Filler substances are primarily utilized to restore volume to focal areas of the face; thus, they are applicable to treating facial wrinkles and loss of subcutaneous volume resulting from a variety of causes. To properly use these substances to achieve the maximal cosmetic improvement while minimizing the risk of complications, the physician must have a thorough understanding of facial esthetics and the changes that occur as the patient ages.

Gender Differences in Aesthetic Facial Appearances

The word *aesthetic* is derived from the Greek word *aisthesis*, which means having a sense or love of that which is beautiful. The attractive, idealized face tends to exhibit several general characteristics, with slightly different proportions and shapes between women and men. While there are exceptions to every rule, these trends tend to be universally perceived across different cultures and across the ages. The idealized female face tends to exhibit:

- A larger, smooth forehead with a smaller nose
- Eyebrows that have an arch or gull-wing shape
- Eyes that are set wider apart, creating a bigger look
- Prominent cheekbones
- A heart-shaped taper to the lower face, with a smaller lower-to-upper face ratio
- Full, vermilion lips

The attractive masculine face tends to have:

- An overhanging, horizontal brow with minimal arch
- Deeper set eyes that appear closer together
- A somewhat larger nose
- A wider mouth
- A squared lower face with a more equal ratio of lower-to-upper face proportions
- A beard or coarser texture to the lower facial skin

Esthetics is a scientific attempt to explain a subjective concept by assigning proportions to various components of the face. Although these proportions may be used to define the 'ideal', 'attractive', or 'perfect' face, the real value in studying these principles lies in clarifying the range of normal relationships that exist between facial units. Harmony and balance of the face exists through a wide range of sizes, shapes, and configurations of the individual parts. The cosmetic surgeon must appreciate this in order to understand the changes the face develops and endures over time.

Etiology of the aging face

The face ages in response to a number of factors, which may appear to varying degrees among individuals. Sun exposure and smoking tend to accelerate these changes.

Chronic ultraviolet light damage to the skin: Photoaging adds to the inevitable changes seen with intrinsic chronologic aging; indeed, cumulative sun exposure is the single largest factor involved in our clinical perception of aging skin, and it is responsible for a large portion of the unwanted aesthetic effects.

Loss of subcutaneous fat: In general, with age there is a loss of the fullness and roundness of the facial contours of youth, resulting in a flattened or sunken appearance to facial structures.

Changes in the intrinsic muscles of facial expression and their influence on the skin: The muscles of facial expression are unique in that they insert directly into the skin. Years of facial expressions constantly folding the skin result in the progressive development of hyperdynamic wrinkles, which initially appear only with facial movement, but may ultimately remain as wrinkles at rest. Hyperdynamic wrinkles are more prominent in areas where the underlying muscles and fascia have more direct attachments to the skin, such as in the frontal, glabellar, nasolabial, perioral, and periocular areas.

Gravitational changes from loss of elasticity of the tissue: With aging, the facial soft tissues lose their inherent resiliency and ability to resist stretching; inevitably, they begin to sag under the effects of gravity.

Remodeling of the underlying bony and cartilaginous structures: Over time, bony resorption may result in a decrease in apparent facial volume, and gravitational stretch of cartilaginous structures may result in the drooping of structures such as the nasal tip. Facial asymmetry due to underlying bony or cartilaginous structural changes is difficult to correct, and pointing out these differences at the initial consultation is important in setting realistic patient expectations.

Photoaging

Over the past few decades, there has been an increase in sun exposure through increased leisure time and outdoor activities. Years of people trying to acquire the 'healthy tan' has produced high rates of prematurely aged skin. Cumulative sun exposure is the greatest factor in aging skin, and is responsible for a large portion of unwanted aesthetic effects, including many of the wrinkles which may be treated with filler substances. Glogau has developed a systematic classification of patient photoaging types (see Box 2.1). Depending upon the degree of sun exposure, these generalizations apply at different ages and to different degrees in patients with more pigmented skin.

Glogau photoaging classification

Type I – 'No wrinkles'

- Early photoaging
  Mild pigmentary changes
  No keratoses
  Minimal wrinkles
- Younger patient – 20s or 30s
- Minimal or no make-up

Type II – 'Wrinkles in motion'

- Early to moderate photoaging
  Early senile lentigines visible
  Keratoses palpable but not visible
  Parallel smile lines beginning to appear lateral to mouth
- Patient age – late 30s or 40s
- Usually wears some foundation

Type III – 'Wrinkles at rest'

- Advanced photoaging
  Obvious dyschromia and telangiectasias
  Visible keratoses
  Wrinkles even when not moving
- Patient age – 50s or older
- Always wears heavy foundation

Type IV – 'Only wrinkles'

- Severe photoaging
  Yellow-gray color of skin
  Prior skin malignancies
  Wrinkled throughout, no normal skin
- Patient age – sixth or seventh decade
  can't wear make-up – 'cakes and cracks'

Adapted from Glogau (1994 and 1996).

Box 2.1 Glogau photoaging classification

Type I patients have early photoaging changes, and are usually in their 20s or 30s. These patients generally have no rhytides at all, even when the face is animated during speaking or expression. Early photoaging, if present, may include mild pigmentary changes causing a disruption in the homogeneity of skin color. These patients generally wear no make-up foundation at all, as they do not require it for either rhytides or pigmentary alterations (see Fig. 2.1).

Type II patients are usually in their late 30s or 40s. These patients have early to moderate photoaging changes, and chronic ultraviolet damage to the elastic fibers impairs the inherent 'snap back' quality of the skin. These patients are without wrinkles while the face is at rest, but wrinkles begin to appear as expression lines when the face is in motion, appearing parallel to the meilolabial fold, the corners of the mouth, the lateral canthal areas, and over the zygomatic arch and malar eminences. Early solar lentigines begin to appear, and patients frequently

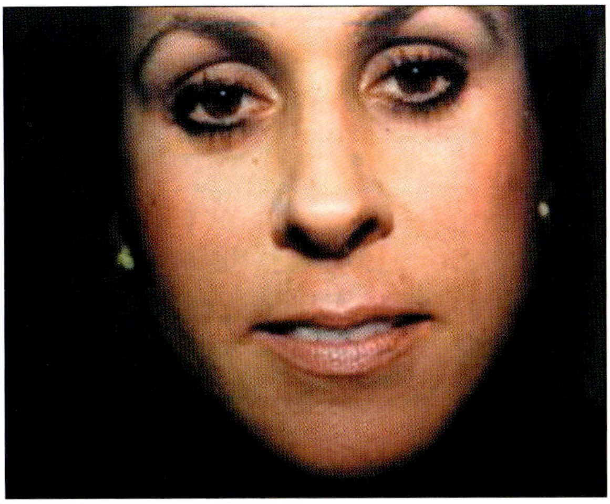

Fig. 2.1 Glogau photoaging Type I. Note the absence of wrinkles and pigmentary alterations

utilize make-up foundation to conceal the pigmentary irregularities (see Fig. 2.2). As these patients only have wrinkles while the face is in motion, they most aptly demonstrate the effects of the underlying musculature on the skin, a critical consideration when contemplating the use of botulinum toxin.

Patients classified as Type III have advanced photoaging changes, and are typically in their 50s or beyond. Damage to the cutaneous elastic fibers becomes more severe, and the wrinkles produced by facial movement eventually persist even at rest. These may present as wrinkles radiating outwards from the lateral canthi, inferiorly from the lower eyelids onto the malar cheeks, parallel to the oral commissures, and vertically radiating outward from the upper and lower lips. Advanced photoaging results in obvious pigmentary dyschromias, telangiectasias, and visible keratoses. Patients commonly wear heavy make-up foundation to conceal these changes (see Fig. 2.3).

Type IV patients have severe photoaging changes and are usually in their 60s or 70s, but may be younger in the most severe cases. Wrinkles gradually spread to cover the majority of facial skin, and these patients may not have any unlined skin remaining on their faces. The dermis becomes engorged with thick debris, rendering a thickened, coarse quality to the skin. Pigmentary dyschromias are present as a yellow-gray sallow color of the skin, and patients have often had prior cutaneous malignancies (see Fig. 2.4). Type IV patients are not able to wear make-up, as the uneven facial surface often causes the make-up to have the texture of 'cracked mud'.

Anatomic Approach to the Aging Face

Physicians should approach a patient seeking cosmetic improvement of the signs of aging from an anatomic standpoint. The determination of *what* is wrong must precede *how* it should be corrected. All too often, physicians develop a preference for one or

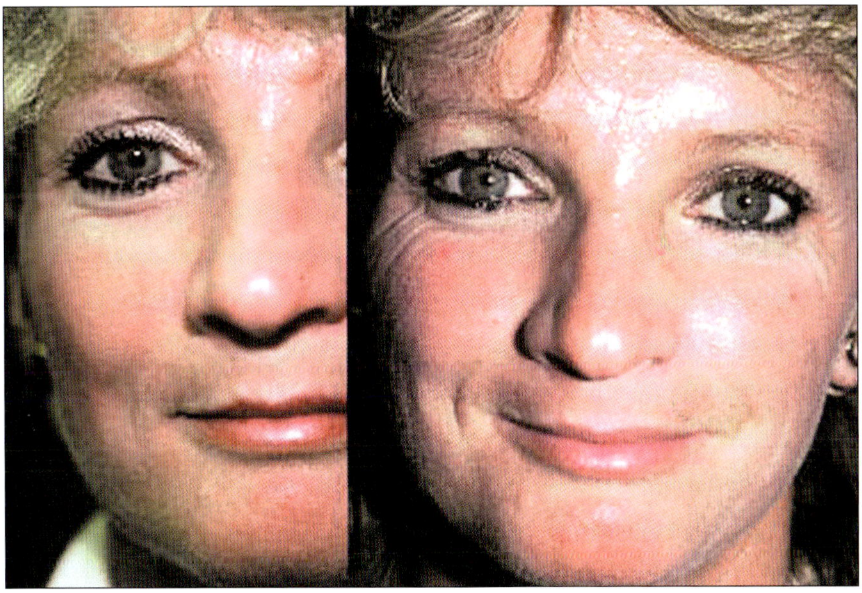

Fig. 2.2 Glogau photoaging Type II. Note the absence of wrinkles while the face is at rest, and the appearance of wrinkles with facial movement

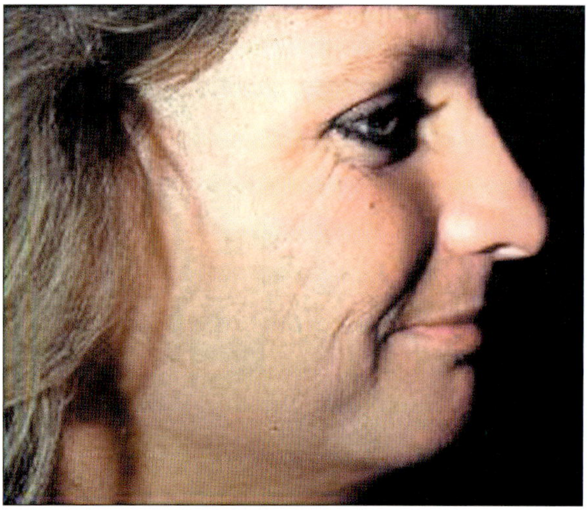

Fig. 2.3 Glogau photoaging Type III. Note that wrinkles are present while the face is at rest

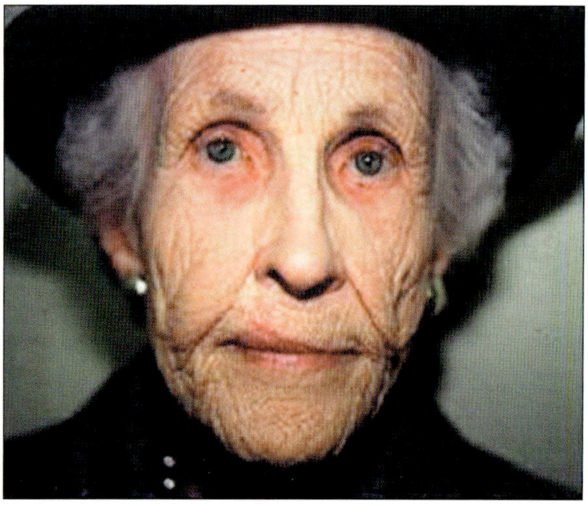

Fig. 2.4 Glogau photoaging Type IV. The facial skin is entirely wrinkled, with no normal skin remaining on the face. Also note the yellow-gray, sallow color of the skin

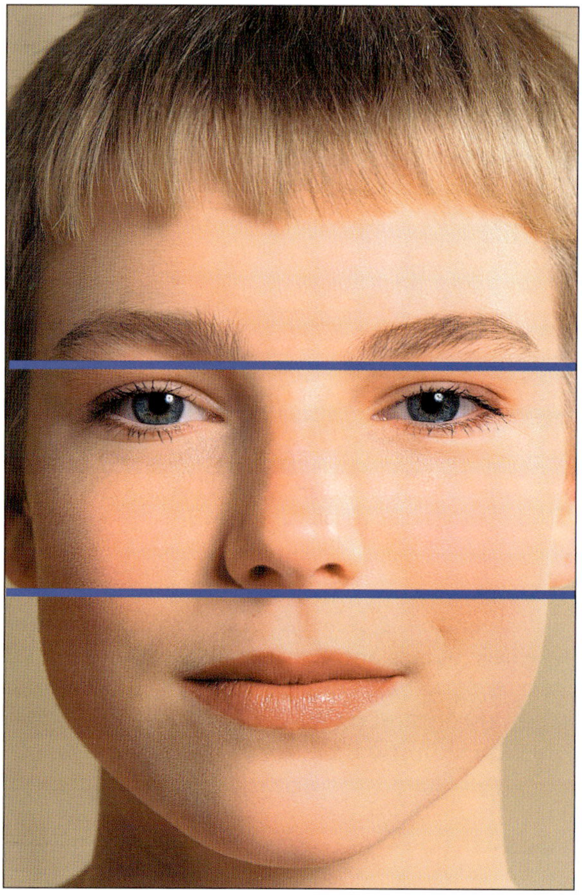

Fig. 2.5 Division of the face into thirds. The upper third ranges from the trichion to the glabella, the middle third from the glabella to the subnasale, and the lower third from the subnasale to the menton

a few cosmetic techniques, and then attempt to apply these to all situations. Inappropriately using a therapeutic technique that does not address the underlying anatomic basis for a cosmetic problem leads to mediocre results at best, and disasters at worst. For example, patients with deep glabellar furrows treated with filler substances may experience transient improvement; however, unless the underlying muscles causing these hyperdynamic lines are weakened with botulinum toxin, the wrinkles will rapidly recur. Thus, an anatomic approach to the aging face is essential, and will allow the physician to rationally select the optimal therapeutic tool from a wide variety of therapeutic options.

To appreciate facial symmetry and balance, one commonly used practice is to divide the face horizontally into thirds (see Fig. 2.5). The upper third ranges from the trichion to the glabella, the middle third from the glabella to the subnasale, and the lower third from the subnasale to the menton. Filler substances are mainly applicable, either alone or in combination with other treatment modalities, to the lower two-thirds of the face, although their effects in the upper face are becoming increasingly appreciated.

Upper third of the aging face

Changes in the upper third of the face are primarily related to chronic ultraviolet light damage, to the

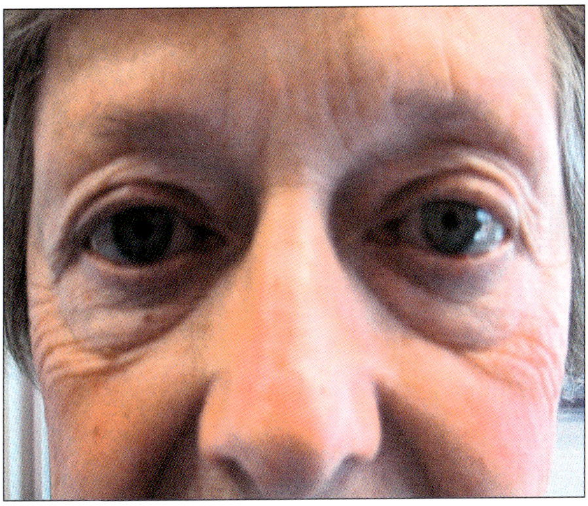

Fig. 2.6 Aging of the periorbital tissues. Note dermatochalasis and protrusion of the lower eyelid subcutaneous tissues

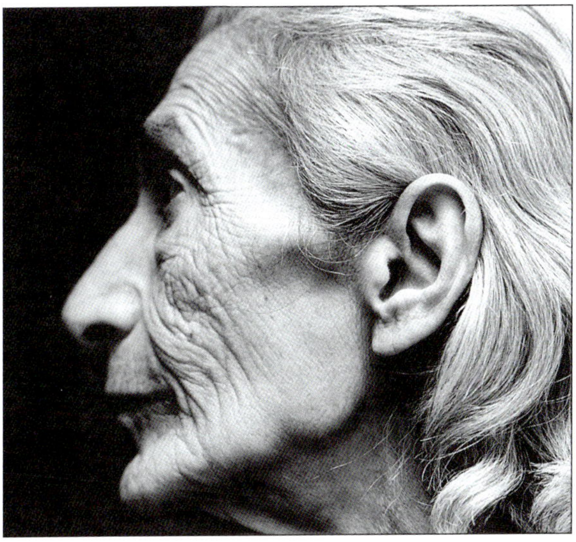

Fig. 2.7 Aging of the cheek. Note the development of a buccal depression, resulting in the appearance of a prominent malar eminence

intrinsic muscles of facial expression and their influence on the skin, and to gravitational changes from loss of elasticity of the tissue. Occasionally, filler substances may be used in conjunction with botulinum toxin to soften hyperdynamic wrinkles after the underlying causative muscles have been paralyzed. For a full description of facial esthetics and aging in the upper third of the face, please see the chapter entitled 'Botox esthetics' within this series.

Middle third of the aging face

Aging of the middle third of the face affects the eyelids and periorbital regions, the cheeks, and the nose. These changes primarily result from a combination of photoaging, loss of subcutaneous tissue, loss of cutaneous elasticity, and remodeling of underlying cartilaginous and bony structures.

Aging of the periorbital tissues results in both cosmetic and functional impairments. Dermatochalasis results from the combination of progressive cutaneous laxity of the eyelid skin and the effects of gravity. In severe cases, the upper eyelid skin may become so redundant that the visual fields are impaired. The canthal tendons and the tarsal plates provide the support structure of the eyelids, and loss of elasticity of these structures results in decreased lid tone and ability to 'snap back' after stretching of the eyelids. In severe cases, stability of eyelid position may be affected, resulting in either ectropion or entropion. The orbital septum may weaken over time, allowing for protrusions of the upper- and lower-lid fat compartments; however, some people may experience a loss of periorbital subcutaneous tissue, resulting in a 'sunken-in' skeletonized appearance to the orbits (see Fig. 2.6).

The cheeks may be affected by volume loss of the buccal fat pad, which is positioned between the masseter muscle anteriorly and the buccinator muscle posteriorly. In childhood, an ample buccal fat pad contributes to the fullness of the cheeks; however, with age this fat pad atrophies. A buccal depression may develop, leading to the appearance of prominent malar eminences (see Fig. 2.7).

Aging of the nose results in both structural and surface changes. The support mechanisms of the nasal tip may become inelastic and stretch with age, resulting in nasal tip ptosis and an apparent elongation of the middle third of the face (see Fig. 2.8). The fibrous attachments between the inferior margin of the upper lateral nasal cartilage and the superior margins of the lateral crura of the alar cartilages elongate from a combination of gravity and remodeling of the underlying bony and cartilaginous tissues. Additionally, the sling supporting the dome area weakens and there is loss of subcutaneous tissue, resulting in nasal ptosis, a downward and posterior rotation of the nasal lobule, retraction of the columella, and prominence of the nasal hump and cartilages. On the surface, enlargement of sebaceous

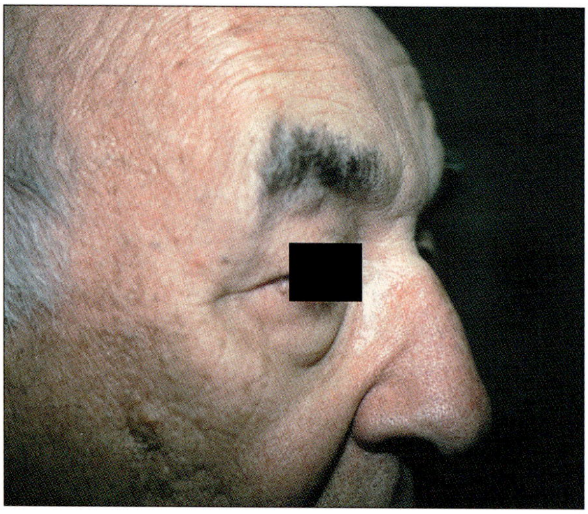

Fig. 2.8 Aging of the nose. Note ptosis of the nasal tip, with downward and posterior rotation of the nasal lobule

glands may alter the skin texture, resulting in a spectrum from widely enlarged pores to a rhinophymatous appearance.

Lower third of the aging face

The aging changes seen in the lower third of the face affect the lips, the chin, the lower cheeks, and the neck. Changes result from a combination of chronic ultraviolet light damage to the skin, loss of subcutaneous fat, changes due to the muscles of facial expression, gravitational changes from loss of elasticity of the tissue, and remodeling of the underlying bony and cartilaginous structures.

Changes in dentition and absorption of maxillary and mandibular bone may result in an overall loss of height and volume. The chin rotates forward, and is seen to sharpen and protrude. These changes may result in the lower third of the face appearing smaller relative to the upper and middle thirds, straying from the ideal, approximately equal proportions. Aging changes from the middle third of the face may contribute to this appearance, as nasal tip ptosis may create the appearance of a shortened upper lip (see Fig. 2.9). The constant effects of gravity combined with loss of elasticity in the tissue may allow for excess skin to droop off the mandible, manifesting as 'jowls' along the mandibular rim and 'wattles' in the anterior neck (see Fig. 2.10).

The origin of the meilolabial fold is unclear. Some authors feel that it is derived from insertions of

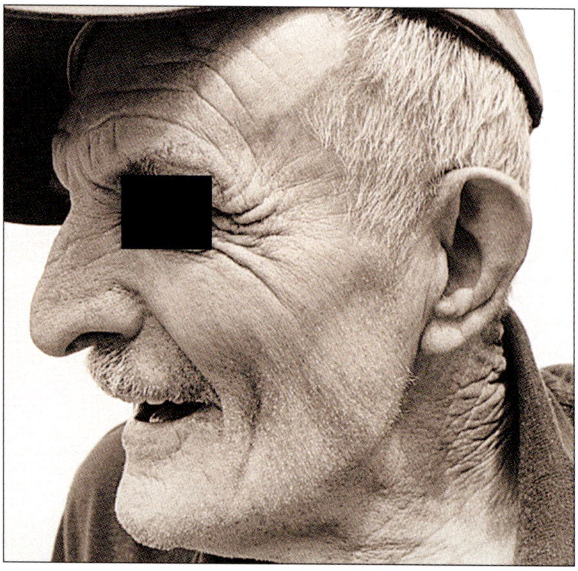

Fig. 2.9 Alterations of the proportions of the face. Note the nasal tip ptosis which elongates the middle third of the face, while the lower third has lost height and volume with maxillary and mandibular bone resorption

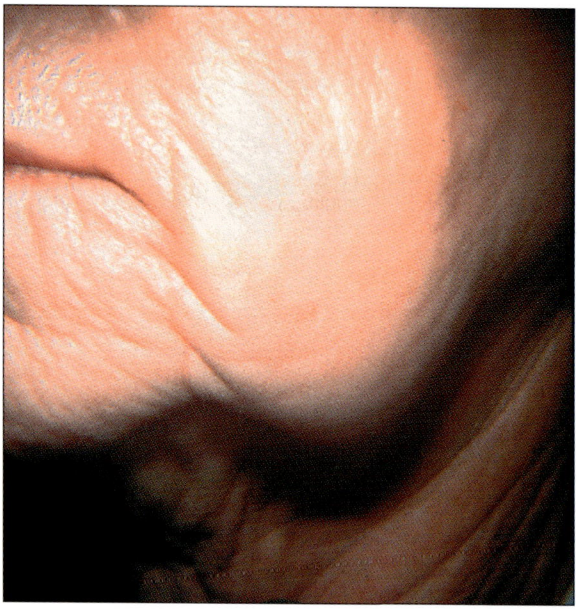

Fig. 2.10 Excess, inelastic skin drapes off the mandible as 'jowls' along the mandibular rim, and 'wattles' in the anterior neck

lip elevator muscles into the skin, whereas others hypothesize that it results from differences in the subcutaneous structure in the cheek and oral areas. In any case, the prominence of this fold varies with age. In childhood, the lips and cheeks contain more

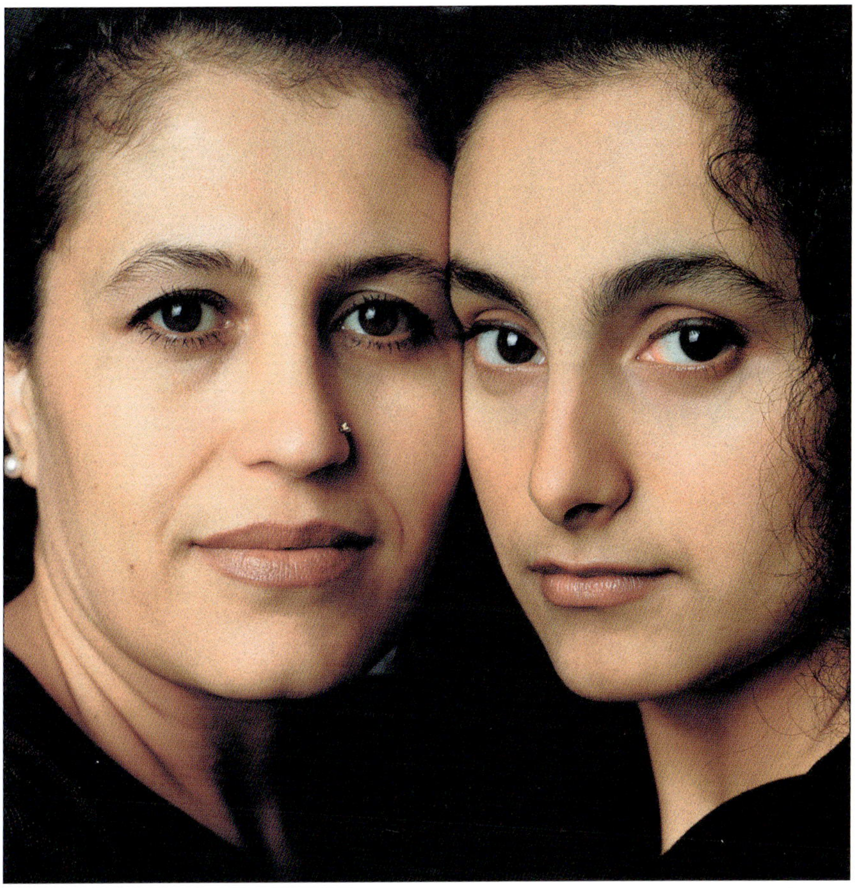

Fig. 2.11 Changes in the meilolabial fold over time. Note the subtle meilolabial fold in young adulthood, followed by the apparent deepening with age

abundant subcutaneous tissue, such that this fold is relatively inapparent; however, age-related loss of subcutaneous fat, combined with the loss of elasticity of the skin, results in the draping of redundant tissue over the muscular insertion point into the groove. Clinically, this results in an apparent deepening of the meilolabial fold (see Fig. 2.11).

Wrinkles form around the lips as a result of the constant pulling of the orbicularis oris muscle on progressively more inelastic upper- and lower-lip skin, creating angular, radial, and vertical wrinkles. Marionette lines may form as vertical wrinkles extending downwards from the oral commissures (see Fig. 2.12). The effects of gravity result in drooping of the oral commissures laterally and downward, which may lead to a tired and sad appearance. Loss of elasticity may lead to lip skin redundancy, enhancing the drooping and vertical elongation (see Fig. 2.13). Fullness of the lips and a strong definition of the philtrum are seen in youth; however, with

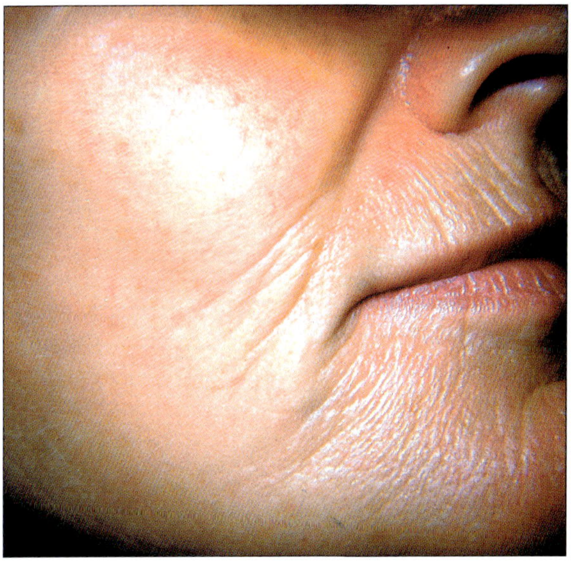

Fig. 2.12 Perioral wrinkles radiating outward from the upper and lower lips. 'Marionette lines' form as vertical wrinkles extending downwards from the oral commissures

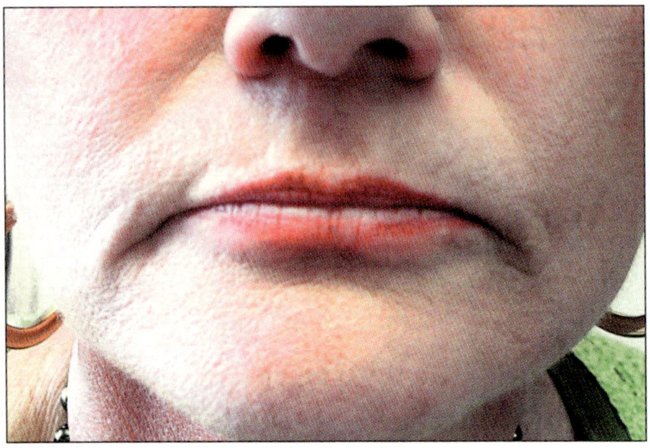

Fig. 2.13 Drooping of the oral commissures with age, leading to a tired and sad appearance

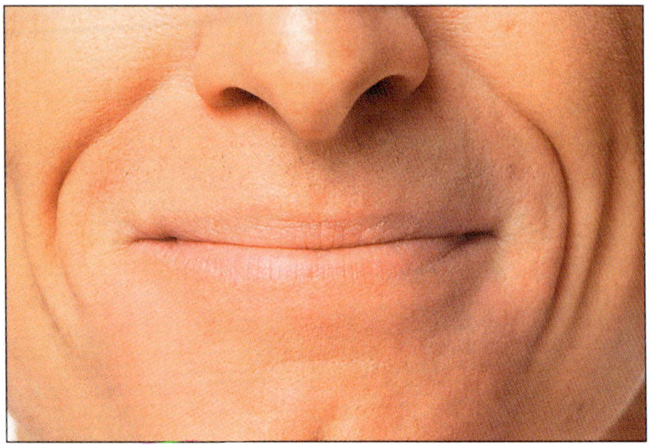

Fig. 2.14 Loss of fullness and flattening of the lips with age. Cupid's bow, the central arch of the upper lip, is flattened

advancing age, there is atrophy of the orbicularis oris muscle and loss of subcutaneous tissue, leading to an overall flattening and loss of fullness in the lips, with less of the vermilion showing. 'Cupid's bow', the central arch of the upper lip, may flatten (see Fig. 2.14). In severe cases, there may be disruption of normal lip position. Loss of subcutaneous tissue and hypotonic lip musculature may allow the lips to invert, creating a 'sucked-in' appearance; however, the occasional patient may develop a lip ectropion due to excess tissue and hypotonic lip musculature.

Conclusion

The desire to restore the focal loss of facial volume that occurs with age has driven the development of numerous filler substances. When approaching a patient seeking cosmetic improvement of these areas, the physician must be able to assess the quality and position of the subcutaneous tissues. Are the lips thin? Have they lost their shape? Are the cheekbones flattened? Is there wasting in the temporal fossae, above the eyebrows, or in the buccal fat pads? With an appreciation of facial esthetics and a working knowledge of the capabilities and limitations of each filler substance, the physician will be able to use the most appropriate filler substance to achieve maximal cosmetic improvement.

Further Reading

Dzubow L. The aging face. In: Coleman WP III, Hanke CW, Alt TH, Asken S, editors. Cosmetic Surgery of the Skin: Principles and Techniques, 2nd edn. St Louis: Mosby, 1997, pp. 7–17.

Gliklich RE. Proportions of the aesthetic face. In: Cheney ML, editor. Facial Surgery: Plastic and Reconstructive. Baltimore, MD: Williams & Wilkins, 1997, pp. 147–157.

Glogau RG. Chemical peeling and aging skin. Journal of Geriatric Dermatology 1994; 2(1): 5–10.

Glogau RG. Aesthetic and anatomic analysis of the aging skin. Seminars in Cutaneous Medicine and Surgery 1996; 15(3): 134–138.

Glogau RG. Evaluation of the aging face. In: Kaminer MS, Dover JS, Arndt KA, editors. Atlas of Cosmetic Surgery. Philadelphia: WB Saunders, 2002, pp. 29–33.

Glogau RG. Systematic evaluation of the aging face. In: Bolognia JL, Jorizzo JL, Rapini RP, editors. Dermatology. London: Mosby, 2003, pp. 2357–2360.

McKinney P, Cunningham BL. Anatomy. In: Aesthetic Facial Surgery. New York: Churchill Livingstone, 1992, pp. 25–51.

Pwell N, Humphreys B. Proportions of the Aesthetic Face. New York: Thieme-Stratton, 1984.

Ridley MB, VanHook SM. Aesthetic facial proportions. In: Papel ID, Frodel J, Park SS, Holt GR, Sykes JM, Larrabee WF et al, editors. Facial Plastic and Reconstructive Surgery, 2nd edn. New York: Thieme, 2002, pp. 96–109.

Salasche SJ, Bernstein G, Senkarik M. Surgical Anatomy of the Skin. Norwalk, CT: Appleton & Lange, 1988.

3 Injectable Collagens

Seth L. Matarasso, Kenneth Beer

Introduction

This chapter will discuss the various available collagen products used to temporarily improve and reduce dermal cutaneous defects. The products approved by the FDA for the glaborous skin of the nasolabial fold and vermilion border are primarily used in the lower third of the face. Augmentation of the lips and bolstering the lateral oral commisures are perhaps the most frequent uses of these products and may be used as off label indications. Other areas amenable to soft tissue augmentation with collagen include marionette lines, soft atrophic scars, and static rhytides unresponsive to chemodenervation with botulinum toxin preparations in the forehead, glabella, and periocular regions.

Historical perspective

Fueled by the overwhelming success of botulinum toxin chemodenervation for dynamic rhytides, and patients' demand for ambulatory procedures with little recuperation time, the field of soft tissue augmentation continues to gain momentum and popularity. This minimally invasive modality remains a treatment of choice and the cornerstone treatments for many facial imperfections.

Soft tissue fillers have been used for more than a century to improve contours, soften rhytides, blunt depressed scars, and enhance lips. The history of soft tissue augmentation dates back to 1893, when Neuberg first attempted to use autologous fat transfer for tissue augmentation. He utilized blocks of free fat harvested from the arms to reconstruct depressed facial defects. In 1899 Gersvny injected paraffin into the scrotum as a testicular prosthesis for a patient with advanced tuberculosis. Lexor, in 1910, used large-block grafts to treat malar depressions associated with chin recession. This was followed by Brunings who, in 1911, first described using the syringe technique to transfer free fat. In 1950, Peer reported 50% survival of transplanted fat using syringe aspiration. Baronders published a review of permanent soft tissue augmentation with liquid silicone in 1953 (Table 3.1). Although useful

Historical milestones of filler substances		
Year	**Physician**	**Milestone**
1893	Neuberg	First to use autologous fat for tissue augmentation
1899	Gersvny	First to use bioinjectable paraffin to correct cosmetic deformities
1910	Lexor	First to use large-block grafts to treat malar depression with chin recession
1911	Brunings	First described transfer of free fat employing the syringe technique
1950	Peer	Reported 50% survival of syringe-aspirated transplanted fat at 1 year
1953	Baronders	Use of liquid silicone in medicine
1976	Fischer	Cellusuctiome extraction of fat
1978	Ilous	Liposuction as a fat source
1981		FDA approval of Zyderm I
1986	Fournier	Microliposuction
2003		FDA approval of human based collagen (CosmoDerm 1 and CosmoPlast)
2004		FDA approval of hyaluronic acids (Restylane and Hylaform)

Table 3.1 Historical milestones of filler substances

Partial list of characteristics of the ideal filler substance

Material
- Nonallergenic (decreased risk of hypersensitivity)
- FDA approved
- Noncarcinogenic/nonteratogenic
- No migration
- Minimal inflammation
- No overt cutaneous change (undetectable)
- Reproducible
- Durable
- Minimal adverse sequelae
- Stable (inert)
- Affordable

Administration
- Basic administration
- Painless
- Outpatient (minimal recuperation)
- User friendly
- Large amount available
- Easy storage

Box 3.1 Partial list of characteristics of the ideal filler substance

when injected by an experienced physician, this product has had a tumultuous history and continues to be controversial. Pure injectable grade liquid silicone (350 centistokes) was never approved by the US Food and Drug Administration (FDA) and remains prohibited. However, silicone is approved for retinal tamponade in patients with retinal detachments. Out of necessity for lack of an acceptable alternative, there is an ongoing multicenter study exploring the benefits of injectable microdroplet silicone (Silikon 1000) for patients suffering from facial lipoatrophy due to infection with the human immunodeficiency virus. Two forms of silicone (AdatoSil 5000 centistoke, Escalon Medical, Chicago, IL, USA; Silikon 1000, Richard-James Company, Peabody, MA, USA) have both been used for off label indications with increasing frequency for permanent soft tissue augmentation. However, when administering these products, physicians should discuss their use with their medical malpractice carriers because the administration of silicone may not be covered in the event of legal action.

Arguably one of the most significant advances in soft tissue augmentation was the introduction of bovine collagen. Initial investigations began in earnest in 1958 and continued through the next two decades. In 1981 Zyderm I (Collagen Corporation, Santa Barbara, CA, USA) became the first FDA approved xenogenic agent for soft tissue augmentation. Following this the two additional formulations of bovine collagen, Zyderm II and Zyplast, were granted FDA approval. In the United States, while many materials and substances are available, the most commonly used injectables remain bovine collagen and autologous fat. It is perhaps the success and availability of these products that ushered in a renewed quest for the ideal formulation for soft tissue augmentation (Box 3.1).

No wrinkle is created equal as they come in many shapes and sizes, and as such there is no one filler agent that is suitable for all defects. Treatment should be predicated on the defect and individualized to each patient's needs. The selection of the appropriate implant (whether dermal or subcutaneous, temporary or permanent; liquid, semisolid, or solid) requires knowledge of the available materials and their characteristics. Furthermore filler substances may be used as monotherapy or combined with resurfacing, chemodenervation, or surgery.

Filler Materials

There is an ever-expanding menu of materials and devices for soft tissue augmentation and they can be classified, based on either derivation or site of cutaneous placement. Autologous materials (adipose) are harvested from the same patient and hence have no risk of immunologic reaction, but do require an initial harvesting procedure and potentially have a limited donor reservoir. Xenografts are semisynthetic formulations harvested from a different species (bovine collagen, and some avian hyaluronic acid derivatives) that are readily available and carry a low risk of infection and rejection. Allograft materials (Dermalogen, Cymetra) are harvested from human cadaveric tissue, have a minimal risk of hypersensitivity reaction, but pose a theoretic risk of infection. While synthetic substances (such as expanded polytetrafluoroethylene) provide longer lasting results they require insertion, as opposed to injection, and because they are foreign bodies, may be extruded. The collagen products meet many of the criteria of the ideal product for soft tissue augmentation (ambulatory, reproducible, FDA approved) and they have an extensive safety profile.

Collagen products

There are many forms of injectable collagen but the two that have maintained the widest appeal and diversity are the bovine derived Zyderm family of products, and the human bioengineered form, the CosmoDerm family (Table 3.2). Both are manufactured by Inamed Esthetics (Santa Barbara, CA, USA) and are further subdivided into three categories based upon the viscosity of the material and their corresponding indication. They are available in boxes of six preloaded single use syringes containing white-opaque collagen suspended in phosphate buffered physiologic saline with 0.3% lidocaine (Lignocaine), and are stable for up to a year when stored in a refrigerator (4°C). The manufacturer recommends that any unused collagen should be disposed of and not be stored between patient visits. Should there be any separation of the microfibrils and there is not a uniform consistency of the material the syringe should not be used and it should be returned to the manufacturer. The single use syringes are accompanied by labels with a lot number and expiration date that can be affixed to the patient's chart for tracking purposes and 30 gauge 0.5 inch or adjustable depth gauge needles (ADG). The latter have the ability to be adjusted to alter the distance between the distal end of the needle and the skin surface.

Bovine collagen

The bovine derived collagen products are Zyderm I, Zyderm II, and Zyplast. These collagen products have been used safely and effectively as biomaterials since 1982 due to their unique physical properties and weak immunogenicity. To date over two million patients have been treated with highly purified reconstituted bovine collagen. All three Zyderm collagen implants are 95–98% type I collagen, with the remainder being type III. Zyderm I is the least concentrated and contains 35 mg/mL of collagen and generally is used for very superficial rhytides or to layer on top of another filling agent. Placement of Zyderm I should be in the superficial papillary

FDA approved collagens					
Type of collagen	**Concentration of collagen**	**Indications**	**Size of syringe available**	**Placement**	**Degree of overcorrection**
Zyderm I	35 mg/mL Bovine	Fine lines: perioral periocular glabellar	0.5, 1.0, 1.5 mL	Superficial papillary dermis	150–200×
Zyderm II	65 mg/mL Bovine	Mild-moderate rhytides: scars perioral	0.5, 1.0 mL	Mid dermis	100–150×
Zyplast	35 mg/mL crosslinked with glutaraldehyde Bovine	Deeper rhytides and folds: nasolabial vermilion marionette lines	1, 1.5, 2, 2.5 mL	Deep dermis	No overcorrection
CosmoDerm 1	35 mg/mL Human derived	Fine lines: perioral periocular glabellar	1 mL	Superficial papillary dermis	150–200×
CosmoDerm 2 (pending)					
Cosmoplast	35 mg/mL crosslinked with gluteraldehyde Human derived	Deeper rhytides and folds: nasolabial vermilion border marionette lines	1, 1.5 mL	Deep dermis	No overcorrection

Table 3.2 FDA approved collagens

dermis. Because a significant portion of Zyderm I is saline, which is rapidly resorbed, the defect should be overcorrected by 150–200% imparting a white blanch or peau d'orange appearance to the epidermis. Zyderm II is a more concentrated and viscous form of Zyderm I and contains 65 mg/mL of collagen and is intermediate in durability between Zyderm I and the more robust form Zyplast. Zyderm II is appropriate for deeper lines and wrinkles and is placed deeper in the papillary dermis with about 100–150% overcorrection. Zyplast has a concentration of 35 mg/mL but it has the longest duration because it is cross linked by the addition of 0.0075% glutaraldehyde. This characteristic decreases proteolytic degradation by collagenase and enhances its in vivo stability, lasting longer than the 3 months generally anticipated for the Zyderm products. Typically Zyplast is placed deeper in the dermis and is recommended for deep rhytides and folds and there should be no overcorrection upon injection.

Prior to therapy with any of the three bovine products, potential allergic response to the products must be excluded. Hypersensitivity can be reduced with double skin testing. The skin test is available in 1.0 mL tuberculin syringes that contain 0.3 mL of Zyderm I, which screens for all three forms of bovine collagen. Approximately 0.1 mL is injected subcutaneously in an inconspicuous area, such as the volar aspect of the forearm or upperarm. Hypersensitivity is characterized by swelling, induration, tenderness, pruritus, and/or erythema at the injection site and resolves with time as the implant is absorbed. This has been found in approximately 3% of patients and indicates a pre-existing allergy to bovine collagen. Despite a negative preliminary test, an additional 1–2% of patients will develop allergic reactions to the products at subsequent treatments. Therefore, it is generally the standard of practice to perform a second challenge 2 weeks after the initial skin test. This test, using a similar volume, can be injected on the contralateral arm and should be monitored for two additional weeks. A positive reaction occurring with either of the tests is a contraindication and conversely negative skin testing allows the patient to proceed with treatment 4 weeks after the initial test or 2 weeks after the second. An amended protocol is recommended for patients who have previously been successfully treated with bovine collagen, but have not had soft tissue augmentation for a year or more. If these patients do not wish to switch to the newer form of human derived collagen and elect to continue with bovine products, to reduce the risk of bovine hypersensitivity, a single retest with a 2 week observation period is suggested prior to commencing treatment.

Synthetic human collagen

The development of human derived collagen was prompted by the need for a product that would eliminate hypersensitivity reactions and the required skin testing. Based on the safety profile following their use in burns and wounds, the CosmoDerm family of products was granted approval by the FDA for soft tissue augmentation in March of 2003. There are currently only two forms; CosmoDerm 1 and CosmoPlast, the third, CosmoDerm 2, is still pending final FDA approval. They have the same consistency and injection properties as Zyderm and Zyplast but are grown from a single human fibroblast cell culture and, unlike other human derived products (Dermalogen and Cymetra), are not cadaveric in nature. They are the result of tissue engineered technology and have undergone extensive pathogen screening for viral and bacterial contamination to avoid the possibility of disease transmission. As these products are nonanimal based they have the significant advantage that they do not require initial skin testing to exclude the risk of hypersensitivity prior to administration and hence can be injected on the same day as the initial consultation. Similar to its bovine counterpart Zyderm I, CosmoDerm 1 has a concentration of 35 mg/mL and is placed into the superficial papillary dermis with a comparable degree of blanching and overcorrection, and is also primarily indicated for superficial lines and defects. Cosmoplast, like Zyplast, is the more robust of the two and contains 35 mg/mL of human derived collagen cross-linked with glutaraldehyde, which not only increases its durability but also makes it less immunogenic. It is a deeper dermal implant, to a depth of approximately 2 mm, and does not require overcorrection to improve deep folds and wrinkles.

Human cadaveric collagens

In the late 1980s research began on extracting intact human collagen fibers and acellular dermal matrix from cadavers for human dermal implantation. These products, Dermalogen and Cymetra, were available as injectables in preloaded syringes and implantable grafts. However with the introduction and availability of the newer forms of bioengineered human collagen these products seem to have lost some of their initial appeal.

Dermalogen (Collagenesis, Inc., Beverely, MA, USA) is an injectable allograft material of human tissue collagen matrix origin. It is composed primarily of intact collagen and elastin fibers and glycosaminoglycans harvested from the dermal layer of human cadaveric skin. Tissue is obtained from accredited American Association of Tissue Banks (AATBs) facilities. Extensive screening is done on the donor tissue for human immunodeficiency virus, T-lymphotrophic virus-1, hepatitis B and C, syphilis, and bacterial contamination. It is processed to ensure safety by rupture and removal of cells, two viral inactivation steps, a prion inactivation step, and sterilization. The material, a 3.5% concentration, is supplied in 0.50 or 1.0 mL syringes with a 30 gauge needle. Dermalogen does not contain lidocaine (lignocaine), and injections tend to be rather painful. Discomfort should be reduced by local anesthesia with nerve blocks, topical anesthetics, and/or local anesthesia with lidocaine placed at the injection sites. Unlike bovine collagen which should be kept refrigerated until used, it is suggested that Dermalogen be allowed to equilibrate to room temperature for 1 hour prior to injection to improve flow characteristics and make it more pliable and easier to inject. The injections are carried out in the dermal plane. Some overcorrection is appropriate and a temporary blanch can occur. Because there is some evidence of neovascularization and host collagen deposition in sites injected with Dermalogen, early reports suggested that correction may be long lasting; however, this has yet to be substantiated. Although skin testing was originally recommended, Dermalogen does not carry the risk of hypersensitivity, and no skin test is currently supplied. Therefore consultation, evaluation, and augmentation can occur on the first visit. In addition to technique sensitive adverse events, prolonged erythema and hyperpigmentation have been reported at the injection site. In 2003, Dermalogen was removed from the US market pending further study.

Cymetra, manufactured by Lifecell Corporation (Branchburg, NJ, USA) and distributed by OMP (Long Beach, CA, USA), consists primarily of micronized human collagen fibers. It is comparable to other injectable allogragfts (Dermalogen) and is similar in composition and processing, with screening carried out by the American Association of Tissue Banks. Furthermore, its acellular nature mitigates skin testing, and to date there have been no reports of hypersensitivity reactions. This feature provides a major advantage for patients with a prior history of bovine collagen hypersensitivity.

The primary distinction of Cymetra is that it is in powdered form which translates to both a prolonged shelf-life, and the necessity of reconstitution before injection. 1.0 mL of 1% lidocaine (lignocaine) is used to rehydrate the product; it is mixed for approximately 3 minutes in a 3.0 mL syringe attached via a Luer tip to a 5.0 mL syringe. Once completely saturated the product changes from a white powder to a cream color with a paste-like consistency. The viscous, semiliquid substance can be injected with the 3.0 mL syringe or transferred to a tuberculin syringe. The latter, smaller syringe requires less pressure to evacuate the contents. Although lidocaine is used for rehydration, the placement of the first injection requires some form of anesthesia. The product is supplied with both a 0.5 and 1.0 inch 23 gauge needle, which allows access to the deep dermis. The large size of the needle generally would mandate injection with a single puncture. Creating a dermal pocket with a needle prior to administration further aids in placement. There may be a transient blanch, but of more consequence is the profound distension and subsequent postinjection edema. This swelling can be readily apparent and may not subside for many hours, and massage, ice compresses, and systemic anti-inflammatory medications may be necessary to reduce the edema (Fig. 3.1).

Isolagen

No chapter about collagens would be complete without mention of Isolagen (Isolagen Inc., Houston, Texas, USA). Isolagen is derived not from bovine, cadaveric or cultured unrelated fibroblasts, but rather from autologous fibroblasts. This process utilizes skin harvested from the patient, which is cultured at Isolagen Inc. and then injected back into the patient.

The process of using Isolagen begins with a 3 mm punch biopsy to harvest skin. Typically, the donor site chosen is from the posterior auricular area. This area is thought to be ideal because it has not had sun damage, is well vascularized, and is a good site in which to create a small scar. Using local anesthetic, the biopsy is obtained and the donor site is closed with a suture or adhesive. The specimen is then transported to Isolagen Inc. where it is cultured.

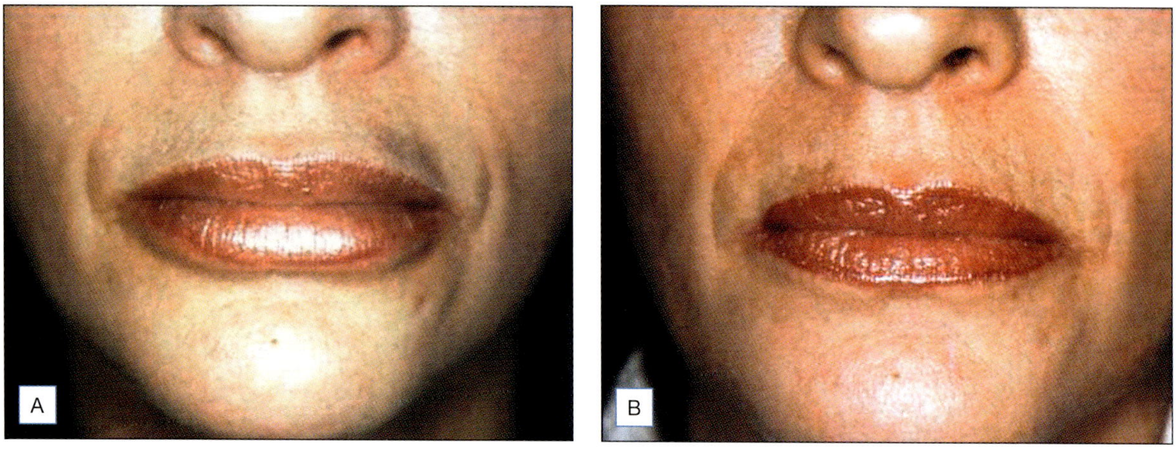

Fig. 3.1 1 week postinjection of Cymetra into the vermilion border (**A**), and at approximately 2 months following injection (**B**)

From the single biopsy, fibroblasts that will produce collagen are stimulated to produce tens of millions of cells. After a period of weeks, the harvest is ready for injection. After the patented harvesting technique has been performed, the yield of product is between 1 and 1.5 cm^3. This is injected into areas that are traditionally treated with collagen, such as the nasolabial creases, lips, marionette lines, etc. The company recommends that the procedure be repeated three times, each about 2 weeks apart.

Once injected back into the body, it is hoped that the fibroblasts will continue to produce collagen that will be long lasting.

Potential benefits of this procedure seem to be attractive: no risk of rejection from foreign proteins, no risk of infections from an animal or unrelated human donor, and continuous production of collagen from living fibroblasts. Theoretically, however, the potential for the introduction of infectious organisms and contamination exists in any tissue culture environment. The extent to which the fibroblasts continue to produce collagen and affect a soft tissue correction needs to be defined in clinical trials which are (according to the company) underway.

At the present time, it may be said that Isolagen appears to be a promising collagen treatment. Clinical trials will be very helpful in determining where this product fits into the range of soft tissue augmentation products offered by the dermatologic surgeon.

Patient Selection

Patients seeking treatment with soft tissue augmentation often do not adequately appreciate the nature of their defect and hence should be educated about the underlying 'anatomy of a wrinkle'. The distinction must be made between dynamic versus static lines, and those secondary to chronology and gravitational pull. Although these defects are not mutually exclusive and, in fact, often appear in combination, their treatment mandates individual evaluation.

While the type of defect is clearly important, so too is its size, depth, and location, as well as the appearance and integrity of the adjacent tissue (Box 3.2). The patient must also be informed of the many different means for improving them. A

Soft tissue augmentation preinjection considerations

Defect parameters

- Medications (anticoagulants)
- History of hypersensitivity reaction
- History of herpes labialis
- Volume required
- Location
- Alternative/simultaneous treatments
- Medical history
- Pregnancy/lactation
- Autoimmune disease

Patient goals

- Expectations (longevity)
- Degree of improvement (what is of concern to the patient?)
- Morbidity patient is willing to sustain
- Risk/benefit ratio

Box 3.2 Soft tissue augmentation preinjection considerations discussion regarding therapeutic options should include the alternatives of surgery: rhytidectomy, excision, punch grafting, and resurfacing and chemodenervating agents (botulinum toxin), as well as no intervention at all. Patients should have an adequate comprehension of the indications and technique, advantages and disadvantages, and inherent risks of each procedure, with an estimate of the time needed for full recuperation. As with any treatment, the success is largely proportional to the extent of realistic and appropriate goals and expectations set by both the physician and the patient. Patients undergoing soft tissue augmentation must be especially aware of the temporary nature and primary purpose of replacing lost or atrophic subcutaneous tissue. It is the physician's responsibility to critically evaluate the defect, determine its etiology, and provide treatment parameters.

Treatment Guidelines

Prior to any form of soft tissue augmentation it is recommended that patients abstain from medications that can inhibit platelet aggregation and potentiate ecchymosis for approximately 10–14 days before their appointment. After an informed consent form is signed that is applicable specifically to fillers, the area should be photographed and the pretreatment photographs viewed by both physician and patient. Corroboration by the patient with a hand held mirror is essential. The area to be treated is cleansed of all soaps and make-up with either alcohol or a clear surgical antiseptic solution. When necessary the area to be addressed can be delineated with a surgical marker and topical anesthesia can be applied. Percutaneous injections can be painful, especially in the central face and perioral areas, and anesthesia should be offered to patients. Cutaneous anesthesia can be obtained with various creams (LMX, topicaine, or betacaine) and local anesthesia and nerve blocks are unnecessary. For adequate pain management the topical anesthetics should be applied liberally and left intact for 15–30 minutes. They also have enhanced penetration when used under occlusion. Although not mandatory, to aid in diminishing patient discomfort/anxiety, it is also helpful to have auditory (music) and tactile (a soft rubber ball placed in their hand) diversions.

Patients should be in a dependant or seated position with their heads upright so that their lines and folds are accentuated and not obliterated upon reclining. To further appreciate the defects overhead lighting and magnification are helpful.

Before penetrating the skin surface any topical preparations and anesthetics should be removed in a nonabrasive manner with gauze and then the filler can be injected. It is preferable to bend the needle to a 45 degree angle and insert it with the bevel up gently through a pilosebaceous opening. The material can then be placed in the proper dermal location with the serial puncture technique, linear threading, or a combination of the two. The former, serial puncture, is preformed by applying small discrete amounts of material at the leading edge of the previously injected deposit, the later threading is one continuous uninterrupted injection. Massage and ice applied to the treated area can reduce erythema and edema. Unlike many other facial procedures the results are immediate with few postprocedural restrictions and patients can reapply make-up and promptly resume their normal daily activities.

Indications

Areas that are amenable to treatment with Zyderm I or CosmoDerm 1 include the superficial periorbital and perioral lines that radiate from the eyes and lips (lipstick lines). Lines in the glabella and forehead may be treated with Zyderm I or II or CosmoDerm 1. The oral commissures, vermilion borders, and nasolabial creases are best suited to the thicker products; Zyplast or CosmoPlast as the non-cross linked products do not provide sufficient long term augmentation. Shallow soft distensible scars due to trauma, surgery or infection such as varicella or acne vulgaris respond well to any of the forms of collagen. While there are few absolutes with respect to selection of collagen, and there can be a great deal of personal physician preference, the one irrefutable contraindication is the use of the thicker fillers, Zyplast and CosmoPlast, in the glabellar complex. The deeper placement required of these products has been associated with vascular compromise and sloughing of the skin (Fig. 3.2).

Scars

Patients that are good candidates for scar correction with collagen include those who acknowledge that the results are temporary and will need multiple visits for optimal outcomes. Anatomically the indications are shallow scars that are approximately

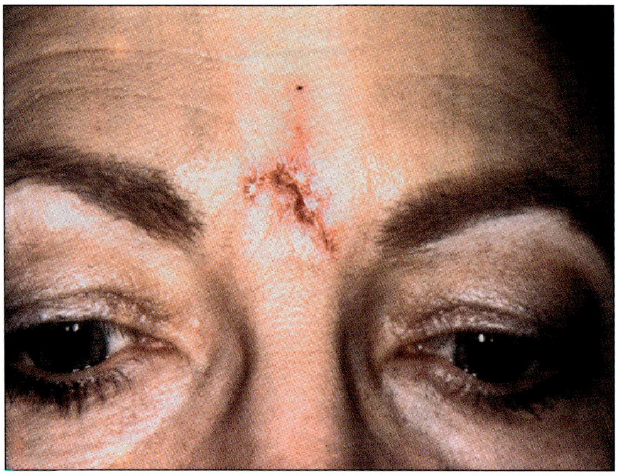

Fig. 3.2 Slough of the skin following vascular embarrassment from deep placement of Zyplast into the glabellar region. The use of any cross-linked products is an absolute contraindication in this area

1–2 mm in depth, 2–4 mm in width, and are not prominent. Patients with a history of keloidal scarring should be treated cautiously since the injection of collagen can theoretically precipitate new keloid formation.

It is important to appreciate the thickness and amount of sebaceous glands of a patient's skin prior to selecting the collagen to be used. For patients with thin or translucent skin (underlying blood vessels can be seen), a non-cross-linked collagen such as Zyderm or CosmoDerm is adequate. Men, and in general patients with thicker skin with a greater density of sebaceous glands, should be treated with a crosslinked collagen such as Zyplast or CosmoPlast.

Prior to injecting collagen into a scar some have advocated 'subcising' the area. Under local anesthesia using an 18 gauge needle and a windshield like action, a dermal pocket can be created where the material can be deposited. This serves to trap and immobilize the implanted material and eliminates mechanical forces that could lead to early degradation. The collagen injection should begin at the junction between the scar and adjacent uninvolved skin. Several injections made from differing angles release any remaining subcutaneous fibrous attachments that may exist and assists in uniform and homogenous placement. Correction of small annular scars should be directed towards the center, and with linear scars, injections should be oriented at about 45 degrees with the long axis of the scar.

Lip augmentation

The injection of collagen in the circumoral area is one of the most frequently requested regions for enhancement and there is a wide range of acceptable candidates. Commonly they are patients with atrophy of the lip secondary to age, those with vertical rhytides emanating from the vermilion ('smokers lines'), and those desiring augmentation simply for enhanced cosmesis. Unlike other areas, the lips are the central focus of the face and patients express very strong feelings about their size and shape. It is wise to have a frank discussion of what can reasonably be achieved. While patients often will provide photographs from lay publications of what they may consider their 'ideal lip', it would be prudent to maintain appropriate goals as the most significant contraindication is patients with unrealistic expectations. A relative contraindication is patients with recurrent herpes labialis, and these patients require prophylaxis with oral antiviral medications.

The basic issues of lip augmentation are: definition of the vermilion border, oral commissure elevation, volume replacement, and vertical rhytide correction, and all are interrelated as improvement of one directly impacts the others. The vermilion is the only FDA sanctioned indication and the thickest forms of collagen, Zyplast and CosmoPlast, are used here and in the angles of the mouth. For volume and perioral rhytides the non-cross-linked formulations such as Zyderm I and II and CosmoDerm 1 are recommended.

Understanding lip anatomy and the esthetics and ratios of the lower face are essential for optimum lip augmentation. The lip should not be perceived as a homogenous, linear structure, rather, it is has different contours, volumes, and inflection points. The proportions of the lip change with time and in a youthful lip the ideal ratio of the upper lip to the lower lip is 0.6 : 1 and it is important to attempt to restore the lower lip to a more youthful dominant proportion. The two constants of lip augmentation are that the lip should have transition points and there should be no downward slope, but rather an elevation of the lateral commissures.

Prior to injection, any pre-existing asymmetries should be identified and pointed out in the pretreatment photographs to the patient. In combination with the lidocaine (lignocaine) already mixed in with the collagen the discomfort can be adequately managed with various topical preparations. Regional nerve blocks (infraorbital, mental) are effective in completely eliminating pain, but are generally not needed as they can distort the oral anatomy and impart a false sense of fullness to the patient.

To accentuate the vermilion border and define the lip, Zyplast or CosmoPlast is injected in a threading manner into the potential space that runs continuously along the lip edge. This small channel runs the entire length of the lip and allows collagen to flow uniformly with minimal pressure on the syringe plunger. This by itself creates a demarcation that defines the lip margin, stops lipstick from 'bleeding' from the lips, and restores some volume. However, when one of the goals is to further increase the volume of the lip, it is recommended to place 0.1 mL aliquots of Zyderm I or CosmoDerm 1 with the serial puncture technique along the 'wet/dry' (epidermal–mucosal) junction. This however is an area where the Fordyce glands are typically located and showing them to patients prior to injection prevents concerns that the collagen caused them. Although not an FDA approved location for collagen implantation, when a patient requests more volume, everting the lips slightly and injecting directly to the labial mucosa will produce a slight eversion and give the appearance of a fuller lip. Upon injection it is important to monitor both the amount being used to maintain symmetry and to avoid deep placement that would interfere with the labial artery. The 'cupids bow' may better be defined by adding additional Zyplast or CosmoPlast in that midline curvilinear structure and injecting directly into the philtral columns. Patients who require treatment of perioral rhytides tend to be women whose genetics, musculature, smoking habits, or photodamage have resulted in moderate vertical lines. A typical patient is a woman in her mid thirties to late forties with a complaint that her lipstick is bleeding into the surrounding skin. Patients with severe perioral rhytides will do better with resurfacing rather than with soft tissue augmentation. In order to correct these lines a non-cross-linked material such as Zyderm I or II or CosmoDerm 1 is used. The cross-linked products have a tendency to produce contour irregularities and bumps. The needle is placed at the vermilion border pointing away from the mouth and is inserted under the entire length of the rhytide and the collagen is injected in a retrograde manner as the needle is slowly withdrawn. This allows for an even distribution. Alternatively the collagen can be injected in a serial puncture manner. However, using this technique, careful control of the plunger must be exercised to ensure that very small amounts are placed with each injection or beading will occur. Following either injection technique, gentle massage is performed.

Correction of ptosis of the triangular area at the angle of the mouth, the lateral commissure, is an ideal indication for collagen as it bolsters up the lower lip and acts like a buttress restoring the 'drool area' to a more neutral position. Since the goal is volume replacement and not line reduction the material selected for this region should be one of the crosslinked products. Adding volume is done with serial injections of about 0.05–0.1 cc of Zyplast or CosmoPlast. Beginning inferiorly just above the edge of the mandible these injections address the marionette lines that extend down from the lateral oral commissure. Then the second leg of the triangle is addressed, which is located at an angle of about 60 degrees from the marionette line and points towards the corner of the mouth. Finally, the third leg of the triangle of the oral commissure is the line that connects the two, and is the horizontal border of the lower lip vermilion. Filling all three aspects of this triangle raises the corner of the lip (Figs 3.3 and 3.4).

In many cases, the lip position, texture and volume can be softened with collagen but the patient may continue to have deep perioral rhytides or malposition of the angles of the mouth. This is often secondary to hypertrophy or hyperkinetic movement of the perioral musculature. An advanced injectable technique that can improve the appearance of the senescent mouth is the adjunctive use of chemodenervation with botulinum toxin (Botox Aesthetic, Allergan Inc., Irvine, CA, USA). To prevent unwanted migration, upon completion of soft tissue augmentation of the lips, reconstituted Botox (2.5 mL preserved normal saline/100 unit vial; 4 units/0.1 mL) can be injected into the orbicularis oris muscle. The patient is instructed to purse their lips to visualize maximum muscle mass and 1–2 units are superficially injected into each quadrant of the upper and lower lips. Crossing the midline is contraindicated as it can result in blunting of the Cupid's bow. Reducing the perioral lines with Botox has the added benefit of simultaneously weakening the sphincter activity of the orbicularis oris muscle which everts the lip and gives the appearance of a fuller lip (pseudoaugmentation) (Fig. 3.5). Similarly, inducing paresis of one of the lower lip depressors,

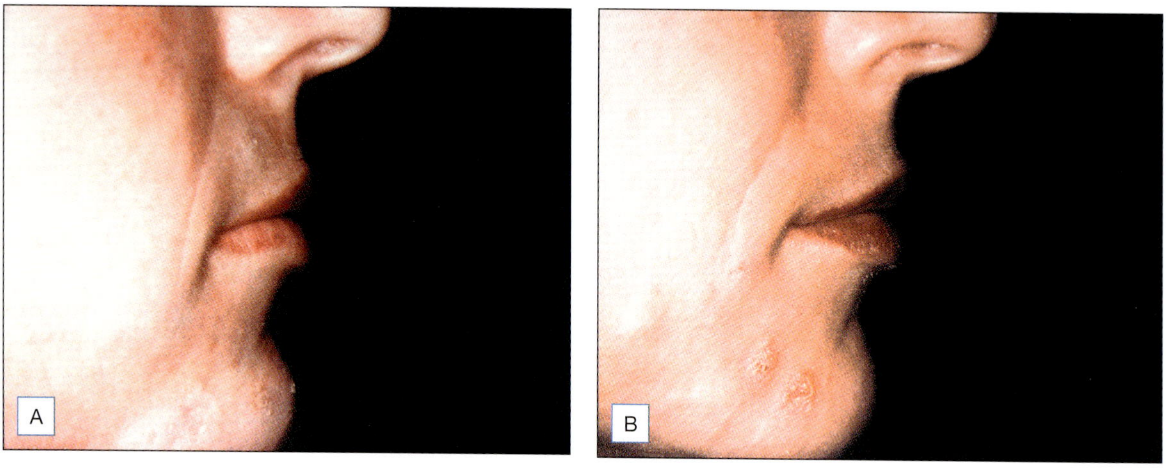

Fig. 3.3 Profile before (**A**) and after (**B**) lip augmentation with Zyplast collagen into the vermilion border and oral comissures

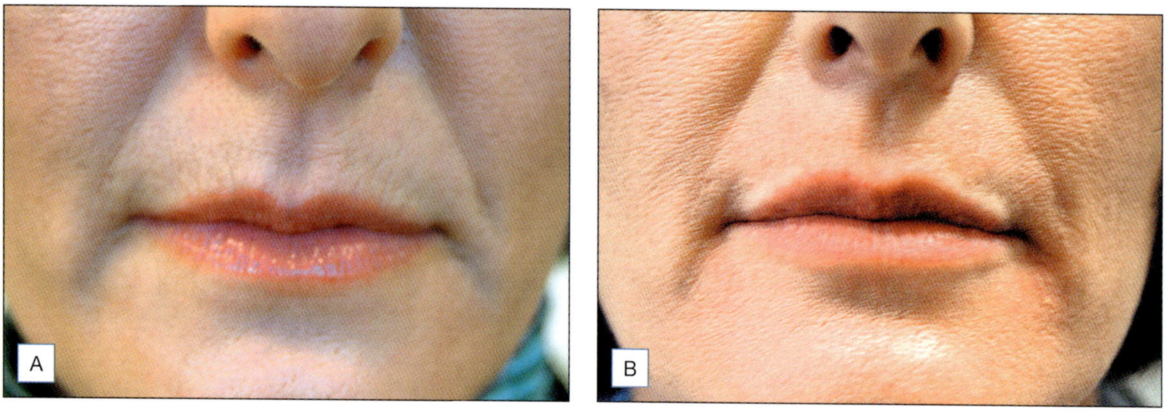

Fig. 3.4 Before (**A**) and after (**B**) frontal photographs of vermilion augmentation with CosmoPlast

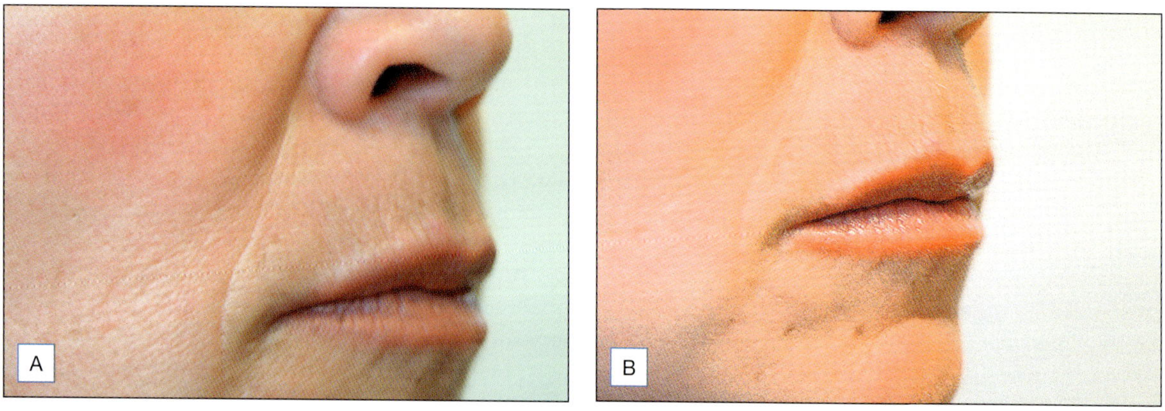

Fig. 3.5 Combination therapy:before (**A**) and after (**B**) three quarters view using CosmoPlast into the vermillion border and CosmoDerm 1 and Botox for the perioral rhytides

the depressor anguli oris muscle, with 2–3 units of Botox eliminates its downward pull and aids in elevation of the lateral commisure. This small muscle can be located just anterior to the masseter muscle as it crosses the mandible. Relaxing this muscle bilaterally in conjunction with collagen augmentation elevates the angles of the mouth. An additional injection pearl for those wishing to combine different filler products is to initially flow one of the collagens along the vermilion border. The lidocaine (lignocaine) in the collagen will provide some degree of anesthesia so that a second agent such as one of the recently approved hyaluronic acids that does not contain lidocaine can be injected with less discomfort. As in other areas the ideal patient for soft tissue augmentation in the perioral region is an individual who is willing to accept short term correction. When addressing the lip area it is of particular importance that realistic expectations about durability of correction should be reinforced and it is preferable to err in the conservative range of 3–4 months.

Nasolabial fold

Smile lines, wrinkles that extend from the angle of the nose to the corner of the upper lip, are a frequent site for soft tissue replacement and the criteria for selecting patients for treating this area are similar to those for other regions. Treatment of nasolabial creases is performed in order to correct volume defects in the deep dermis and the amount required should be predicated on the depth of the fold. To ensure patient satisfaction, placement of adequate volume is important. There is no perfect filler for all defects, and when very large volumes are necessary for adequate volumetric correction and collagen would not be sufficient, an alternative such as autologous fat transplantation should be discussed with the patient (Table 3.2).

Effacing the nasolabial creases involves injections with a needle at a depth of about 1.0–2.0 mm. The material, Zyplast or CosmoPlast, should be placed medial to the crease to avoid lateral extravasation. Beginning at the distal portion of the crease, collagen is injected in a cephalad direction. It is wise to evaluate the symmetry and predict the total quantity that will be needed and divide half of the allotted material for the contralateral fold. One area that often is neglected when correcting nasolabial creases is the triangle at the nasal sill immediately adjacent to the ala. If this is not treated adequately, the entire cosmetic unit will appear undercorrected. Injection should involve injecting the entire expanse of the nasolabial crease to its termination at the nasal ala. Care must be taken as the facial vein and artery are located in this triangle and deep injections can eventuate into profound bruising and intravascular placement can result in tissue necrosis and slough. Following treatment of the nasolabial fold with collagen, one gloved finger can be inserted into the mouth and another finger placed on the outside and gentle massage of the two opposing digits may reduce bumps and locate any areas that have been skipped.

Periorbital rhytides

Treatment of periocular rhytides, those radiating from the lateral ocular canthus (crows' feet) and infraocularly in the nasojugal groove, are more challenging uses of collagen. The periorbital skin is very thin with a rich superficial vascular plexus and treating this region with fillers is unforgiving, often resulting in visible beading and significant eccyhmosis. It is routinely considered as an ancillary treatment to Botox, resurfacing procedures, and blepharoplasty surgery.

Since many of these lines are dynamic, due to activity of the underlying orbicularis oculi muscle, Botox is considered the primary treatment of choice. The subsequent addition of fillers primarily addresses any of the remaining static and photodynamic lines.

Selectively inactivating fibers of the large annular orbicularis oculi muscle that encircles the eye sustains and preserves the benefits of collagen in this area. Between 10 and 15 units of Botox placed lateral to the ocular rim eliminates many of the mimetic horizontal crows' feet lines. An additional 2–4 units at the lateral canthus and approximately 3 mm below the ciliary margin at the midpupillary line will greatly improve the appearance of the lower eyelid rhytides. Any of the remaining fine lines can be treated with collagen. The collagen used for periocular rhytides should be a thin product such as Zyderm I or CosmoDerm 1. When placing collagen around the eyes, the technique is similar to that used for the vertical perioral rhytides. The needle should be very superficial and with minimal force on the plunger serial injections of about 0.05 mL should be used to gradually fill the rhytides. Treating the infraorbital sulcus with collagen should also be done cautiously but the results for treating this 'hollow' at the infraorbital rim can be dramatic.

When injecting collagen around the eyes, patients should be forewarned that swelling may be significant. Additionally significant bruising can occur and may last between 5 and 7 days. This can be minimized by limiting products that anticoagulate blood (aspirin, homeopathic medications, and vitamins) for 10 days prior to treatment. Should ecchymosis occur cool compresses with ice and massage can reduce their size and green based make-ups can ultimately camouflage them.

Adverse sequelae and complications associated with collagen

Bovine and human derived

- Temporary concerns: erythema, edema, ecchymosis
- Infection: herpetic, acneiform eruption
- Contour irregularity: superficial placement, beading
- Intravascular injection: tissue necrosis, vision loss

Bovine collagen

- Localized hypersensitivity reaction: granulomatous, cystic

Box 3.3 Adverse sequelae and complications associated with collagen

Glabellar complex

The etiology of glabellar wrinkles is mainly due to hypertrophy of the bilateral corrugator supercilli and midline procerus muscles. Paralysis of these muscles with 20–35 units of Botox eliminates much of the muscular movement and eliminates the lines in the region. However despite adequate muscular immobility, often due to both chronic photodamage and repetitive movement, there remains a pair of superimposed deeply etched parallel lines in the skin. Zyderm I or CosmoDerm 1, non-cross-linked products, is used to soften these residual static lines. Zyplast and Cosmoplast are absolutely contraindicated for this area due to their deep placement and the risk of vascular embarrassment and subsequent skin necrosis. The injecting technique for the glabellar lines is analogous to those in the periocular and perioral regions.

Complications

A common source of frustration for patients receiving collagen injections is the temporary nature of the correction. Duration of implanted dermal filling substances is dependent on the volume used, the type of defect, and the mechanical stresses at the implantation site. Patient satisfaction is a combination not only of anatomic defect and physician expertise, but also managing expectations. This can be tempered if patients are provided with an idea about the time range over which augmentation can be sustained. In general, patients can anticipate 3–6 months of improvement with gradual diminution of results; however, patients can receive additional treatment or maintenance therapy at any time. It has also been anecdotally noted that while the CosmoDerm family of products has better flow characteristics, which is advantageous for the physician, it has also been allegedly found to have a briefer duration of augmentation.

The adverse events for both classes of injectable collagen can be nonhypersensitive, and additionally for bovine collagen hypersensitive reaction patterns may occur (Box 3.3). Many of the former nonhypersensitive reactions are technique dependent, and include injection site ecchymosis, superficial placement with apparent beading, and deep placement with intravascular injury. Vascular occlusion following dermal placement of collagen, a rare occurrence, presents as an immediate cutaneous blanch associated with pain. Immediate vasodilation with warm compresses and topical nitroglycerin can reduce the vasospasm. Ultimately, if tissue necrosis and slough occur, sustained emotional support and appropriate wound care are essential to expedite resolution.

With bovine collagen there are two forms of true classic type IV hypersensitivity to the implants. They develop in about 1% of those whose two skin tests are negative and who subsequently receive treatment. Due primarily to Zyderm I and occurring at approximately 2 weeks after treatment, the more common reaction is manifested by swollen, indurated granulomas at both the treatment and test sites. Although they resolve spontaneously and without permanent scarring, they can take up to 1 year to completely dissipate. In addition to reassurance, treatment has included nonsteroidal anti-inflammatory drugs and intralesional injections of dilute corticosteroids (triamcinalone).

There has been anecdotal evidence that oral cyclosporin and topical immune modulators (tacrolimus) have expedited resolution. Sterile abscesses are the second form of delayed hypersensitivity that has been associated with bovine collagen. The incidence is low, approximately 1–4 in 10 000 treatments, and is due in large part to Zyplast. Adverse reactions are characterized by the sudden onset of pain, usually a few weeks after injection, followed by tense edema and erythema with fluctuant nodules. The lesions can be treated by incision and drainage, intralesional steroids, and oral antibiotics. However scarring can occur. The circulating antibovine-collagen antibodies that occur in these reactions do not cross-react with human collagen products, and there has not been any statistical association between bovine collagen and autoimmune connective tissue disease.

It should also be noted that the bovine collagens are all derived from the hides of a closed herd of American cattle, and therefore do not come in contact with animals exposed to the prions that cause bovine spongiform encephalopathy.

Conclusion

Facial soft tissue deformities and age related cutaneous changes have a great impact on psychosocial interactions. There are many causes for these defects, and in our quest for enhancing the appearance of the facial skin envelope there is a correspondingly wide range of techniques for improving them. The vast arrays of available filler products, and those still on the horizon, are safe and effective means to provide volume and improve contour irregularities associated with aging and trauma.

Further Reading

Aschinoff R 2000 Overview: soft tissue augmentation. Clinics in Plastic Surgery 274:479–487

Bauman L, Kerdel F 1999 The treatment of bovine collagen allergy with cyclosporine. Dermatologic Surgery 25:247–249

Drake L, Dinehart S, Farmer E, et al 1996 Guidelines of care for soft tissue augmentation. Journal of the American Academy of Dermatology 34:695–697

Elson ML 1989 The role of skin testing in the use of collagen-injectable materials. Journal of Dermatologic Surgery and Oncology 15:301–303

Kaminer MS, Kraus MC 1998 Filler substances in the treatment of facial aging. Medical and Surgical Dermatology 15:215–221

Matarasso SL, Matarasso A 2001 Treatment guidelines for botulinum toxin type A for the periocular region and a report on partial upper lip ptosis following injections to the lateral canthal rhytides. Plastic and Reconstructive Surgery 108:208–214

Matarasso SL, Sadick NS 2003 Soft tissue augmentation. In: Bolognia J, Jorizzo JL, Rapini RV, Horn T (eds) Dermatology. Mosby/Harcourt Health Sciences, London, pp 2439–2449

Moody BR, Sengelmann RD 2001 Topical Tacrolimus in the treatment of bovine hypersensitivity. Dermatologic Surgery 27:789–791

Orentreich DS, Orentreich NO 1988 Injectable fluid silicone. In: Roenigk RK, Roenigk HH (eds) Dermatologic Surgery: Principles and Practice, Marcel-Dekker, New York, pp 1349–1395

Rohrer TE 2001 Soft tissue filler substances. Current Problems in Dermatology 13: 54–60

Stegman SJ, Chu S, Armstrong RC 1988 Adverse reactions to bovine collagen implant: clinical and histologic features. Journal of Dermatologic Surgery and Oncology 79:39

Toman DP, Egbart BE, Thomas JA, DeLustro FA 2004 Development of a novel nonantigenic dermal implant composed of human placental collagen. Plastic and Reconstructive Surgery 113:1015–1023

4 Hylans and Soft Tissue Augmentation

Paul H. Bowman, Rhoda S. Narins

Introduction

Recent advances in soft tissue augmentation have expanded our options in the search for an ideal filling agent. Since the 1980s, collagen (Zyderm and Zyplast, Collagen Corporation, Palo Alto, CA) has been the most popular filler in the USA, the 'gold standard' against which all other fillers are judged. Hylans, derivatives of hyaluronic acid, are exciting new filler substances with significant advantages compared to collagen, including higher biocompatibility and longer residence times in the skin (Table 4.1). There are several forms in clinical use as soft tissue fillers (Box 4.1), and more are being developed as experience with this new class of filler grows. This chapter will review the most commonly used agents, their indications (Box 4.2), safety, efficacy, advantages compared to other fillers such as collagen, and techniques of implantation.

Hylans are ideal for patients who like the results of temporary tissue fillers, but desire something longer lasting than collagen. As with other fillers, folds and wrinkles that are readily distensible will respond the best. Deep, nondistensible, and 'ice-pick'-type scars that do not easily efface with gentle, manual stretching of adjacent skin will not respond well (Box 4.3). Rejuvenation of age-related facial changes, such as static rhytids, deepened nasolabial folds (NLFs), and atrophy of the lips and oral commissures (causing a downturn of the corners of the mouth and a resultant aged appearance) can also be addressed well with hylans.

Contraindications are similar to other soft tissue fillers (Box 4.4). As these are relatively new agents, there is limited experience combining them with other implants (especially permanent fillers such as silicone, Goretex, Artecoll, etc.). Patients allergic to bovine collagen, and first-time patients who want treatment 'today' (no skin test required) will especially welcome these derivatives of hyaluronic acid.

Hylans compared to collagen as soft tissue fillers

	Collagen	Hyaluronic acid
Compatibility	Species and tissue specific	Identical in all species and tissues
Duration in tissue	Lasts 3–5 months	Lasts 6–12 months[a]
Origin	Bovine or human	Animal or bacterial
Pattern of loss	Steady volume loss	Isovolemic degradation[a]
Viscosity	Constant viscosity	Dynamic (shear-thinning) viscosity
Anesthesia	0.3% lidocaine included	No lidocaine included
Discomfort	Slightly less injection pain	Slightly more injection pain
Target correction	50–100% overcorrection	No overcorrection
Pre-op skin test?	Double skin test required[b]	No skin test required
Allergy prevalence	3% population allergic[b]	< 0.4% population allergic[c]
Shipping & storage	Refrigerated	Room temperature

[a]*When in HA gel (hylan) form,* [b]*For bovine collagen,* [c]*(Lowe 2001).*

Table 4.1 Hylans compared to collagen as soft tissue fillers

Hyaluronic acid preparations in clinical use as soft tissue fillers					
Hylaform	Restylane	Restylane Fine Lines	Perlane	Juvéderm	Hylan Rofilan Gel
Achyal	Dermalive	DermaDeep	Hyacell	Viscontour	

Box 4.1 Hyaluronic acid preparations in clinical use as soft tissue fillers

Conditions treated with hylans			
Static facial rhytids	**Lip sculpture**	**Facial contouring**	**NLFs**
Forehead ('worry' lines)	Volume enhancement	Cheek augmentation	Distensible scars
Periorbital lines ('crow's feet')	Vermilion border definition	Chin augmentation	
Perioral (upper lip and smile) lines	Philtral crest definition	Temporal augmentation	
Glabellar lines	Oral commissure effacement	Infraorbital augmentation	

Box 4.2 Conditions treated with hylans

Hylans **not** indicated for:	
	Better options
Dynamic rhytids	Botox
'Ice pick' & other nondistensible scars	Surgery
Striae & widened surgical scars	Surgery or laser
Actinic damage of lips	Laser or topical chemotherapy creams
Extensive facial rhytids	Laser resurfacing, chemical peel, rhytidectomy

Box 4.3 Conditions for which hylans are not indicated

Contraindications to treatment with hylan soft tissue fillers	
Absolute	**Relative**
Previous serious reaction to hyaluronic acid derivatives	History of hypertrophic or keloid scars
Patients with severe allergies manifested by history of anaphylaxis	Active inflammation at site to be treated (acne, rashes, etc.)
Patients with multiple severe allergies	Active disease which koebnerizes (pyoderma gangrenosum, etc.)
Implantation for breast augmentation	Patient has important social function in next 72 hours (erythema)
Implantation into muscle, bone, tendon, blood vessels	Unrealistic expectations of patient

Box 4.4 Contraindications to treatment with hylan soft tissue fillers

Hyaluronic acid (hyaluronan, sodium hyaluronate, HA) is a naturally occurring linear polysaccharide composed of alternating residues of the monosaccharides D-glucuronic acid and N-acetyl-D-glucosamine (Fig. 4.1). It is widely distributed in the extracellular matrix of connective tissues, synovial fluid, the aqueous and vitreous humor of the eye, and other tissues. Unlike collagen, it exhibits no species or tissue specificity; its chemical structure is uniform throughout nature, and it thus has no potential for immunogenicity in its pure form. In the skin, it forms the elastoviscous fluid matrix in which collagen fibers, elastic fibers, and other intercellular structures are embedded. Synthesized on cell membranes and then extruded into the extracellular space, HA is the largest (mass of 50 kDa) and most plentiful glycosaminoglycan (GAG) in the extracellular matrix of the dermis. Unlike other GAGs (chondroitin sulfate, heparin sulfate), it is not sulfated or bound to a core protein. It is negatively charged and binds enormous amounts of water; multiple chains of hyaluronic acid entangle and interpenetrate each other to produce highly elastoviscous solutions, giving the skin its supple, resilient quality.

The amount of hyaluronic acid in the skin decreases with age, resulting in reduced dermal hydration and increased wrinkling.

Owing to its lubricating and cushioning properties, HA and its derivatives have been used in ophthalmologic surgery for over 2 decades. More recently, intra-articular injection has had promising results in the treatment of osteoarthritis. With its stabilizing, hydrating, cushioning properties and high biocompatibility, it would seem to also be an ideal soft tissue filler material. However, in contrast to the earlier mentioned applications, soft tissue augmentation requires a sustained presence at the site of deposition. Since the half-life of natural HA in tissue is only 1–2 days (exogenous HA is rapidly cleared from the dermis and degraded in the liver to carbon dioxide and water), it is a poor candidate for soft tissue augmentation in its unmodified form.

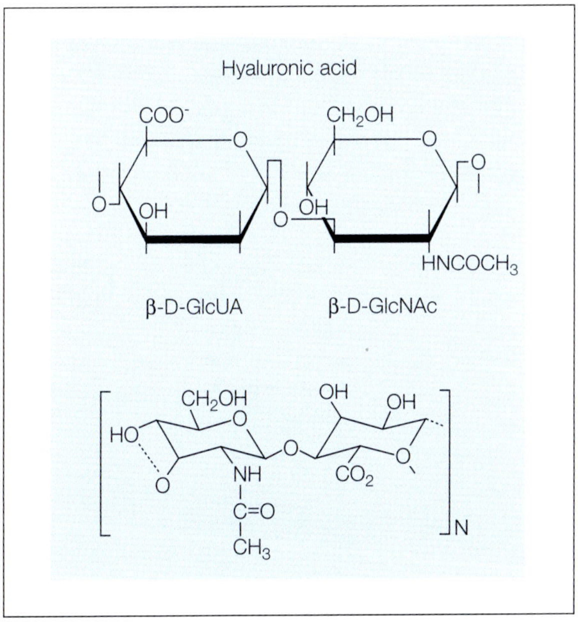

Fig. 4.1 Chemical structure of hyaluronic acid

By chemically cross-linking molecules of HA, more stable macromolecules are formed which have the same biocompatibility as native HA, but are water-insoluble and thus have prolonged tissue residence time after injection. Since they retain their affinity for water, they swell to form a three-dimensional network known as a gel. Hyaluronic acid gels (hylans) are classified as **chemical** gels, since the gel network is connected by covalent bonds, and also as **hydrogels** since they are swollen with water (95% of weight) rather than an organic solvent.

In addition to their high biocompatibility and prolonged stability in tissue, hylans have several other physicochemical attributes that make them especially attractive as soft tissue fillers. Hylans are 'shear-thinning' gels that have the unique attribute of dynamic viscosity, which decreases with increasing shearing force (Fig. 4.2). Under pressure of injection (high shear rate) the gel can pass through a relatively small gauge needle. Upon removal of the shearing force, viscosity increases, forming a thick gel at the site of tissue implantation, which is unlikely to migrate. Viscosity also decreases with increasing temperature, another suitable attribute of an injectable filler. These rheological (flow) properties are determined by molecular weight, concentration, and degree of cross-linking, and vary among different hylans.

Since the hylans used in tissue augmentation are water insoluble gels, they remain stable in tissue, being slowly resorbed over months. However, unlike other temporary soft tissue fillers such as collagen,

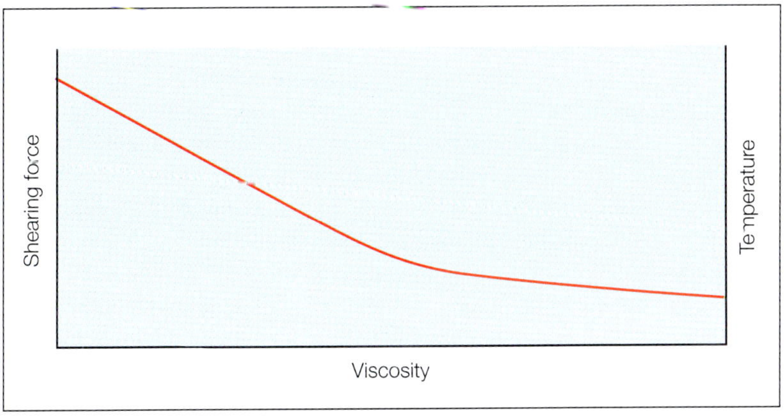

Fig. 4.2 Dynamic viscosity of hylans

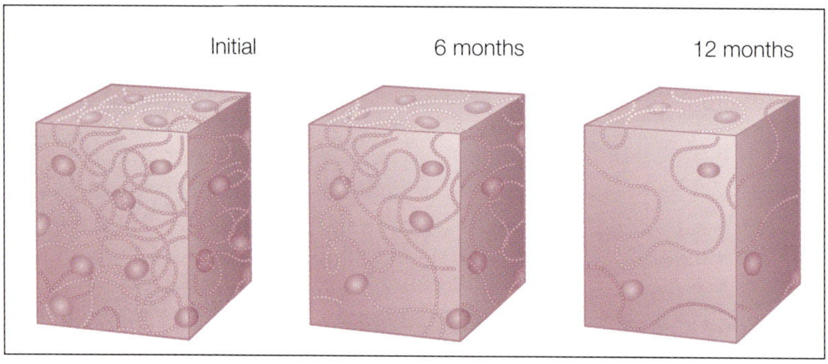

Fig. 4.3 Isovolemic degradation of hylans

their disappearance from tissue may follow **isovolemic degradation**: as individual molecules of HA are degraded, those remaining are able to bind more water, such that the overall volume of the gel remains unchanged. In other words, the concentration of the gel decreases during reabsorption, but volume remains high until the last molecules of HA are degraded. Clinically, this translates to an implant that maintains a high proportion of its initial space-filling volume until the last of the material is completely resorbed (Fig. 4.3). So far this model has not been obvious clinically, with most of the studies showing an initial more rapid loss of correction followed by a slowly declining plateau, in contrast to an initial plateau followed by a sharp drop-off as predicted by the isovolemic model.

Hylaform

Hylans can be classified by their concentration, the method and degree of cross-linking, and the source of the HA. Previous sources of HA have included rooster combs, umbilical cord, vitreous humor, tendons, skin and bacterial cultures. The first preparation widely used for soft tissue augmentation was hylan B gel (Hylaform Gel, Biomatrix Inc., Ridgefield, NJ), which was developed in the mid-1980s. It uses HA derived from the dermis of rooster combs, which is then purified and chemically cross-linked with divinyl sulfone (hydroxyl groups of HA chains react to form an infinite network of sulfonyl-*bis*-ethyl cross-links). It is distributed in Canada by Inamed Corporation (Toronto, Canada) and in Europe by Collagen International, Inc. It has been used in the treatment of soft tissue defects and facial augmentation throughout most of the world (Canada, Europe, Australia, South America, Asia, etc.) for many years, and recently became available in the USA (April 2004).

Preclinical animal studies demonstrated that hylan B gel implants do not elicit clinically significant immunogenic, inflammatory, or foreign-body reactions, and remain stable in tissues over time. Injected into the vocal cords of rabbits, hylan B gel provided durable augmentation in a study by Hallen et al over a study period of 1 year, without inflammatory or other adverse reactions. In a study by Piacquadio et al comparing intradermal injection of hylan B gel and collagen implants in guinea pigs, most of the injected collagen was resorbed after 26 weeks, while 75% of hylan B gel injection sites still showed histologic evidence of residual material even at 52 weeks.

To determine the safety and efficacy of Hylaform Gel for facial scars and wrinkles, Pollack conducted a six-center, open-label, 12-month study. A total of 216 patients enrolled and 177 completed the entire follow-up period of 1 year. Of the 724 treatment sites, 86% were facial folds or wrinkles. Of the sites studied, 53% required a touch-up injection (at 2 weeks), and 17% required a third injection (at 4 weeks) to achieve a baseline of '100% correction.' Treatment success, defined as 60% of all sites showing at least a 33% degree of correction, was noted in both wrinkles/folds and scars at 18 weeks. Through linear regression analysis, the investigators calculated a mean effectiveness of 22 weeks (18–26 weeks) for wrinkles/folds and 23 weeks (13–48 weeks) for scars. Treatment reactions included mild erythema, itching, swelling and pain. Less than 2% of all treatments were associated with persistent erythema, acne, or ecchymoses, all of which resolved without long-term sequelae.

Restylane

Restylane (Q-Med AB, Uppsala, Sweden) is a stabilized, partially cross-linked HA gel. The HA is produced from cultures of *Streptococcus equi* by fermentation in the presence of sugar, which is alcohol precipitated, filtered, and dried. The HA chains are then chemically stabilized through permanent cross-linking with epoxides, altering less than 1% of the hyaluronan molecular network. The material is heat sterilized in its final container and has a shelf life of 1.5 years from the date of manufacture. Since its production does not require an animal source, it has been termed a nonanimal, stabilized hyaluronic acid (NASHA).

There are thus several key differences between the two most commonly used hylans (Table 4.2). Manna et al and Micheels conducted comparative chemical evaluation of both products and found Hylaform to be 'rheologically superior,' behaving as a stronger (more elastic) hydrogel. Low levels of impurities have been detected by Olenius in both products: Avian proteins in Hylaform and fermentation byproducts and additives to enable cross-linking in Restylane. Restylane also contains small, undetermined amounts of phosphate, calcium, and other ions. Restylane was reformulated in 1999 to decrease protein content, and the contaminant levels in both products are now reportedly similar.

In a Swedish study by Olenius of the clinical safety and efficacy of Restylane, 285 facial sites were treated in 113 patients, including glabellar lines, NLFs, and oral commissures. After achieving close to 100% correction of each fold or wrinkle (two-thirds of the sites had a second 'touch-up' injection at week 2), all areas were evaluated at weeks 12 and 26. Physician evaluation revealed that treatment sites maintained an average of 82% and 69% of correction at 12 and 26 weeks, respectively, while subjects self-reported 75% and 61% improvement at these same time points. Twenty of the subjects were randomly selected for evaluation at 1 year, at which time treatment sites still maintained 66% of their original correction by physician evaluation (57% by subject self-evaluation) (Fig. 4.4).

An Italian study by Duranti et al of Restylane's clinical efficacy and tolerability also showed favorable results. In this multicenter evaluation, 158 Caucasian women (average age 37) received intradermal injections in 273 facial areas. Treatment sites included glabellar lines (56), NLFs (99), oral commissure folds (36), lips (78) and depressed acne scars (four). Patients were then evaluated at 1, 2, 4, and 8 months postoperatively. At the 8-month visit, 78% of patients still had moderate to marked improvement in the treated areas, with NLFs and lips maintaining the most improvement (Fig. 4.5). Five of the patients also had injections of Restylane and Zyplast (glutaraldehyde cross-linked bovine collagen, Collagen Corporation Inc., Palo Alto, CA) in the forearms, which were visually and histologically evaluated by biopsy at 1, 3, 6 and 12 months postoperatively to compare their residence times in the tissue. Histologically, staining with toluidine blue for hyaluronic acid and picro-sirius for collagen, all Zyplast implants had been completely resorbed by 6 months, while

Comparison of Hylaform and Restylane		
	Hylaform	**Restylane**
Cross-linking	Divinyl sulfide	Epoxides
HA source	Rooster comb	*Streptococcus* bacteria
Viscoelasticity	More elastic	More viscous
HA concentration	6 mg/mL	20 mg/mL
Supplied in	0.6, 1.2 mL	0.4, 0.7 mL

Table 4.2 Comparison of Hylaform and Restylane

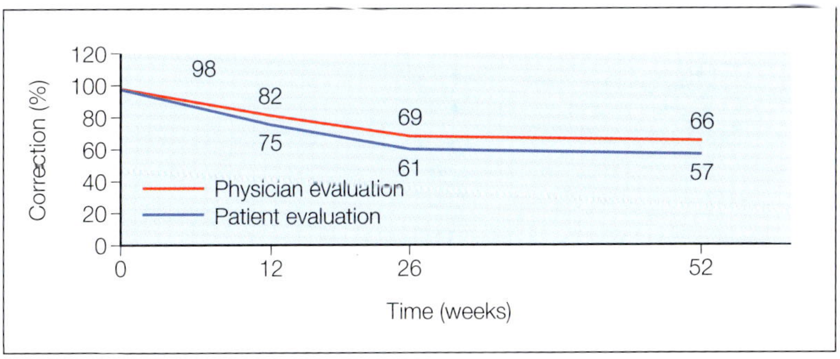

Fig. 4.4 Physician and patient evaluations of correction after Restylane injection. (Data from Olenius 1998)

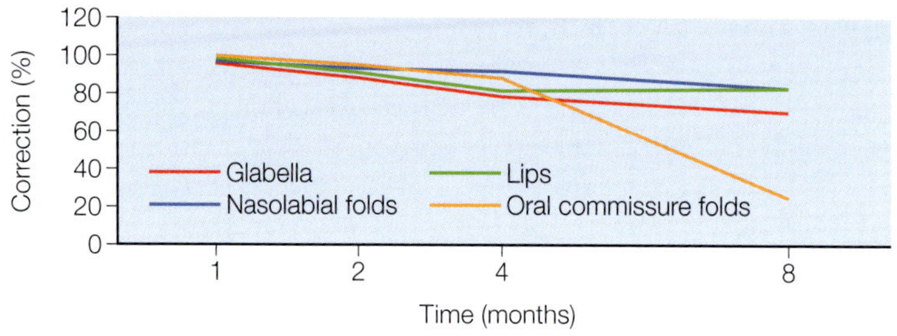

Site	1 month	2 months	4 months	8 months
Glabella	96%	89	79	71
Nasolabial folds	98	96	92	83
Lips	99	91	82	85
Oral comm. Folds	100	97	89	25

Fig. 4.5 Persistence of Restylane correction by implantation site. (Data from Duranti et al 1998)

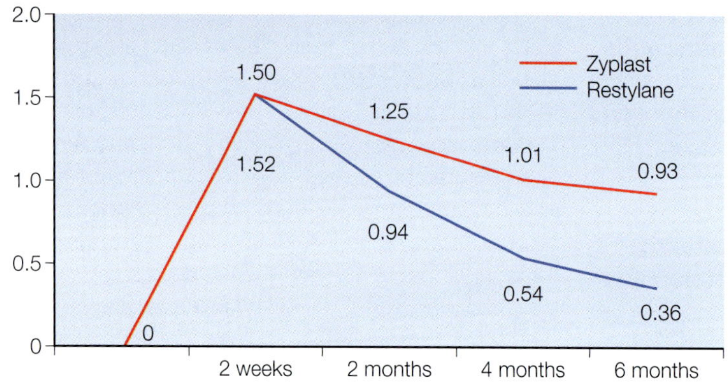

Fig. 4.6 Maintenance of improvement in NLFs after treatment with Restylane vs Zyplast. Mean change from pretreatment in WSRS over 6 months. WSRS is a method of quantifying facial folds, in which 1 = absent, 2 = mild, 3 = moderate, 4 = severe and 5 = extreme

four of the five Restylane implants were still apparent at 12 months. The authors noted that the later biopsies of Restylane sites showed the hylan implant to have a more 'watery' appearance than the earlier samples, consistent with its property of isovolemic degradation, binding more water as its concentration decreases. Some Restylane implants had a slight inflammatory reaction, although none showed fibrosis or 'severe foreign body reaction.'

A more recent study by Narins et al in the USA compared treatment of NLFs with Restylane to Zyplast. In this six-center double-blinded study, 138 patients with moderate to severe NLFs were randomized to treatment with Restylane and Zyplast on contralateral sides of the face. After undergoing 'touch-up' injections at 2-week intervals as required to achieve an 'optimal cosmetic result' baseline, subjects were evaluated at 2, 4, and 6 months for maintenance of improvement. Using a wrinkle severity rating scale (WSRS), investigators found Restylane to be superior to Zyplast at maintaining correction at all post-baseline time points (Fig. 4.6). At the 6-month visit, investigators reported Restylane to be superior to Zyplast in 56.9% of patients, Zyplast to be superior in 9.5%, and both fillers to be equal in 33.6%. At the same time point, 52.6% of

Implant-related adverse events (AEs) associated with Restylane[a]			
Event	**Duranti (% sites)**	**Olenius (% sites)**	**Narins (% patients)**
Intermittent swelling	4.8%		87.0%
Erythema	2.6	6.6%[b]	84.8
Edema	1.8		NR
Discomfort	1.8	NR	NR
Tenderness	1.1	NR	77.5
Bruising/dark area	1.1	3.2[d]	52.2
Itching	0.4	NR	30.4
Pain	0.4	0.4	57.2
Other[c]	NR	NR	24.6
Overall AE rate	12.5%	13.4%	93.5%[e]

NR = not reported. [a]In Duranti & Olenius studies AEs were directly observed by investigators; in Narins' study they were recorded from daily patient diaries. [b]Includes erythema, swelling, and edema. [c]'Other' includes injection site stiffness, nodules, and pimples. [d](1.4% injection related, 1.8% technique related). [e]In comparison, local injection site reactions to Zyplast during the same time period were reported in 90.6% of diaries. Most were mild or moderate in intensity such that at the investigator evaluation at 2 weeks, less than 15% of all reactions were still clinically apparent, similar to the other two studies.

Table 4.3 Implant-related adverse events (AEs) associated with Restylane[a]

Reports of incidence of delayed hypersensitivity from hylan implants			
Implant	**Incidence (No. of cases/total)**	**Time period**	**Source**
H or R	0.42% (3/709)	1996–2000	Lowe[a]
H or R	3.7% (8/219)	1997–2001	Micheels[a]
R	0.07% (104/144 000)	1999	Friedman[b]
R	0.02% (52/262 000)	2000	Friedman[b]

H = Hylaform, R = Restylane. [a]From personal observation. [b]From retrospective review of adverse event database of Q Med Esthetics.

Table 4.4 Reports of incidence of delayed hypersensitivity from hylan implants

subjects felt that Restylane was superior to Zyplast, while 41.6% felt they were equivalent. At 6 months, 67.2% of Zyplast-treated folds had returned to their pretreatment condition compared with only 29.9% of Restylane-treated folds. Although the number of treatment sessions required to reach the initial baseline of an 'optimal cosmetic result' did not differ between the two fillers (mean 1.4, range 1–3), the total injection volume needed to produce this effect was lower for Restylane (mean 1.0 mL, range 0.3–2.8 mL) than for Zyplast (mean 1.6 mL, range 0.1–5.0 mL).

Similar mild and transient side effects occurred in all three clinical studies (Table 4.3). Injection-related adverse events included redness, swelling, darkening of the treatment site and slight pain, most of which resolved within 3 days. Red spots, bumps, and hematomas were infrequent and seemed to be associated with injection technique. Several cases of transient swelling of implanted material occurred, particularly after lip augmentation. This was most problematic during the first postoperative week. In some cases the swelling was stimulated by exercise, sun exposure and menstruation and was judged to be due to the hydrophilic properties of the implant. In Duranti et al and Olenius' studies, adverse events were observed by the investigators at an incidence of 13%. Narins et al reported similar mild and transient side effects, although with a much higher incidence, probably because patients were required to keep a daily diary of any adverse events for 2 weeks after each injection session. Injection site pain was slightly higher for Restylane than Zyplast (57.2% compared to 42.0% in patient diaries), perhaps due to the absence of lidocaine and its more viscous character.

Although these early efficacy studies did not demonstrate hypersensitivity or other allergic reactions to hylans, in 2000 Lupton and Alster reported a case of delayed hypersensitivity in a 54-year-old Caucasian woman after having three injections of Restylane over a 14-month period. Two weeks after the last injection into the melolabial folds, she developed multiple acute tender red nodules in the treatment areas. Some exuded coagulated, yellow, stringy, pus-like material, but bacterial cultures were negative. Warm saline compresses bid, minocycline 250 bid × 1 week and 4 mg methylprednisolone q.d. × 1 week and intralesional triamcinolone cleared the reaction. Two weeks later, recurrent inflammation and new tender nodules in previously inactive sites responded to warm compresses and intralesional triamcinolone.

The exact incidence of delayed hypersensitivity reactions has varied among reports (Table 4.4). Lowe et al reported delayed implant site reactions in three of 709 patients (0.42%) treated with hylan implants in London between 1996 and 2000 (438 Hylaform, 271 Restylane). No abnormal skin reactions occurred until 6–8 weeks after injection. In addition, three patients treated elsewhere had similar delayed reactions. Altogether, four patients had reactions to Hylaform and two to Restylane, ranging from mildly inflammatory nodules to firm, tender, edematous abscesses. Several required intralesional triamcinolone injections to reduce induration and inflammation. A punch biopsy of one such reaction in the nasolabial area showed moderate infiltrates of lymphocytes and plasma cells and organizing fibrosis, but no eosinophils or foreign body giant cell reaction. Five of these patients agreed to retrospective skin testing with both agents; four developed inflammatory nodules in 5–7 weeks (to both fillers in three patients, Hylaform alone in one). Positive skin testing to both agents implies causes other than avian protein reactivity, which would be expected only with Hylaform.

Micheels treated 219 patients with Hylaform (106) or Restylane (133) between 1997 and 2001; in that time, eight patients (3.7%) developed delayed inflammatory reactions of redness, pruritus, painful swelling, or 'nettle-like rash' reactions. These reactions lasted up to 4.5 months without oral treatment. Subsequent intradermal testing resulted in positive inflammatory reactions in five in response to Hylaform and six in response to Restylane. Biopsies in four of these patients revealed strong granulomatous foreign-body reactions with giant cells, including reactions to both agents. Several patients also developed anti-Restylane and/or anti-Hylaform antibodies.

A retrospective review by Friedman et al of reactions to Restylane in particular was performed by examining the worldwide adverse events database of Q-Med Esthetics. This included patients treated in Europe, Canada, Australia, South America and Asia in 1999 and 2000. Based on the number of syringes sold, an estimated 144 000 patients were treated in 1999, of which one out of every 650 (0.15%) reported an adverse event. These were temporary events and included redness, swelling, localized granulomatous reactions, bacterial infection and acneiform and cystic lesions. One out of every 1400 patients (0.07%) treated developed a localized hypersensitivity reaction of swelling, erythema, and induration at the implant site; none had systemic symptoms or anaphylaxis. One of every 2100 patients treated developed injection site inflammation/reaction shortly after injection, consisting of redness, edema, and tenderness that resolved spontaneously after an average of 4 days. In 2000, an estimated 262 000 patients were treated, of which one out of every 5000 developed a localized cutaneous hypersensitivity, appearing on average 22 days after injection, and lasting 15 days. Injection site inflammation occurred in 49 patients, including erythema, swelling, pain, itching, discoloration, tenderness or temporary palpable lumpiness; spontaneous resolution occurred within 1–2 days of injection into the skin or 1 week after injection into the lips. Two cases of injection site necrosis were recorded, both of the glabellar area. The decreased incidence of side effects in 2000 was judged to be due to the reformulating of Restylane in mid-1999, as well as increased experience with the product and possibly decreased reporting.

Case reports of other reactions have also occurred, including abscess-like swellings, tender nodules, arterial embolization, venous occlusion resulting in a varix of the lip, and granulomatous reactions. A list of reported side effects from hylans appears in Box 4.5.

Side effects reported from use of hylans

Common	Rare
Erythema	Delayed local hypersensitivity
Swelling/edema	Granulomatous reaction
Pain	Abscess-like swelling
Tenderness at injection site	Arterial embolization
Bruising	Venous occlusion resulting in lip varix
Itching	Acneiform eruption

Box 4.5 Side effects reported from use of hylans

Overview of Treatment Strategy

Evaluate defect to be treated/patient interview

The first step in performing any sort of soft tissue augmentation is having a detailed discussion about what the patient wants to change. Do they see a fold, wrinkle, or scar that is bothersome? Having the patient hold a hand mirror so both of you can see and discuss individual lines or lesions is helpful. Make sure you are talking about the same thing, and fully understand their request. Consider using a

Patient interview questions

Does the patient have:

- Experience with soft tissue fillers in the past?
- History of hypertrophic scars or keloids?
- History of herpes simplex infection?
- History of easy bruising/bleeding?
- Dermatologic condition that exhibits pathergy (pyoderma gangrenosum, Sweet's syndrome)?
- Any active inflammation (acne, rash, etc.) in area to be treated?
- High pain tolerance (need for anesthesia)?
- Important social plans in next 3–7 days?
- Realistic expectations?

Box 4.6 Patient interview questions

pointer (wooden end of a cotton-tipped applicator, etc.) to precisely indicate the item of concern. Many of the changes the patient requests may be better served by other treatment approaches (Box 4.3). Dynamic rhytids (present only when patient furrows brow, smiles, purses lips, etc.) are the most common, and are best addressed with botulinum toxin (Botox). In general, Botox is the most useful agent for rhytids in the upper face (glabella, crow's feet) and fillers are second. In the lower face (NLFs, oral commissures) this situation is reversed. One approach is to treat an area (e.g. glabella) with Botox to eliminate any dynamic rhytids and soften any static ones. Later, any residual static lines can be eliminated with fillers. Lips and nasolabial folds respond best to fillers, and hylans in particular. Use manual stretching of skin to estimate how well a certain wrinkle, fold or scar will or will not respond. Sometimes demonstrating this to the patient as they look on in a mirror is helpful.

Ask questions to confirm the patient's understanding of the filler and its potential, as well as what it **cannot** do (Box 4.6). Discuss that hylans are temporary (although longer lasting than collagen) fillers. Determine if the patient is at increased risk for scarring (history of hypertrophic scars, keloids, etc.) Do they have any experience with soft tissue augmentation, and if so, were they pleased with the results? Do they have a history of herpes simplex in the area to be treated (lips) that could be reactivated with the trauma of an injection? Injections should also be deferred until any active inflammation in the area (acne, rash, etc.) has resolved.

Injection-related hematomas, which result from the entrapment of hemoglobin from small bleeders during injection, can leave dark spots that may remain for a time if they become entrapped in the implant. Consider having the patient discontinue the use of aspirin, nonsteroidal anti-inflammatory medications, St John's Wort, vitamin E and other blood-thinners for 7–10 days prior to procedure if this is a concern; in patients who should not discontinue these, discuss the increased likelihood of ecchymoses.

Finally, as of the time of this writing, Restylane and Hylaform are the only FDA-approved hylans available in the USA, and are only indicated for the treatment of moderate to severe facial wrinkles and folds, such as the NLFs. All other uses are currently considered off-label. They have not been studied in patients who are pregnant, breastfeeding, under 18 years of age, or on immunosuppressive therapy.

Choose implant agent

As more hylans become available, there will be a greater opportunity to match specific hylan preparations to treatment areas and defects. In general, fine, superficial wrinkles and distensible scars respond best to thin fillers placed at the mid to upper dermal level. Deeper, more substantial wrinkles, such as the NLFs, require a thicker filler to be placed more deeply in the dermis. Areas requiring true volume augmentation, such as the cheeks or temples, need the most robust filler, with placement at the dermal/subcutaneous interface. Some wrinkles may have both a superficial and a deep component, and require both to be addressed to achieve optimal results.

The Restylane family of products is a good example of different hylan formulations which are designed for use at different dermal depths: Restylane, Restylane Fine Lines, and Restylane Perlane (Table 4.5). The concentration of HA is identical in all three preparations at 20 mg/mL. What differs is the size of the HA particles, expressed in number of gel particles per mL, and the target depth for implantation (Fig. 4.7). Restylane Fine Lines has the smallest particles, and therefore is the least viscous. It is injected through a 31 gauge needle and is designed for use in the most superficial dermis, to correct fine lines and superficial, easily distensible defects. Restylane, with larger particles that are injected through a 30 gauge needle, is placed in the mid-dermis to correct moderate NLFs and provide lip augmentation. Perlane has the largest particle size, making it the most viscous of the three

Comparison of three forms of Restylane			
	Restylane	**Restylane Fine Lines**	**Perlane**
Composition	20 mg/mL stabilized HA	20 mg/mL stabilized HA	20 mg/mL stabilized HA
No. of gel particles/mL	100 000	200 000	10 000
Indications	Wrinkles, lips	Thin superficial lines	Deep folds (e.g. nasolabial), lip augmentation, facial contouring
Target depth	Mid-dermis	Upper dermis	Deep dermis/upper subcutis
Degree correction	100%	100%	100%
Syringe volume	0.7, 0.4 mL	0.4 mL	0.7 mL
Needle size	30 gauge	31 gauge	27 gauge

Table 4.5 Comparison of three forms of Restylane

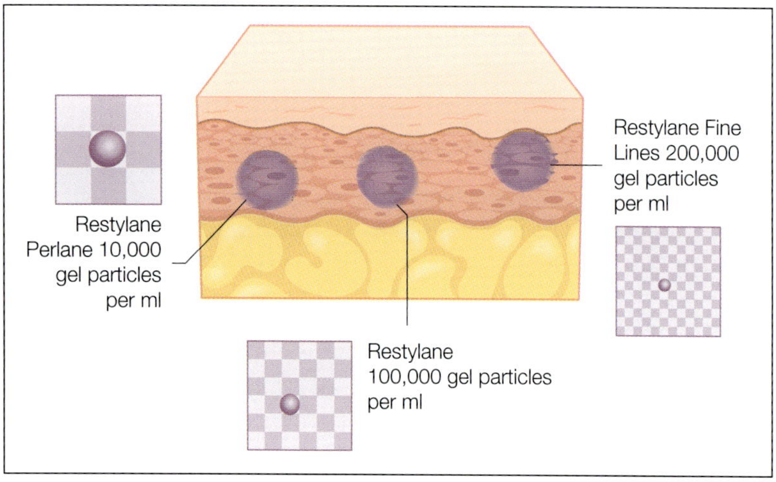

Fig. 4.7 Comparative gel particle sizes and suggested sites of implantation for Restylane Fine Lines, Restylane, and Restylane Perlane

preparations, and requires a 27 gauge needle for injection. It is designed for implantation into the deep dermis and superficial subcutaneous tissue to treat deep folds and provide facial contouring (cheek and chin augmentation, etc.). Restylane was first marketed in Europe in 1996; the other two preparations were introduced in 2000. The three different products can be used in concert, layering one over another for optimal clinical results. Currently, only Restylane is FDA approved for use in the USA (marketed through Medicis Esthetics, Scottsdale, AZ, since December 2003), and is officially indicated only for the treatment of moderate to severe facial wrinkles and folds, such as NLFs. Restylane Fine Lines and Perlane are available in Europe, Asia, and Latin America but have not yet been approved in the USA. As these and other hylans become available in the USA more tailored agents can be matched to individual defects (Fig. 4.8).

Treatment Techniques

General implantation technique

After removing any make-up, the area to be treated should be cleansed with an alcohol prep pad or some other antiseptic. It is useful for the patient to sit upright during treatment, as the contour of some facial folds and tissues changes when the patient is reclining. Some patients prefer to sit in a chair against a wall, so they can rest their head against it during injection.

None of the hylan preparations include lidocaine (unlike collagen products such as Zyderm and Zyplast), and may require separate anesthesia prior to treatment. Topical anesthetics (LMX (Elamax), etc.) can be useful but must be thickly applied for 15 minutes before injection, and the degree of pain reduction provided may not warrant the preparation time involved. Instead, injecting small amounts of

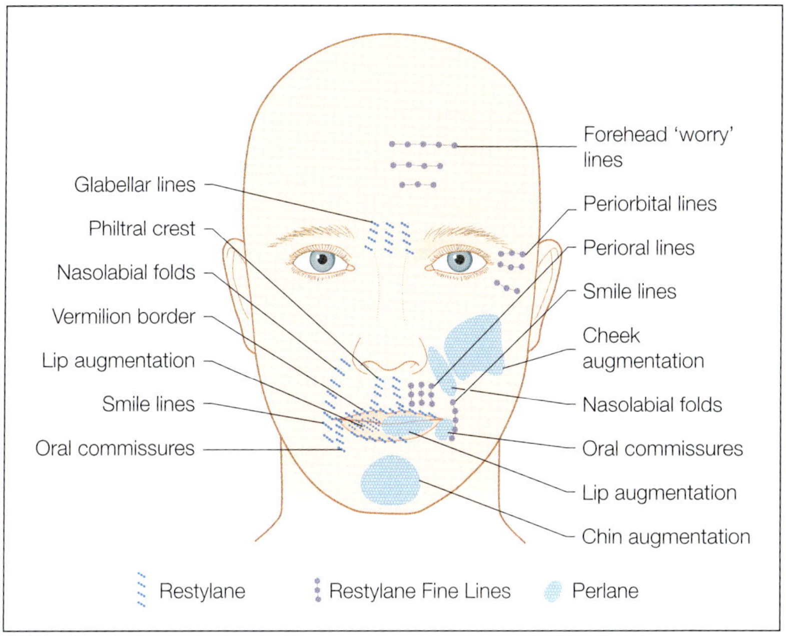

Fig. 4.8 Suggested uses for Restylane preparations based on site and defect to be treated

local anesthetic around the area to be treated in a 'field block' fashion may be preferable. If this is performed, care must be taken to not alter the defect itself with the tumescence of the anesthetic. Finally, a peripheral nerve block can be performed, which provides the deepest anesthesia and does not alter the structure being treated, but is technique dependent and requires 10–20 minutes to achieve complete effect. Some patients can tolerate treatment of NLFs, oral commissures, or the glabellar area without any anesthesia. For injections of the lips, however, peripheral nerve and/or field blocks are usually needed. In any area, the thicker the filler, the deeper the implantation depth, the larger the needle required, and the more likely anesthesia is required.

Hylans are thicker and more viscous than collagen, and take more injection pressure to be pushed out of the syringe and through a needle. Since their viscosity decreases with increasing temperature (the dynamic viscosity of 'shear-thinning' gels), warming the syringe in the hand prior to injection may help. Before injecting the patient, push the plunger forward to feel the intrinsic resistance of the filler moving through the needle, until a small droplet appears at the needle tip. This can be wiped off and injection can begin.

Four different implantation techniques have been suggested: linear threading, serial puncture, fanning, and cross-hatching (Fig. 4.9). These are similar to implantation methods for collagen and other soft tissue fillers. The serial puncture technique is technically easiest (since the needle tip doesn't move during injection), and is often preferred by beginners. Here the needle enters the skin to the desired depth, deposits a small aliquot of filler, and is withdrawn. Individual injections of this type work well to fill distensible acne scars, while successive injections can be used to efface a wrinkle.

The linear threading technique is probably the most commonly used: holding the syringe parallel to the length of the wrinkle or fold to be treated, pierce the skin and advance the needle to its fullest extent. Then, while slowly withdrawing the needle, apply even pressure on the plunger to dispense material into dermis. (For very fine, superficial wrinkles, picture the extrusion of material from the needle tip pushing the needle backwards.) Relieve pressure just before withdrawing the needle from the skin to avoid leakage and wastage of gel. Short, superficial lines and wrinkles can be ablated with a single injection; several successive 'threads' below, above, or beside previous injections may be required to fill larger folds, lines, or wrinkles. Deeper defects may require layering with thicker preparations (Restylane Perlane).

Some practitioners enter the skin with a needle angle of 30° or 45°, others prefer it more parallel to

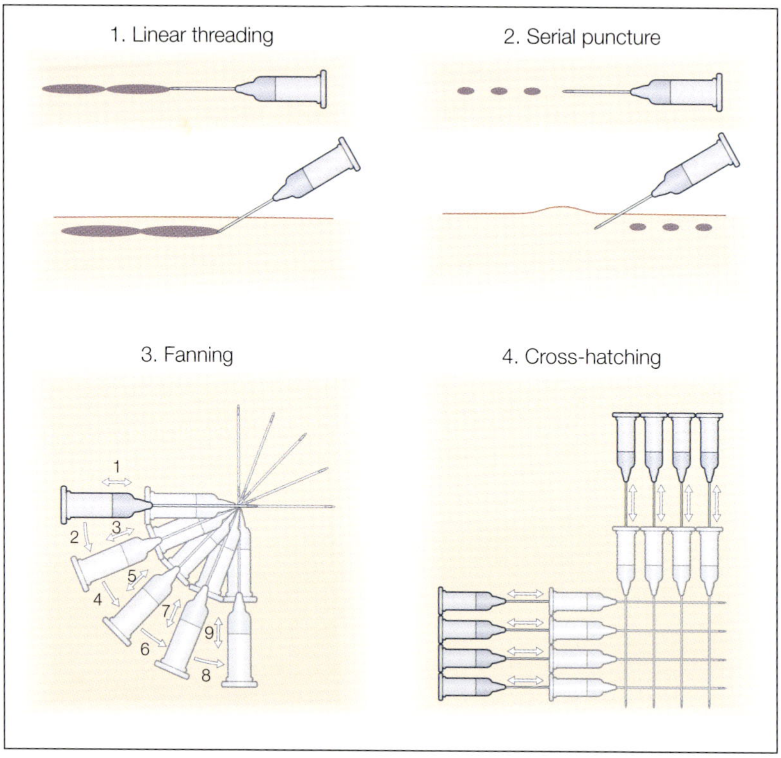

Fig. 4.9 Hylan implantation techniques

the skin; it is really a matter of personal preference. Most authors recommend keeping the needle bevel up, but this is not essential. Studies have shown that the direction of the bevel does not influence the direction of the flow of the material, which follows the course of least resistance. The current authors like to start with the bevel up so the tip of the needle is seen and more precisely controlled where the skin is pierced.

Keep the tip of the needle at constant depth during implantation, depositing all filler material within the same plane to get even results. The depth of needle placement (and thus filler implantation) should be high dermis for superficial lines, mid-dermis for more substantial wrinkles, and deep dermis/subcutaneous border for heavy folds. A rule of thumb to gauge needle depth is that for mid-dermis placement, the needle's contour should be visible, but not its color. Guide treatment while injecting by **visual** response with thinner material placed high in dermis (Restylane Fine Lines) and **tactile** response when placing thicker material more deeply (Perlane). Resistance should be felt placing thicker substances into deep dermis; a sudden drop in such resistance may indicate injection into the subcutaneous plane. The fanning and cross-hatching techniques are merely variations on the linear threading technique, most often used when placing a larger amount of filler more deeply.

The most difficult part of the technique for beginners is developing a feel for needle depth. It is better to err on the side of injecting too deeply, which will simply not give as much benefit. In contrast, injecting too superficially can overcorrect defects and leave surface irregularities. Although the clear hylan gels are not as unsightly as collagen (visible as white material) when placed too superficially, they can tend to make the epidermis transparent, leading to red or gray spots.

After injection, some practitioners manually massage the area gently to smooth out any nodular or uneven areas, and ensure the implanted material conforms to the contour of surrounding tissues. Using an ice pack or other cold compress can help to minimize swelling (on lips especially); some patients also feel it alleviates postinjection discomfort. Unlike collagen implants, which lose some volume after injection due to the accompanying lidocaine, hylans should only correct to 100% of the desired volume. If overcorrected, massage firmly between fingers or against underlying bone to obtain optimal results. Approximately 20% overcorrection can be massaged out; more will lead to a persistent unwanted cosmetic result. Patients can return to normal activities almost immediately after treatment (they can apply make-up if desired.) The duration of correction depends on the character of the defect being treated, tissue stress at the implant site (frequency of muscular activity), implant depth, and injection technique. Most authors suggest a limit of 1.5–2.0 mL per treatment session, and planning a 'touch-up' 2–4 weeks later.

Approach to Selected Anatomic Areas

Lips

Patients/indications

Lip enhancement has increased in popularity to the point that it is now the most sought-after procedure in soft tissue augmentation. There are actually several separate aspects to lip enhancement. The first is improvement of lip line definition, achieved by injecting along the cutaneous/vermilion border. The second is augmentation, produced by direct injection into the bulk of the vermilion of the lip to produce actual enlargement of one or both lips. The former is useful for patients who complain that lipstick bleeds into vertical wrinkles of the upper lip, or simply need more lip definition, while the latter is used in patients who want bigger, more robust lips. Atrophy of the lips is a natural change as we age, and (re)enlargement can provide a rejuvenating effect. Finally, enhancement of the natural philtrum of the upper cutaneous lip can provide aesthetic improvement. One such approach, called the Paris Lip, creates a 'pouting' look.

Equipment (Restylane, Perlane)

One syringe of either Restylane or Perlane is adequate for initial treatment of two lips, with a touch-up performed in 2–4 weeks. Enhancement lasts 4–6 months following one to two treatments, although occasional patients maintain improvement for 6–9 months.

Treatment algorithm (linear threading)

The lips are one of the most sensitive areas of the entire face; unlike other areas, most patients will

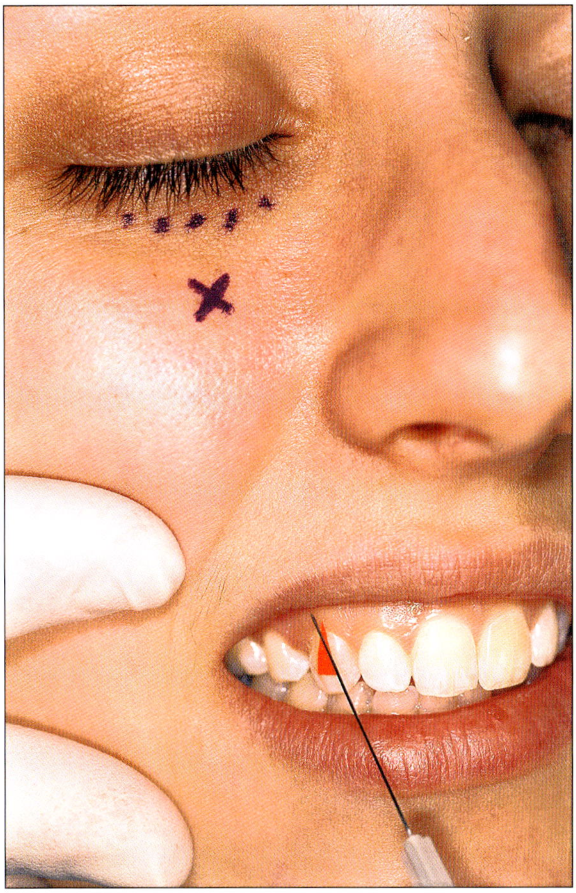

Fig. 4.10 Infraorbital block, intraoral approach (infraorbital foramen indicated by purple 'X', canine indicated by red triangle)

require a nerve block for all but the most minimal treatments here. The infraorbital nerves, which supply sensation to the upper lip, can be blocked with two intraoral injections (one on each side) (Fig. 4.10). Using a 1 in needle at the base of the upper canine tooth, 0.5–1.0 mL of plain 1% lidocaine is injected toward the infraorbital foramen, which is located approximately 6 mm below the infraorbital rim in the mid-pupillary line. The mental nerves, which innervate the lower lip, can be similarly blocked by injecting at the base of each 2nd premolar inferiorly toward the mental foramen, also in the mid-pupillary line (Fig. 4.11). If full nerve blockade is performed, it may take 10–15 minutes for complete anesthesia to ensue. Some practitioners prefer to replace these blocks by injecting anesthetic around the distal nerve fascicles as they approach the posterior (mucosal) aspect of the upper and lower lips. In these 'miniblocks', a small amount of anesthesia

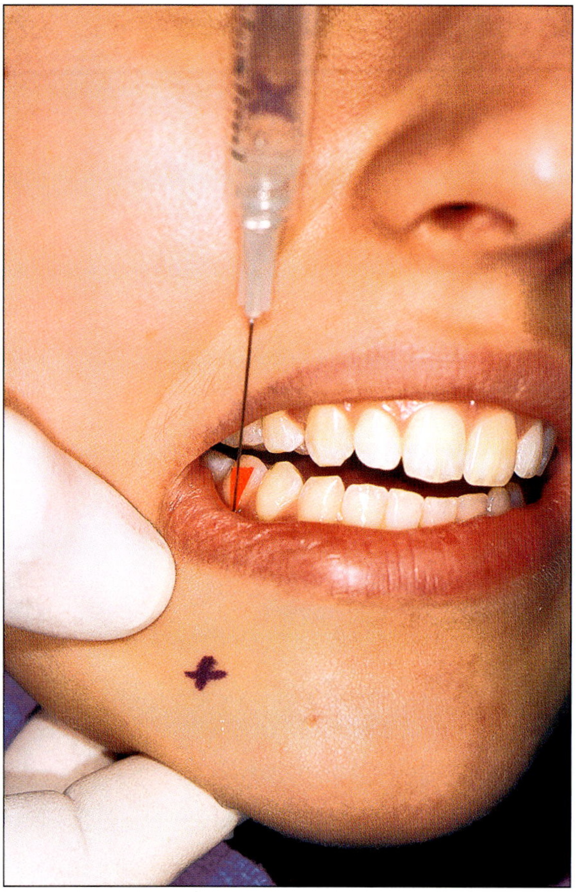

Fig. 4.11 Mental block, intraoral approach (mental foramen indicated by purple 'X', second premolar indicated by red triangle)

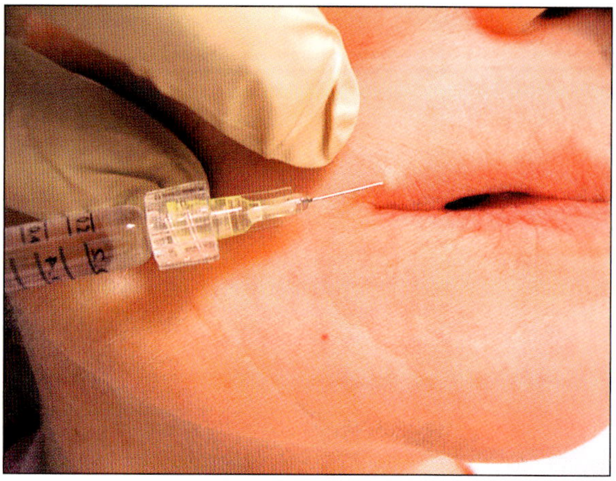

Fig. 4.12 Syringe is held parallel to the long axis of the lip for injection of vermilion border

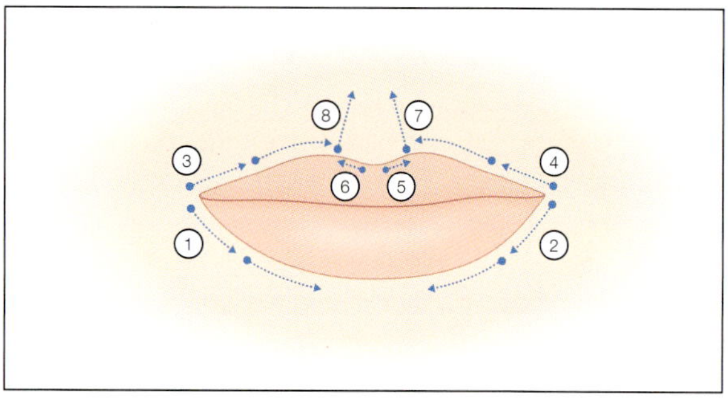

Fig. 4.13 Schematic of injection sequence for lip line enhancement

is injected just under the mucosa in the sulcus adjacent to each canine tooth.

The linear threading technique is used for implantation in essentially all lip injections. To improve lip line definition, inject into the potential space between the lip mucosa and the skin, along the vermilion border (Fig. 4.12). Any sequence of lip injections can be used; the specific approach is one of personal preference. Many physicians begin at the right corner of the lower lip (Fig. 4.13). Standing beside the patient, the thumb of the noninjecting hand is placed at the corner of the mouth, gently stretching the lip posteriorly to keep it taut. Holding the syringe parallel to the lower lip with the other hand, pierce the vermilion just anterior to the oral commissure, and advance it medially along the vermilion border. Using a threading technique, inject the implant into the potential space between the lip mucosa and skin. Continue with successive threads onward toward the center of the lip. Then repeat the process from the left corner of the lower lip toward the center. A 0.5 in needle will reach 20–25% of the lip line in most patients, so four or five threading injections should cover the entire lip. Placing filler in the lateral aspects of the lower lip will also serve to lift the corners of the mouth and provide a rejuvenating effect. The vermilion border of the upper lip is then treated in a similar fashion, although some physicians prefer to enter centrally and proceed laterally to the corners to preserve the patient's natural cupid's bow. Holding the syringe vertically, perpendicular to the upper lip, the philtrum of the lip can also be made more defined by implanting threads of filler below each philtral crest.

If volume augmentation of the lip is also desired, outlining the vermilion border is followed by injection into the mucosa itself. Roughly equal amounts of material are normally used for lip margin enhancement and volume expansion (for example, half a syringe for each). Holding the syringe parallel to the long axis of the lip and using a threading technique, inject along the 'wet line' of the red of the lip, at which the dry outer mucosa meets the moist inner mucosa. Inject uniformly as the needle is withdrawn from the track to create a smooth and even enlargement of the bulk of the lip. Be sure to cease injection just prior to needle withdrawal in order to avoid superficial placement of the gel. Massage gently throughout the treatment to ensure a smooth final contour.

Troubleshooting

Owing to the thin, distensible tissue of the lips, patients may develop localized swelling during treatment. This can make it difficult to judge lip symmetry and the overall degree of augmentation that is appropriate or desired by the patient. It is best to invite the patient to return for a touch-up in 1–2 weeks, rather than risk overcorrection by continually trying to 'equalize' the two sides. Each patient will have a different idea of what is 'too much' lip enhancement, and most will not appreciate over-augmentation.

A history of herpes simplex infection should be sought before treatment to determine if a pretreatment and post-treatment course of antivirals is indicated (acyclovir or equivalent).

Side effects, complications, and alternative approaches

Significant postinjection swelling and bruising are the most common side effects of lip injection. Immediate postoperative ice packs can help minimize the swelling ('kiss the ice'), as can keeping the head elevated after injection. The swelling will decrease in a day or two, but bruising can last 7–10 days. Some advocate applying 1% vitamin K cream twice daily to any areas that are bruised to speed resolution. A short course of systemic steroids can also be used if needed.

A rare complication is reactivation of labial herpes infection, which should respond to an appropriate course of systemic antivirals.

The lips are very vascular structures, supplied by the superior and inferior labial arteries, branches of the facial artery. The most concerning complication of lip augmentation is inadvertent injection into or near a vessel to the point of occlusion with resultant localized necrosis. While this can occur with any injectable filler, it is more likely with thicker substances (Zyplast, Perlane). Since blood cannot be easily drawn back through a 30 gauge needle to ensure a vessel has not been entered, the best insurance is to keep the needle moving during injection to minimize implantation in any single perivascular location. Also, watch for signs of occlusion (pain, blanching) during implantation so injection can be quickly discontinued if needed. The facial artery bifurcates from the angle of the mouth to ascend toward the nose, cheek, and eye on each side; partial or complete occlusion during lip augmentation has been reported to lead to symptoms in those areas as well.

If localized pain or blanching does develop acutely during treatment, immediately discontinue injection and manually massage the area until color returns. If blanching remains, apply warm water compresses to the area and have the patient take an aspirin. Some authors also suggest applying nitroglycerin paste every 2 hours for 24 hours and then every 4–6 hours until resolution, although this has obviously not been studied. Follow the patient daily for 5 days and then weekly until this is resolved. Do not reinject the area with any type of augmentation material until the problem is completely resolved.

Upper lip rhytids

Patients/indications

Many patients have vertical rhytids of the upper cutaneous lip that can be improved with hylan fillers. If a patient is also interested in lip enhancement, however, perform it first as many of the radial lines may soften as they are effaced by the increased volume of the adjacent vermilion. Another consideration is botulinum toxin, which will not do much to remove current lines but can prevent future ones.

Equipment (Restylane, Restylane Fine Lines/Touch)

Most of the lines of the upper cutaneous lip are superficial, and are best treated with thinner fillers such as Restylane and Restylane Fine Lines. The smaller needles (30 gauge and smaller) supplied are also advantageous. Few patients will require more than 0.3 mL in a single treatment session.

Treatment algorithm (linear threading, serial puncture)

Unlike the vermilion of the lips, patients often tolerate injection of the cutaneous portion of the upper lip after topical anesthesia only (LMX, etc.) Allow an adequate amount of time for the topical anesthetic to take effect before injection. The patient can also use an ice pack ('kiss the ice') before and inbetween injections to supplement anesthesia. Treatment is easily performed by standing in front of the patient and holding the syringe upright to inject into the vertical rhytids (Fig. 4.14). Linear threading and serial punture techniques both work well in this area, but take care not to overcorrect. Persistent beading will be evident if material is injected too superficially. Between injections, the implant may be kneaded gently along the line of injection to ensure that it is smooth and uniform.

Troubleshooting

In this area, the most important issues are ensuring adequate anesthesia so the patient can remain still during implant placement, and not injecting the filler too superficially, which can lead to unsightly beading. If this does occur, massage the implant firmly between two fingers (one inside and one outside the lip) or against the underlying bone to try to salvage an acceptable result.

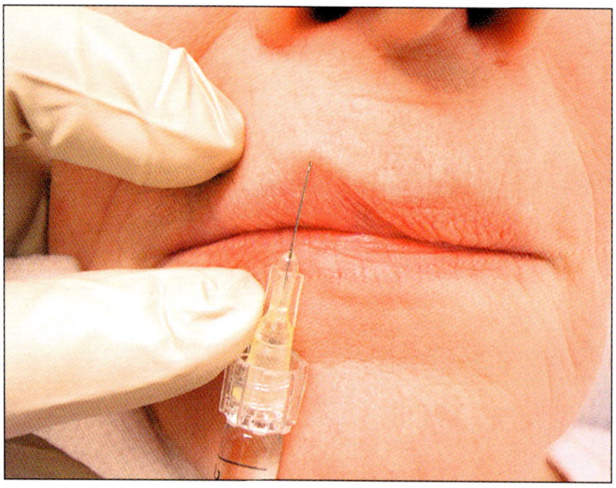

Fig. 4.14 Syringe is held perpendicular to the long axis of the lip (parallel to rhytid being filled) for injection of static upper lip rhytids

Side effects, complications, and alternative approaches

As with injections of the vermilion, necrosis is a possibility with any filler material, but is much less likely here as the plane of injection should be very superficial, and the orientation of the needle is perpendicular to the underlying vessels.

Nasolabial folds

Patients/indications

Patients who would like to diminish prominent NLFs can attain significant improvement with hylan fillers.

Equipment (Restylane, Perlane)

Restylane, Restylane Perlane, or a similar agent will work well for NLFs. If the fold is shallow, Restylane alone may do well, using a 30 gauge needle. If it is more pronounced, a thicker agent (Perlane, etc.) may be required for deeper filling, followed by Restylane layered on top. For many patients with moderate NLFs, one syringe will be adequate. For very deep folds, a second treatment should be scheduled 2–4 weeks later. With less prominent folds, there may be enough left in one syringe to also treat mild oral commissures, glabellar frown lines, or other mild lines.

Treatment algorithm (linear threading, serial puncture, fanning)

Many patients do not require more than topical anesthesia for treatment of NLFs, though some may prefer injection of anesthetic around the area. Using the nondominant hand to apply gentle downward traction to the inferiormost aspect of the fold to immobilize it, the dominant hand is used to inject filler. Steadying the injecting hand on the mandible or the other hand, the linear threading technique is most easily used to deposit the filler beneath the fold and efface it. The peri-alar sulcus, a triangular-shaped concavity at the upper end of the fold, may be more effectively filled with the fanning technique of implantation, where two or three threads are deposited in a fan-like array. Wide portions of the fold may require several threads placed side by side, with gentle massage after each thread is placed.

Troubleshooting

Treatment of this area is generally easy and straightforward, and satisfying for patients and practitioners. Notice that the fold is partially formed by prominent cheek tissue that is lateral to it, with the fold becoming more prominent as the cheek becomes more protuberant. Therefore, injections should stay **medial** to the fold to fill it; injecting lateral to it (in the excessive cheek tissue) can actually tend to accentuate the fold.

Side effects, complications, and alternative approaches

Bruising is the most common side effect in this area and usually resolves in 5–7 days. The facial artery runs below the fold and necrosis is possible, though rare.

Glabellar lines

Patients/indications

Patients with static glabellar lines can have a good response to hylan fillers. Many practitioners will first maximize treatment with botulinum toxin to improve these 'frown' lines, dispelling dynamic rhytids and softening static ones. Then the residual lines can be effaced with fillers.

Equipment (Restylane, Restylane Fine Lines)

Depending on the severity of the rhytid, Restylane, Restylane Fine Lines, or an equivalent hylan can be used to treat fine to moderate wrinkles in this area. Thicker preparations such as Perlane should be used with caution, due to the rare but concerning risk of vascular occlusion in this area (thicker, cross-linked collagen preparations such as Zyplast are contraindicated in the glabellar area for this reason).

Treatment algorithm (linear threading, serial puncture)

Most patients do well with only topical anesthetic (LMX, etc.) in the glabellar area. With the patient seated, immobilize the area to be treated with the noninjecting hand. Since most lines in this area are in a vertical orientation, it is easy to stand directly in front of the patient, holding the syringe upright and angling at 45° to the skin surface (Fig. 4.15). Gentle pressure of the needle tip through the skin surface followed by implantation using the linear threading and/or serial puncture techniques will produce good results. A sudden decrease in resistance during injection may mean the needle tip has advanced too deeply and penetrated the subcutaneous tissue. Postinjection pressure and ice may help to minimize swelling and bruising.

Troubleshooting

Using the thinnest possible filler substance will minimize concerns of vascular occlusion.

Side effects, complications, and alternative approaches

The most concerning side effect of treatment of the glabella is localized necrosis from partial or total occlusion of a vessel. Owing to the limited collateral circulation in this area, 56% of all necrotic events from collagen injection (mostly Zyplast) occur here. If symptoms of vascular occlusion (pain, blanching) occur during treatment, stop the injection immediately. Although the value of massage, warm compresses, and nitroglycerin paste is unsubstantiated in the improvement of outcome, most practitioners suggest trying them (as discussed earlier under lip treatment).

Oral commissure lines (marionette lines)

Patients/indications

Patients with lines extending down from the mouth or depressed oral commissures can benefit from

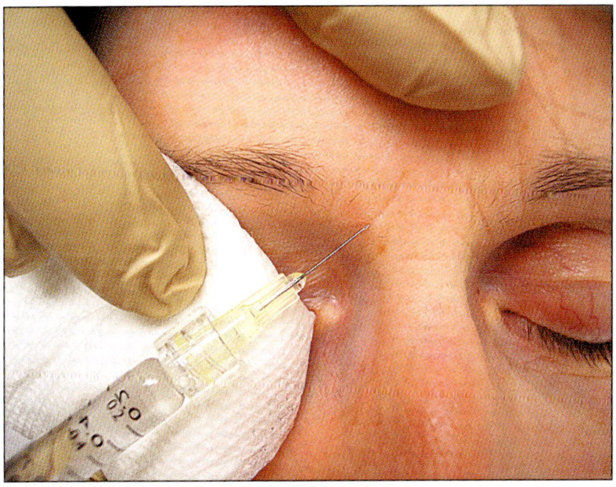

Fig. 4.15 Injection of glabellar lines

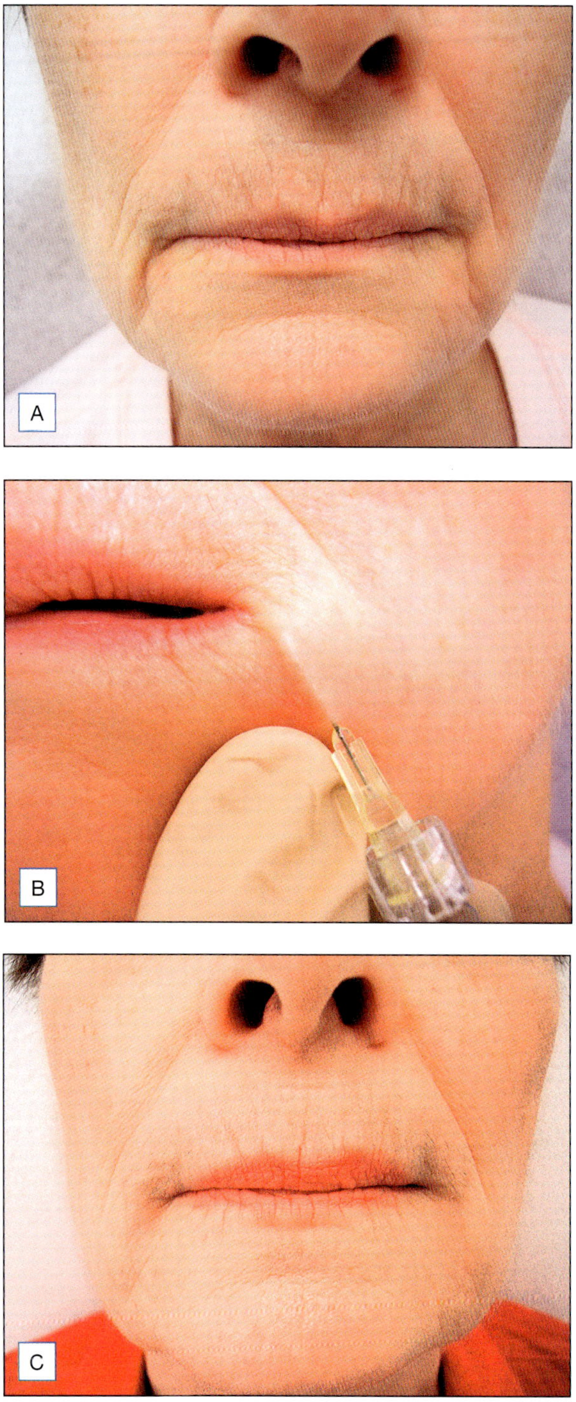

Fig. 4.16 (**A**) Before treatment of bilateral melolabial folds with 0.7 mL Restylane gel. (**B**) Technique used. (**C**) Two weeks after treatment

hylan implants (Fig. 4.16). Many of these patients also have significant NLFs.

Equipment (Restylane, Perlane)

Restylane and Perlane or similar implants will work well for this area; one to two syringes will treat the great majority of patients.

Treatment algorithm (linear threading, serial puncture, fanning)

Patients may or may not require injectable anesthesia in this area; be careful not to efface the area with the lidocaine injection! Another approach is to anesthetize from the mucosal side of the commissure. The serial puncture, linear threading, or fanning techniques can all be useful in treating oral commissures. The noninjecting hand can help to immobilize the skin for the initial puncture of the needle, though during injection take care not to alter the area with such traction. Injecting filler into both lower lateral oral commissures can elevate the corner of the mouth and give a rejuvenated look. Linear 'marionette' lines usually respond well to linear threading implantation.

Troubleshooting

Make sure the patient has been adequately anesthetized, as injections adjacent to the vermilion can be quite painful.

Side effects, complications, and alternative approaches

As with other injections near the lips, swelling and bruising can be significant, and may be minimized by immediate postoperative ice or cold compresses.

Facial contouring of cheeks/chin

Patients/indications

Patients who desire filling of 'sunken' areas of the midface, as from HIV lipodystrophy or other atrophic losses, or those who desire true augmentation of the chin or cheekbones to change facial contour, are appropriate candidates for hylan implantation. Results should last at least 6 months.

Equipment (Perlane)

Since deeper augmentation is required here, more robust fillers such as Perlane are most appropriate. Several syringes may be needed to achieve the desired result, as the area to be treated can have a significant depth and cross-sectional area.

Treatment algorithm (linear threading, fanning, cross-hatching)

Since the thicker fillers such as Perlane require larger (27 gauge) needles, patients may require injection of lidocaine in a 'field block' fashion surrounding the area to be treated. A surgical marking pen may be used to highlight the area to be treated prior to anesthesia so anesthetic fluid will not alter the contour. Rarely patients may get by with topical anesthesia only.

To deposit the large volumes of filler needed for facial contouring, the fanning and cross-hatching implantation techniques are useful. They will also require fewer needle punctures through the skin than the linear threading or the serial puncture techniques. The target depth of implantation is the deep dermis and the dermal/subcutaneous junction; layering of subsequent threads of filler is often needed to achieve a 100% correction.

Troubleshooting

The most difficult aspect of facial contouring with fillers is estimating how much material will be required. The good news is that it is difficult to overcorrect if good technique is observed.

Side effects, complications, and alternative approaches

Most patients do well using hylans for facial contouring. If they are pleased with the results using temporary fillers and want to avoid repeated injections, they may want to consider treatment with more permanent fillers instead (Radiance, Artecoll, Silicone, etc.)

Advanced Topics

Combination techniques

Many of the static rhytids requiring treatment with hylan fillers would not be as prominent had they been treated with botulinum toxin earlier in their evolution. Thus it makes sense to consider combination treatment with both agents to most effectively combat facial rhytids. One retrospective study by Carruthers et al of 16 female patients with moderate to severe glabellar rhytids that had not resolved completely after multiple treatments with botulinum toxin A (BTX-A) documented the usefulness of such a combination. Simultaneous treatment using BTX-A and hylan B (Hylaform) resulted in superior improvement – 94% achieved mild rhytids and 6% (one patient) had moderate ones. No significant interactions or complications occurred. Another approach is to treat an area with Botox to eliminate all dynamic rhytids and soften the static ones, then after several weeks fill any remaining lines with hylans.

The question of skin testing

One of the major advantages of hylans over collagen is the decreased incidence of delayed hypersensitivity reactions. However, while this incidence is very low, sporadic case reports of hypersensitivity reactions show it is not zero. Since it should be impossible to react to pure hyaluronic acid, which is identical in all species and tissue types, any such reactions are thought to be due to impurities in hylan production: residual avian proteins (Hylaform) or byproducts of bacterial fermentation (Restylane). Some authors have therefore suggested pretreatment skin testing, as is performed with collagen implants. Others have pointed out that this would still not prevent all reactions, as some patients do not react until after their third treatment session. In addition, the incidence of such reactions seems to be dropping as the manufacturing process of hylans becomes more refined, resulting in purer products.

Other fillers containing hyaluronic acid or its derivatives

Many fillers now contain hyaluronic acid as a major or minor constituent. The hyaluronic acid may or may not be cross-linked, and may or may not be the substance responsible for volume augmentation. Following is a list of the more common fillers containing hyaluronic acid in current use.

Achyal is a 1% solution of the sodium salt of hyaluronic acid. Since it is not cross-linked, it is not considered a hylan (does not form a gel). It is distributed in 2.5 mL pre-filled syringes with 30 gauge needles, and can be stored at room temperature for up to 3 years. Similar to the hylans, it is used for wrinkles, scars, lip and contour deformities. It is manufactured by Tedec Meiji Farma, S.A., Madrid, Spain, and is not available in the USA.

DermaLive (see also Chapter 7) is a semi-permanent nonanimal filler composed of hyaluronic acid and acrylic hydrogel fragments. Here the hyaluronic acid is merely the delivery system (which accounts for 60% of the volume); the acrylic hydrogel filler is a copolymer of hydroxyethylmethacrylate (HEMA) and ethylmethacrylate (EMA), a nonbiodegradable material belonging to the acrylate family that has demonstrated a good level of tolerance for many years in eye surgery (same acrylic hydrogel as used in intraocular lens implants in cataract surgery). The smooth-walled 45–65 micron hydrogel particles are intentionally irregular (nonspherical), which is thought to help integrate them into newly formed collagen fibers and prevent concentric fibrosis. It is supplied in 0.8 mL syringes and delivered through a 27.5 gauge needle. Produced by Dermatech, the product was first marketed in France 1998 and has now become very popular throughout Europe. The manufacturer suggests several treatment sessions, each separated by a minimum of 3 months. There have been reports of granulomatous reactions from the acrylic particles, manifesting as palpable nodules appearing about 6 months after injection. As with other HA products, no pre-operative skin tests are required.

DermaDeep (see also Chapter 7) is similar to DermaLive, except that the acrylic particle sizes are larger, from 80–110 μm. It is provided in 1.2 mL syringes and delivered through a 26.5 gauge needle. One study describing the use of DermaLive and DermaDeep in 455 patients (859 syringes) over 3 years reports that patients were satisfied in 88% of cases, with 20% developing transient redness or edema at the injection site.

Hyacell is an HA derivative which is widely used in India and Latin America. In addition to hyaluronic acid, it contains zinc, selenium, vanadium, and unspecified 'embryonic extracts'. Its illicit use by a non-physician was suspected to have caused nine cases of *Mycobacterium abscessus* infection in New York city in 2002, although it is unknown whether the material was contaminated during manufacture or from the individual who injected it with unclean technique.

Hylan Rofilan Gel is a hyaluronic acid gel cross-linked with a natural acid instead of a chemical compound. It has not been FDA approved for use in the USA. It is manufactured and distributed by Rofil Medical International B.V., Breda, The Netherlands.

Juvéderm is similar to Restylane in that it represents a range of products based on nonanimal, lightly cross-linked hyaluronic acid technology. The homogeneous nature of Juvéderm gel is touted to create less surface area for the body's enzymes to attack and therefore degrade the hyaluronic acid. It is currently available in three formulations: Juvéderm 18, Juvéderm 24, and Juvéderm 30, which contain 18 mg, 24 mg, and 30 mg of hyaluronic acid, respectively, per 1 g of phosphate buffer. They are pre-packaged with a 27 gauge or 30 gauge needle and are formulated to a pH of 7.2. They are produced in France and are not currently available in the USA.

Viscontour is a sodium hyaluronic acid product which has been developed in three forms to address wrinkles, contour defects, wound healing, and tissue hydration. A noncross-linked injectable version has been marketed in Europe since 2002, and a cross-linked injectable version is being developed by Aventis Dermatology.

Further Reading

Carruthers J, Carruthers A, Maberley D 2003 Deep resting glabellar rhytids respond to BTX-A and Hylan B. Dermatologic Surgery 29:539–544

Duranti F, Salti G, Bovani B, Calandra M, Rosati ML 1998 Injectable hyaluronic acid gel for soft-tissue augmentation. A clinical and histological study. Dermatologic Surgery 24:1317–1325

Fernandez-Acenero MJ, Zamora E, Borbujo J 2003 Granulomatous foreign body reaction against hyaluronic acid: Report of a case after lip augmentation. Dermatologic Surgery 29(12):1225–1226

Friedman PM, Mafong EA, Kauvar AN, Geronemus RG 2002 Safety data of injectable nonanimal stabilized hyaluronic acid gel for soft tissue augmentation. Dermatologic Surgery 28(6):491–494

Hallen L, Johansson C, Laurent C 1999 Cross-linked hyaluronan (hylan B gel): a new injectable remedy for treatment of vocal cord insufficiency – an animal study. Acta Oto-laryngologica (Stockh) 119:107–111

Klein AW 2001 Skin filling: Collagen and other injectables of the skin. Dermatology Clinics 19(3):491–508

Lowe NJ, Maxwell A, Lowe P, Duick MG, Shah K 2001 Hyaluronic acid fillers: Adverse reactions and skin testing. Journal of the American Academy of Dermatologists 45:930–933

Lupton JR, Alster TS 2000 Cutaneous hypersensitivity reaction to injectable hyaluronic acid gel. Dermatologic Surgery 26(2):135–137

Manna F, Dentini M, Desideri P, DePita O, Mortilla E, Maras B 1999 Comparative chemical evaluation of two commercially available derivatives of hyaluronic acid (Hylaform from rooster combs and Restylane from *Streptococcus*) used for soft tissue augmentation. Journal of the European Academy of Dermatological Venereologists 13:183–192

Micheels P 2001 Human anti-hyaluronic acid antibodies: Is it possible? Dermatologic Surgery 27(2):185–191

Narins RS, Brandt F, Leyden J, Lorenc ZP, Rubin M, Smith S 2003 A randomized, double-blind, multicenter comparison of the efficacy and tolerability of restylane versus zyplast for the correction of nasolabial folds. Dermatologic Surgery 29(6):588–595

Olenius M 1998 The first clinical study using a new biodegradable implant for the treatment of lips, wrinkles, and folds. Aesthetic Plastic Surgery 22:97–101

Piacquadio D, Jarcho M, Goltz R 1997 Evaluation of hylan B gel as a soft-tissue augmentation implant material. Journal of the American Academy of Dermatologists 36:544–549

Pollack SV 1999 Some new injectable dermal filler materials: Hylaform, Restylane, and Artecoll. Journal of Cutaneous Medical Surgery 3(suppl 4):27–35

5 Augmentation with Autologous Fat

Lisa M. Donofrio

Introduction

Thorough evaluation and management of the aging face requires that the cosmetic dermasurgeon look past obvious superficial changes that have occurred with photoaging and begin with assessing the changes in morphologic structure that occur as a result of chronologic aging. The purpose of this chapter is to instruct the reader in the differences between surface aging changes such as wrinkles and deeper aging changes that occur in fat and bone that lead to misdraping of the skin envelope.

In the first decade of life the soft tissue structures of the face are round and cherubic. Due to the abundance of fat in the cheek, there is an accentuation of the nasolabial and labiomental creases. Fat distribution is in 'pockets' and easily grabbed between thumb and forefinger. The maxillary height appears short when compared with the orbital height, leading to a visual diminution of the lower third of the face. This bony relationship as well as the abundance of fat seen in the medial cheeks is responsible for the presence of jowls seen in infants and young children (Fig. 5.1). In the young adult, however, there is an aesthetic balance in the facial bones of the upper and lower cranial skeleton so the soft tissues drape harmoniously. The fat is abundant but unlike the infant face is smoothly and diffusely distributed. There is a continuum of the fat within and between cosmetic units of the face, so the distribution of fat appears balanced and homogeneous. In the youthful face there are many points of highlight and rare areas of shadow. Due to the density of the fat compartments, the face projects away from the underlying bony framework forming light reflecting arcs. In profile two arcs distinguish a young face: the forehead arc which lifts the skin away from the frontal bones diving into the superior lid crease, and the midface arc traveling from the lower lid tarsus through to the mandible acting as a strut to 'tent' the skin of the cheek anteriorly (Fig. 5.2). Additionally the jawline is arced from mastoid to mastoid and curved in its superior to inferior dimensions forming a distinct yet rounded border with the neck (Figs 5.3, 5.4). Animation in the young face shows the mimetic muscles to work independently of the skin. Contraction of the muscles of facial expression results in little if any surface convolutions due to the thickness of the subcutaneous tissue and the proportion of required muscular force (Fig. 5.5).

By contrast, an aging face displays loss of the anterior projection of the forehead, brow, and midface leading to relative skin excess with displacement in the dependent direction (Fig. 5.6). There is

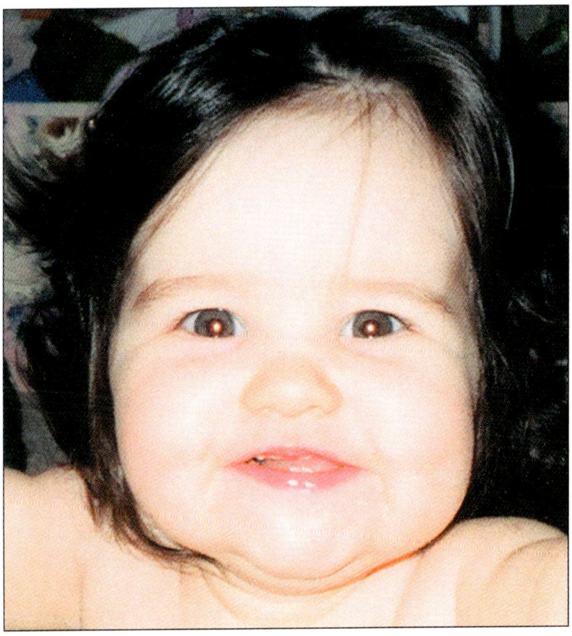

Fig. 5.1 Due to the abundance of cheek fat, a child's face displays prominent nasolabial and labiomental folds

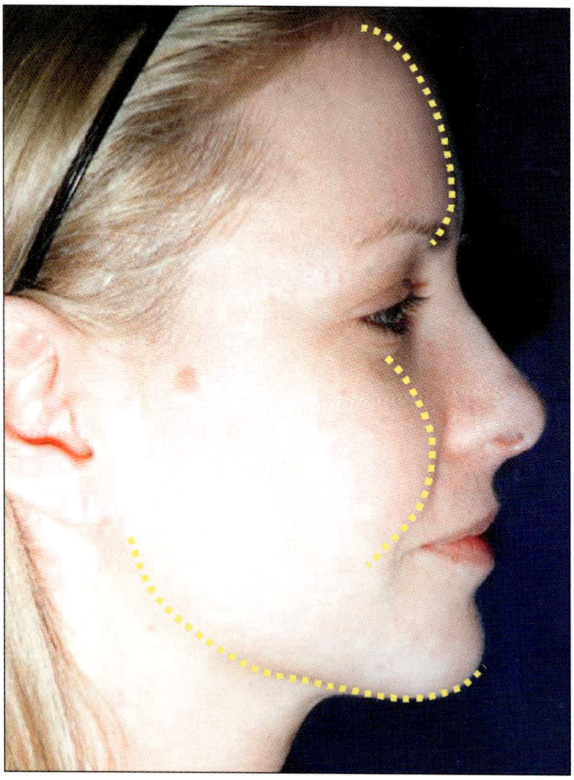

Fig. 5.2 The young face in profile

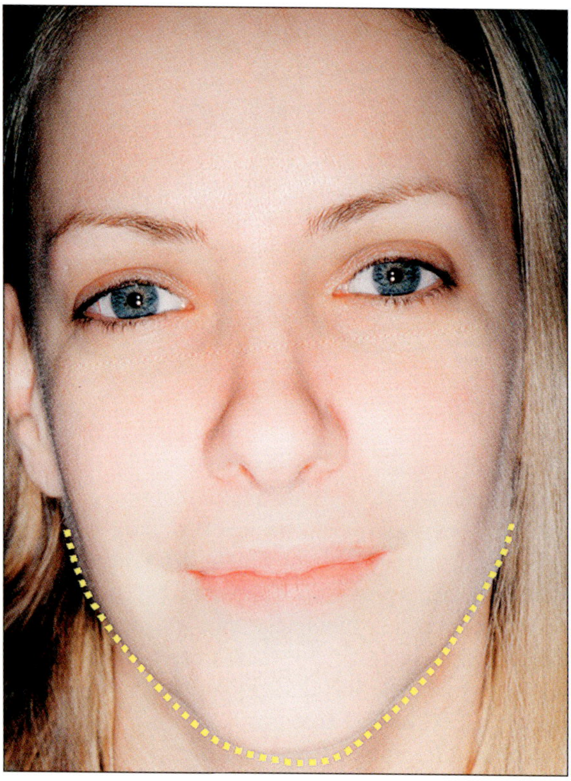

Fig. 5.3 The young face en face

often a discrepancy in areas of the face that appear to have too much or too little fat. This topographically leads to 'hills and valleys', the hills representing areas of fat excess, the valleys fat atrophy. These atrophic/hypertrophic fat patterns are markedly discernible in the aging face of overweight individuals. It seems that with an increase in body fat, the face also stores fat in distinctive areas of the lower midface, lateral malar area, submental area, and lower central cheek lateral to the nasolabial fold. All other areas of the face show atrophic patterns with involution and collapse of soft tissue. Very lean individuals may show panfacial atrophy without any hypertrophy (Fig. 5.7). The suborbital area however can show either an atrophic variant with hollowing and demarcation of the orbital ridge, or a hypertrophic variant with prominent suborbital fullness. It is important to realize that even the hypertrophic pattern of suborbital aging is due to loss in volume of the upper malar fat pad and interruption of the cheek/eye continuum rather than a true hypertrophic event. These suborbital patterns appear to occur independent of total body fat and may instead represent a genetic variant. The combined visual effect of areas of hollowing bordering areas of

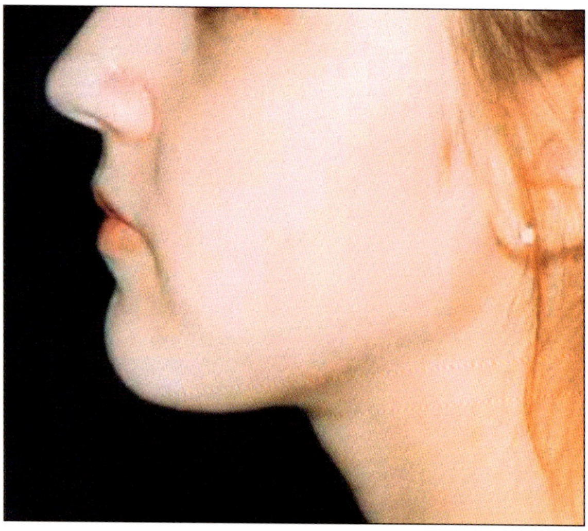

Fig. 5.4 A young neck displays 'rounded angularity' as it dives into the neck

fullness is to give the aged face a shift in shape from the roundness and arcs of youth to a face replete in shadows and irregular contours. These overall morphologic patterns are so important in our ability to determine the age of a person that we use them

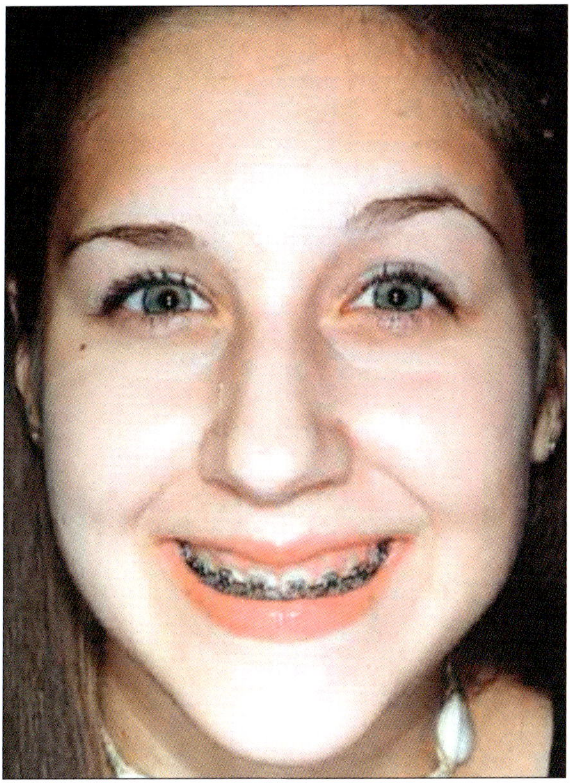

Fig. 5.5 Animation in the young face

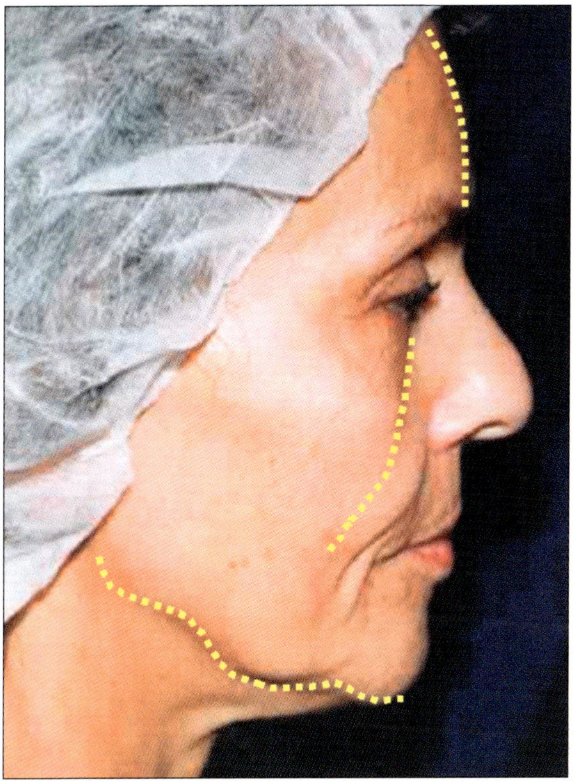

Fig. 5.6 The aging face in profile

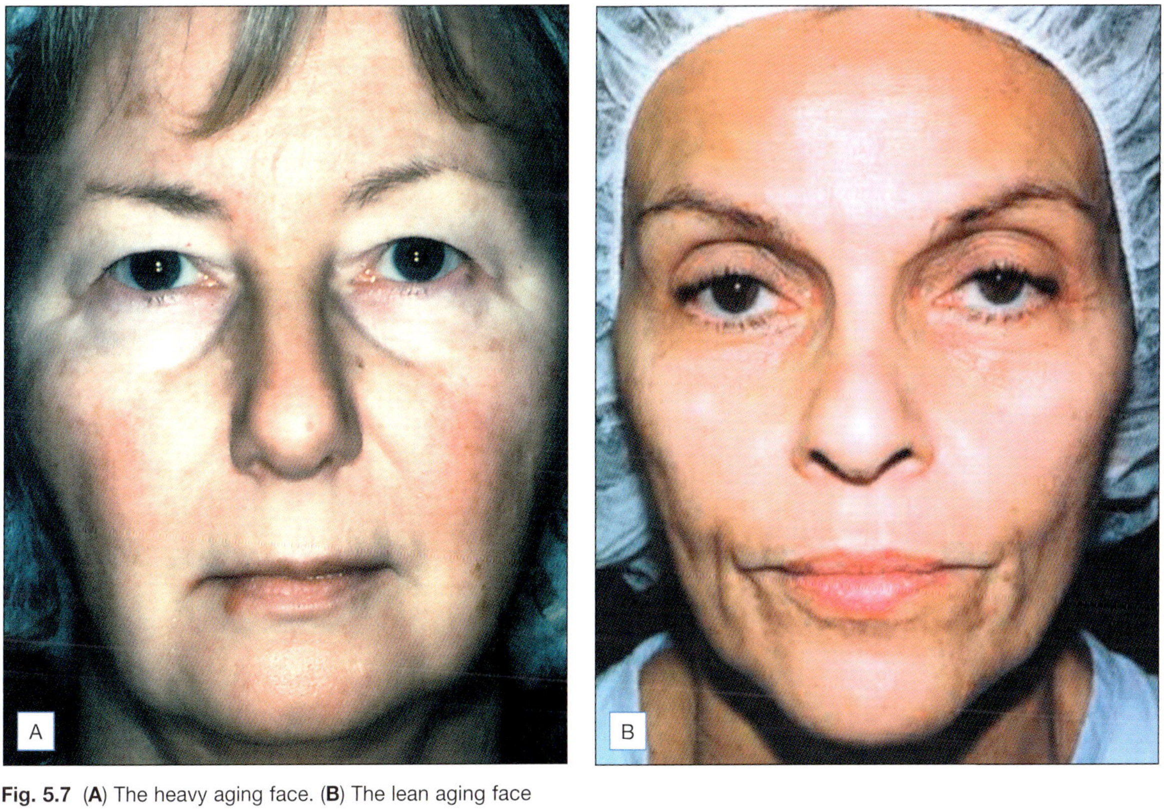

Fig. 5.7 (A) The heavy aging face. (B) The lean aging face

independent of surface characteristics such as wrinkles and photoaging. The interaction between the mimetic muscles and the skin is intimate in the aging face. Due to the diminution in the thickness of the subcutaneous fat, the muscle lies in close juxtaposition with the skin surface. Since the required muscular force relative to the skin thickness is low, the skin tugs along with each contraction (Fig. 5.8). It is interesting to note that the cosmetic use of botulinum toxin decreases the muscular load on the skin, restoring a balanced proportion between the muscular force and the skin thickness reminiscent of that seen in youth.

The above mentioned volumetric changes in facial structure that occur with aging are due mostly to the changes that occur in the fatty compartments of the face. There is no change in the size of facial muscles with age, so mimetic muscles as a structural element play little if any role in the aging process. Since the major morphologic shift in the aging face happens secondarily to changes within the fat, then redistributing fat back to patterns seen in youth is undoubtedly the most reasonable approach to rejuvenate the senescent face. The term 'fat rebalancing' will be used in this chapter to denote the end result of either solely adding fat to atrophic areas of the face or as a combination of microsuction of the hypertrophic areas in combination with transplantation to the atrophic areas. Patients that have a lean frame and therefore a lean face will require only fat transplantation, whereas those patients who are overweight may also require suctioning of the hypertrophic fat distribution areas in the face. Fat transplantation as described in this chapter will take place in the deep tissue planes of the face with the use of blunt cannulas, preferably in a panfacial manner. When using fat in this way the face changes its three dimensional contours returning to a more youthful countenance (Fig. 5.9).

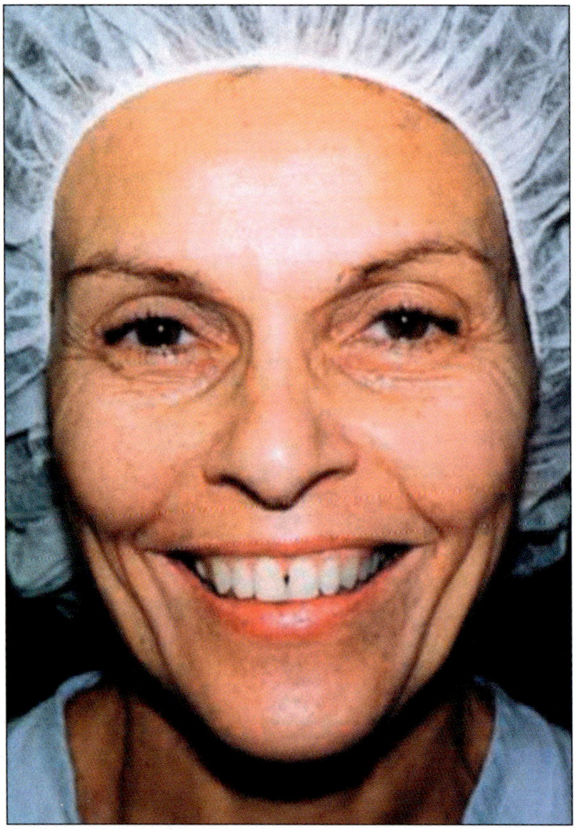

Fig. 5.8 Animation in the aged face

Patient selection

Any patient desiring a more youthful appearance is a candidate for structural fat rebalancing. Because there is no skin excision, there are no telltale scars occurring around the hairline and so fat rebalancing is an excellent rejuvenating treatment for men as well as women (Fig. 5.10). To ensure the selection of patients with a favorable outcome it is important to truly understand how they want to look after a cosmetic procedure. Patients that desire to look like themselves 'only younger', or 'more refreshed', or 'less tired' have excellent expectations and most likely will be happy with fat rebalancing. However patients who apply posterior traction on their facial skin to demonstrate what is desired should be referred out for the more ascetic look of a traditional facelift. Results obtainable with fat rebalancing are much more dramatic if patients can return for between four and six 'touch up' procedures completing the rejuvenation in a staged manner. Patients that can only schedule enough time to do a single procedure will most likely be disappointed unless that procedure is performed in an overly aggressive manner, increasing both the likelihood of misplacement of the fat and long term edema. Since even a mild to moderately aggressive fat rebalancing session can leave the patient bruised and swollen for 1–2 weeks, patient selection should be also based upon their ability to take time off from work or social obligations. Structural fat rebalancing can be successful and dramatic in patients of all ages, however patients in the age range 35–50 are the most ideal candidates for fat rebalancing for the simple reason that they have less to correct. It also stands to

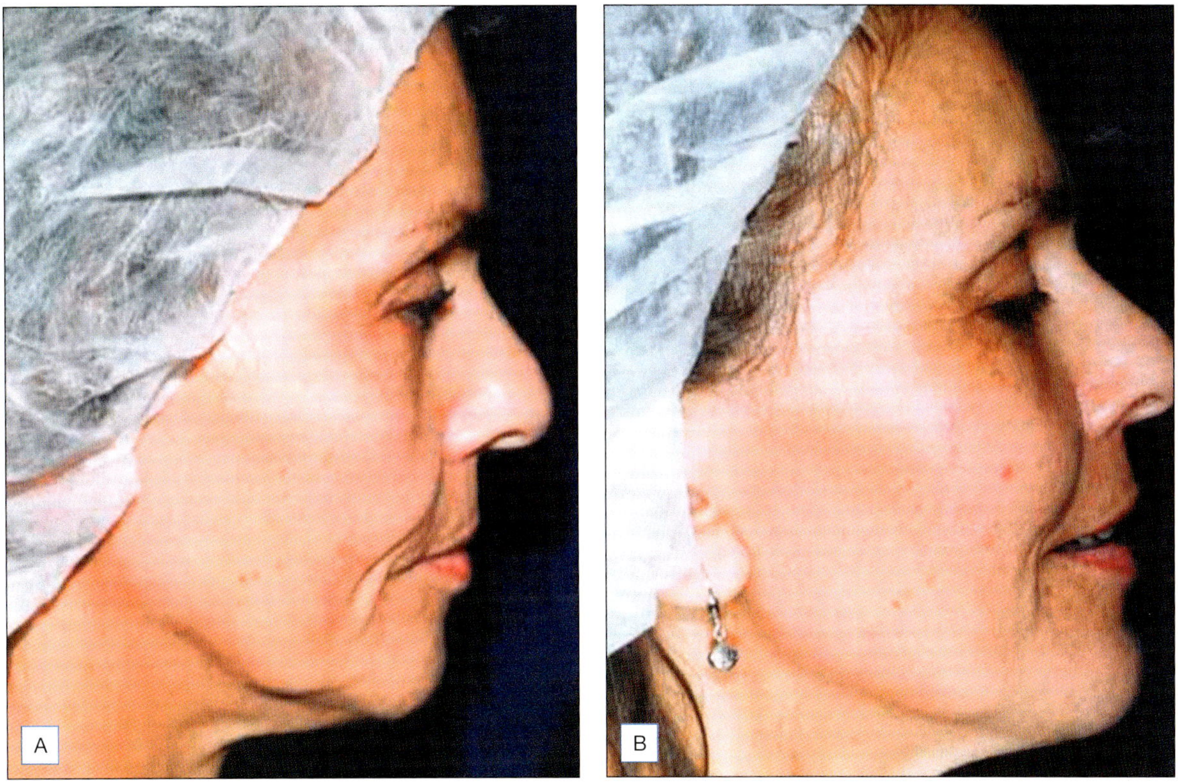

Fig. 5.9 (**A**) Aging patient displaying flattening of forward projection of face. (**B**) Restoration of contours after fat rebalancing

reason that the response of the overlying skin envelope, either to contract if fat is removed or stretch if fat is added, may be much more predictable in a younger aged patient, especially one with minimal photoaging. Severe photoaging is a contraindication to any microsuction since skin with profound solar elastosis tends to show surface irregularities with even the most minimal fat removal. Other contraindications to fat rebalancing are lack of sufficient fat for extraction or poor skin tone in the 'donor' area, and serious chronic medical problems such as advanced organ disease, elevated PT/PTT (natural or iatrogenic), and acute infection. Patients with a past history of pulmonary embolus or deep vein thrombosis need to be evaluated on a case by case basis, taking into account the amount of fat being suctioned, their hormonal status, and their activity level postoperatively.

Expected benefits

Following a series of six to eight structural fat rebalancing sessions, patients can generally expect to capture the shape of their face when they were 10–15 years younger (Fig. 5.11). Segmental use of either microsuction on the face or limited area fat transfer should also be done in a staged, progressive manner and will take a minimum of four sessions to achieve balance. Since most patients can only view themselves in two dimensions it often takes critical analysis by looking at baseline photographs to appreciate the changes in profile after one or two sessions. When structural fat grafting is used to correct iatrogenic defects from facelifts or blepharoplasties, the results are dependent on the degree of fat deficit, the resultant tension on the skin, and the amount of subcutaneous scar tissue. Some deficits may be uncorrectable, for example the case when an overaggressive blepharoplasty has resulted in scleral show from too much skin removal. Fat can replace fat; fat cannot replace skin. Excellent long term retention of fat grafts when placed for structural correction is well documented in the literature, however there are individual patients that do not retain the transplanted fat for unknown reasons. Retention rates vary and are most likely technique and operator dependent. Since there are no objective study designs other than the assessment of

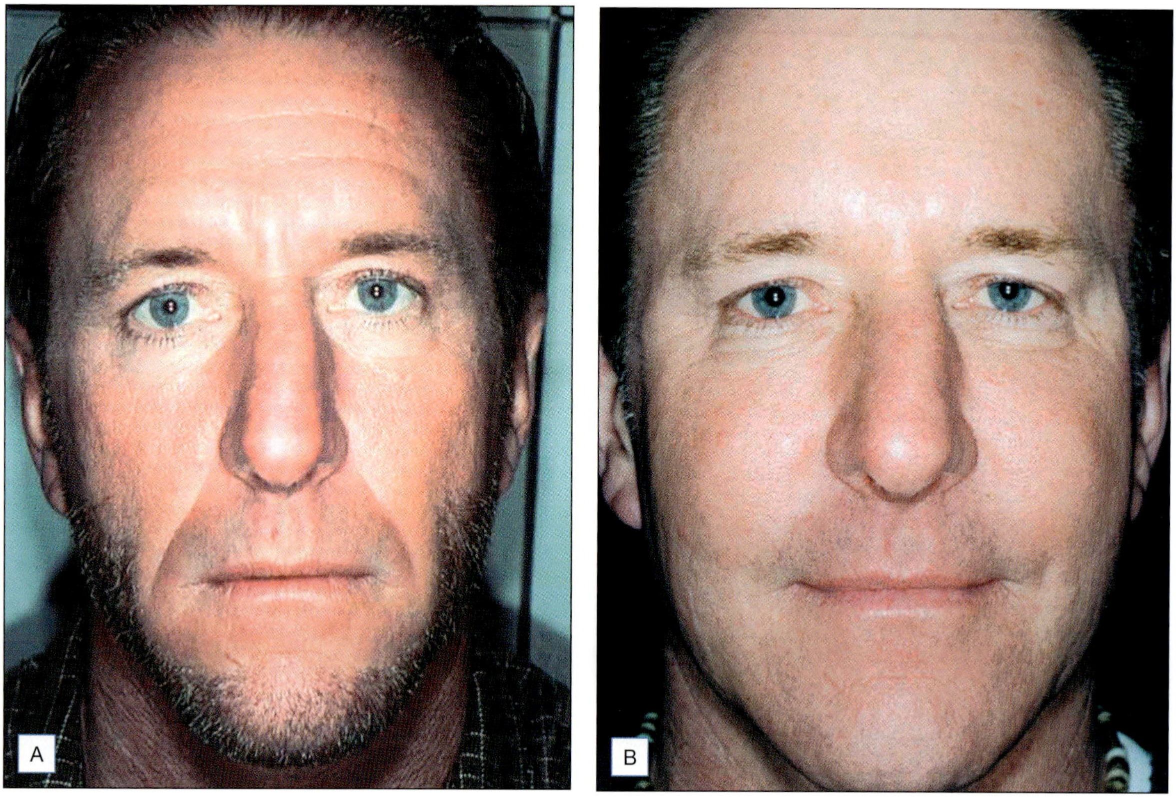

Fig. 5.10 (**A**) 50 year old male. (**B**) Same man now age 55 after fat rebalancing

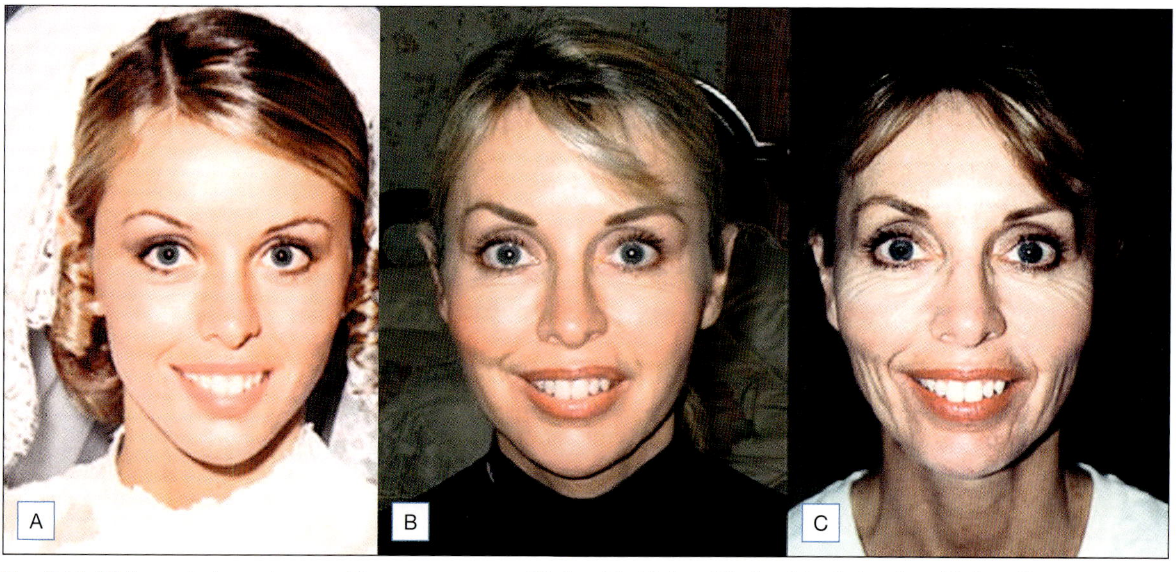

Fig. 5.11 All three photographs are of the same woman. (**A**) Age 20. (**B**) Age 50 after fat rebalancing. (**C**) Age 49

serial photographs, discussion of this nature may at this time be speculative.

Fat restructuring of the face occurs with the help of blunt tipped 17–18 gauge cannulas as described below. Unlike fine placement of dermal fillers, fat infiltration incurs a blunt traumatic injury. Ecchymosis and edema usually lasting 5–10 days is common on the initial fat transplantation procedure or for the touch-ups when fat is placed in the periorbital area. Therefore patients need to be counseled on the expected down-time as well as delayed optimization of cosmetic appearance. Since the final results take between four and eight rebalancing sessions, the amount of total impact on the patient's lifestyle will depend on whether fresh fat is harvested from the body on each transplant visit or whether previously extracted, banked and stored frozen fat is utilized.

Fat extraction takes place via local tumescent anesthesia. Supplemental oral benzodiazepines are helpful to quell preoperative anxiety. Due to the profound safety profile and excellent anesthetic qualities of tumescent anesthesia alone, parenteral anesthetic agents are not recommended. This can be a daunting prospect for the prospective fat rebalancing patient and a certain level of anticipation of discomfort is required. The order of magnitude of discomfort is somewhat dependent on the chosen donor site. Abdomens are the most tender of harvest sites. Since nearly the entire face is addressed, panfacial local anesthesia by the use of nerve blocks or local infiltration will be required. Most patients, however, find the procedure quite tolerable as long as the local anesthesia is buffered, and describe it to be similar in discomfort to a trip to the dentist.

Overview of Treatment Strategy

Treatment approach

The goal of fat rebalancing is to reconstruct the arcs that project the face forward, re-establish the soft curve of the jawline, redraping the skin away from the midface and forming an interface between the mimetic muscles and the skin. Other treatment approaches would be to enhance the cheekbones, reduce the appearance of dark shadows suborbitally caused by tear trough deformities, and redrape the skin of the eyelids via direct infiltration of fat. Fat rebalancing does not address photoaging changes such as skin texture, telangiectasias, or solar lentigos, and these need to be dealt with by other means such as laser rejuvenation or topical retinoids. In addition, ancillary use of botulinum toxin is helpful in decreasing the mobility of underlying musculature in the periorbital area. Although never studied scientifically, this could enhance 'take' of the fat grafts. Off label use of botulinum toxin injections are also suggested when horizontal forehead furrows are present and the patient has neither the desire nor the surplus of fat to address this large surface area with autologous fat grafts.

Major determinants

Patients desiring skin redraping achieved through fat rebalancing are generally looking for a natural appearing rejuvenation procedure and are trying to avoid the 'pulled' or 'done' look of traditional lifts. They may also be quite aware of the loss in volume that has occurred with aging and are concerned that a facelift will hollow them out more. The fact that only local anesthesia is used in fat rebalancing is enormously attractive to many patients afraid of general sedation. Because of the lack of need of anesthesia personnel and operating room time, the cost of fat rebalancing when done in an office setting can be significantly lower than a traditional facelift. Other desirable attributes of the fat rebalancing are the lack of peripheral scars and the gradual nature of the change achieved. Patients choosing facelifts or blepharoplasty are usually looking for a tighter sculpted outcome. They may be overweight with a very full face and the thought of adding any fat to their face appears distasteful to them. The degree of volume enhancement and skin projection achieved with fat transfer is unique and difficult and costly to achieve with 'purchased' injectables such as collagen or hyaluronic acid. However, for simple lip augmentation or superficial correction of either the nasolabial fold or labiomental crease, both collagen and hyaluronic acid are viable choices. The hyaluronic acids may also be used when filling tear trough deformities and superior brow arches. Given the option, the majority of patients opt for filling with fat since it offers a hypoallergenic, natural, large volume, long lasting alternative.

Patient interviews

The patient interview is the most important part of the fat rebalancing procedure. Most patients seek fat rebalancing as a way to rejuvenate their aging face without looking too different or 'operated on'. In addition, many patients seek out fat rebalancing as a way to correct unwanted changes that have occurred to their face as a result of prior cosmetic surgery, especially as a corrective technique for hollowing secondary to blepharoplasty. The most important question to ask the patient is: 'what bothers you about your aging face?' and then come up with a cause–effect treatment strategy from there. For example, a patient who complains about jowling will often display superior and lateral cheek atrophy as well as a corpulent body habitus. Since the hypertrophic fatty changes that occur in the lower third of the face are most times secondary to weight gain with aging, it is unrealistic for the patient to think that she can look as she used to without returning to a similar weight. So the second most important question often becomes: 'how has your weight changed in the last 10–15 years?' Patients who have gained a lot of weight can still benefit from filling atrophic areas of the face with or without microsuction of the hypertrophic areas, but may not obtain the striking results seen in patients whose weight has remained constant. Most patients will explain that they simply 'want to look like they used to look' but more often than not have no real objective idea of what they used to look like. Therefore it is helpful to ask the patient to bring a photograph from a time between 10 and 15 years ago when they liked how they looked. Again, remember to always compare the weight of the patient during the time of that photograph with the current weight. A patient who has had full cheeks her whole life and only through atrophic aging has gained the sculpted look in the buccal area she desires, may ultimately be a better candidate for a traditional face lifting procedure than fat rebalancing. However if the patient and dermasurgeon agree that fat rebalancing is the optimal approach it is still possible to give her what she finds attractive by maintaining the *relative relationship* of the hollowed buccal area to the cheekbone with filling. That way the benefits of anterior projection of the midface can be achieved without making the face look too wide or full. The irony of fat transfer is that the patients who need it most are often the ones with too little to give. Unfortunately very lean patients or those without adequate donor sites due to multiple prior liposuctions must often be turned away from the procedure. However, even small amounts of fat can make a dramatic impact in the periorbital area in the correction of hollowing or in a flat, atrophic central cheek. These areas are often top priority for filling in very thin patients.

Nowhere are young photographs as helpful as when discussing rejuvenation of the periorbital area. Patients often seek skin removal through blepharoplasty as a way to regain the loss of lid show as a result of aging. However, skin redundancy in the upper lids is a result of fat loss with relative skin excess. The truth is that young faces have *less* lid show than their aging counterparts, and the patient interview becomes the perfect opportunity to point this out (Fig. 5.12). Most patients really do want to recapture what they had in youth with fat replacement of the upper lid, however some with very deep set eyes find the added weight of fat in the brows unpleasant. Occasionally these patients need to seek traditional blepharoplasty but often are quite pleased with the brow elevation achieved with filling the forehead alone while avoiding the direct upper lid/brow filling. Evaluation of the suborbital areas requires the patient be classified into one of two aging patterns. Atrophic suborbital aging where the suborbital area is hollow often with apparent demarcation of the bony orbit, and hypertrophic suborbital aging with protrusion of the suborbital fat anterior to the relationship with the inferior cheek mass. Atrophic suborbital aging is true atrophy of the suborbital fat, whereas hypertrophic suborbital aging is actually atrophy of the cheek without atrophy of the orbital fat and is most likely a false relative hypertrophy. Box 5.1 contains key questions to ask patients on the initial interview.

Treatment Techniques

Equipment

The following equipment is recommended when performing fat rebalancing of the face:

- Coleman extractor (Byron, Tucson, AZ, USA).
- 10 mL Luer lock syringes, for manual collection and storage of fat.
- A centrifuge that revolves at 3400 rev/min. Options include older model centrifuges that have removable domes or centrifuges made especially for spinning 10 mL syringes containing fat (Byron).
- Disposable plastic Coleman caps (Byron) or reusable stainless steel caps (Miller Medical,

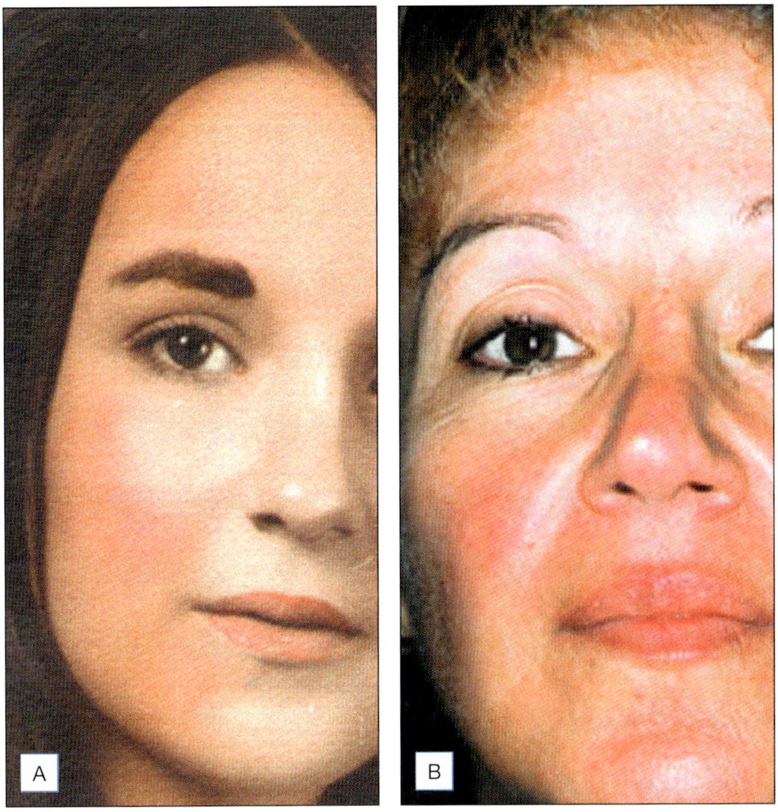

Fig. 5.12 Same woman. (**A**) Age 16. (**B**) Age 50. Note the increase in lid, shown with aging

Key questions to ask at patient interview

- Have you had cosmetic surgery before?
- Were you happy with the results?
- What bothers you about your face as it has aged?
- How has your weight changed over the past 20 years?
- Did you like the way you used to look?
- What didn't you like about your face when it was younger?

Box 5.1 Key questions to ask at patient interview

Mesa, AZ, USA) for centrifugation of 10 mL syringes

- 1 mL Luer lock syringes. These are used exclusively for controlled injection of fat into the face.
- Female–female transfer device.
- 17–18 g blunt infiltration cannulas. Coleman or Donofrio infiltration cannulas (Byron) for placing or removing fat in the face.
- An alarm backed freezer at a temperature of −10 to −30°C (if fat is to be frozen for later use).

Treatment algorithm

Drawing on the face

Following the initial treatment plan determined in the patient interview/consultation the markings are transferred to the face with either a laundry marker or gentian violet pen. It is helpful to also mark out bony landmarks that may assist in local anesthesia infiltration or play a role in the placement of the fat as well as premarking any baseline asymmetry. Having the patient gaze up accentuates the inferior orbital ridge and tear trough if present, facilitating marking these areas. When drawing for upper eyelid filling, the dermasurgeon manually lifts the eyebrow until no lid redundancy remains, then draws a line where the 'new' supratarsal crease is demarcated by the shape of the globe. The mandibular markings are drawn by first palpating and marking the anterior border of the mandible and then drawing a line 1 cm below from mastoid to mastoid. The dermasurgeon may also wish to mark out any fullness in the jowl as a way to avoid this filling or remember to suction this area. At this time the dermasurgeon may wish

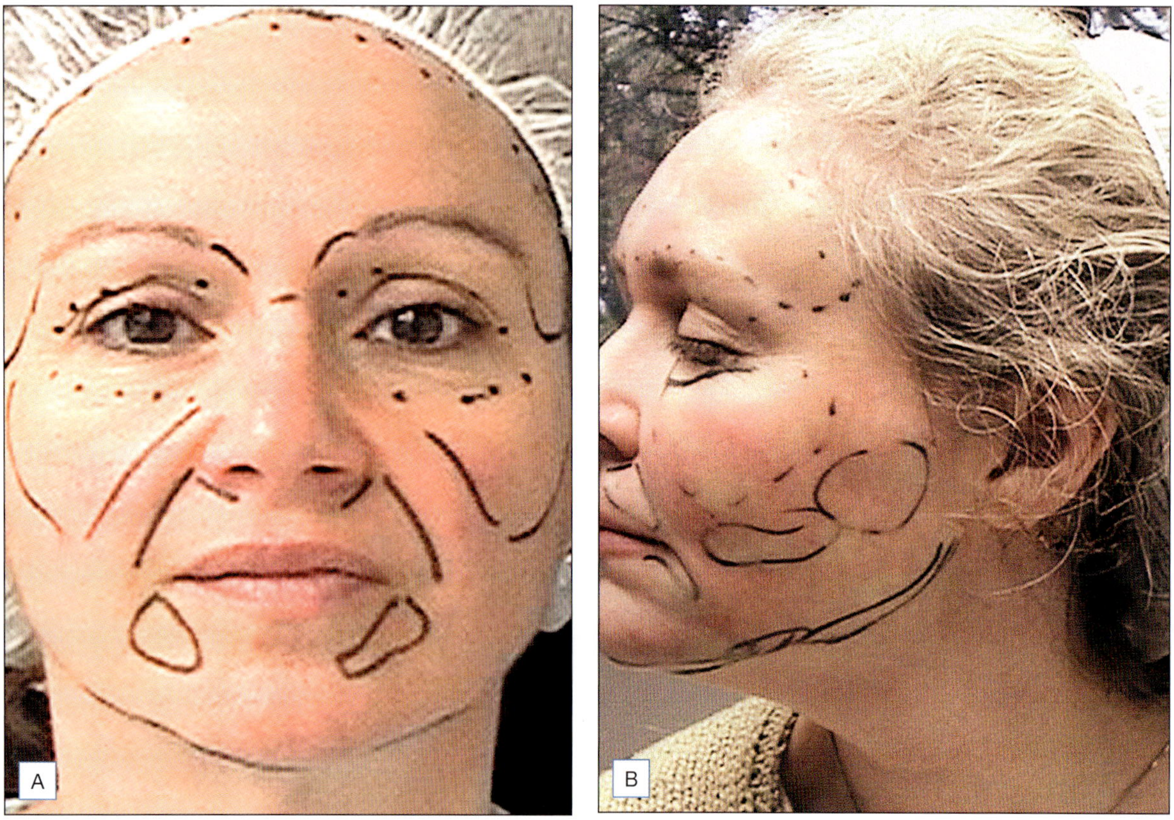

Fig. 5.13 Facial markings for fat rebalancing. (**A**) Front view. (**B**) Side view

to estimate the amount of fat that will be required to fill or advance an area by thinking in terms of elliptical measurements such as teaspoons (5 mL) or tablespoons (15 mL). Some dermasurgeons find it helpful to then transfer these thoughts to the blueprint or onto the face directly. Other markings should include areas of shadow and highlight as they will affect the fat transfer (Fig. 5.13).

Patient preparation

Patients are prophylaxed starting the day before surgery with either cephelexin 500 mg bid or erythromycin 500 mg bid. Ciprofloxacin 500 mg bid can also be used as an appropriate antibiotic. Antibiotics are continued including the day of the procedure and for a total of 7 days. Premedication on the day of the procedure includes 40 mg of prednisone PO and 5–10 mg of oral diazepam if needed. The donor site to be liposuctioned is prepared with a solution of Hibicleans and sterile water and the face is washed with antibacterial soap. Preoperative photographs are taken from multiple angles. It is also helpful to take photographs of the patient in animation and repose. Patients are placed onto a sterile, draped operating table covered with a sterile sheet.

Fat extraction

The patient and dermasurgeon must decide on an appropriate donor site. In females fat from the hips or lateral thighs is preferable to that of the abdomen due to the relative ease of extraction, the greater comfort of the patient, and the paucity of fibrous tissue encountered on extraction. Fat extracted from this area may also have the potential for greater lipogenic activity. The donor site is encircled with a marking pen in a way that would benefit the patient cosmetically. Designated skin markings are done with the patient standing. Autologous fat is harvested for the fat transfer procedure under local tumescent anesthesia. Every effort to make the

Tumescent fluid used for fat rebalancing
■ 500 mg lidocaine (lignocaine) ■ 1 liter lactated Ringers solution ■ 1 mg epinephrine (adrenaline) ■ 12.5 meq sodium bicarbonate

Box 5.2 Tumescent fluid used for fat rebalancing

procedure as sterile as possible is attempted by the use of sterile gloves, gown and mask by the dermasurgeon and a sterilely draped operating table. Lactated ringer's solution is augmented with lidocaine (lignocaine), epinephrine (adrenaline), and sodium bicarbonate in the concentrations specified in Box 5.2. This gives a solution with a final volume of lidocaine of 0.05%. The lidocaine is intentionally kept at a low concentration since it has shown to be inhibitory to the function of adipocytes. With the patient in the recumbent position, entry sites on the skin of the donor area are made with a 1.5 mm punch tool. The tumescent solution is then infiltrated into the adipose tissue of the donor site via a mechanical infiltration pump or by hand infiltration with a 60 mL syringe. Infiltration can be accomplished with a blunt multiholed cannula or with an 18 gauge spinal needle. The end point for true tumescence is tissue turgidity. This also guarantees a bloodless adipose sample. It is necessary to wait for 20 minutes after infiltration for hemostasis to occur before attempting to harvest the fat. Fat collection is accomplished with an open tipped cannula (Coleman extractor, Byron) on a 10 mL syringe (Fig. 5.14). Only manual negative pressure is applied by withdrawing the plunger on the syringe while the cannula is passed back and forth in the deep fat (Fig. 5.15). When the syringe is full, the cannula may be left in place changing only the syringe. Full syringes are left upside down in a sterile test tube tray or specimen cup. For most full face fat rebalancing sessions a total of 50–100 mL of fat is needed. More is collected if surplus fat is to be frozen and stored for later use. It is preferable to briefly centrifuge the syringes of fat for 20 seconds to remove the extracellular tumescent fluid and separate out the supranatant triglyeride layer. Special screw on caps that are disposable (Byron) or autoclavable (Miller Medical) are recommended during centrifugation for a tight seal. After spinning the fat, the infranate is squeezed off and the compacted adipocytes are transferred to 1 mL syringes via a female to female device, stopping short of the triglyceride layer.

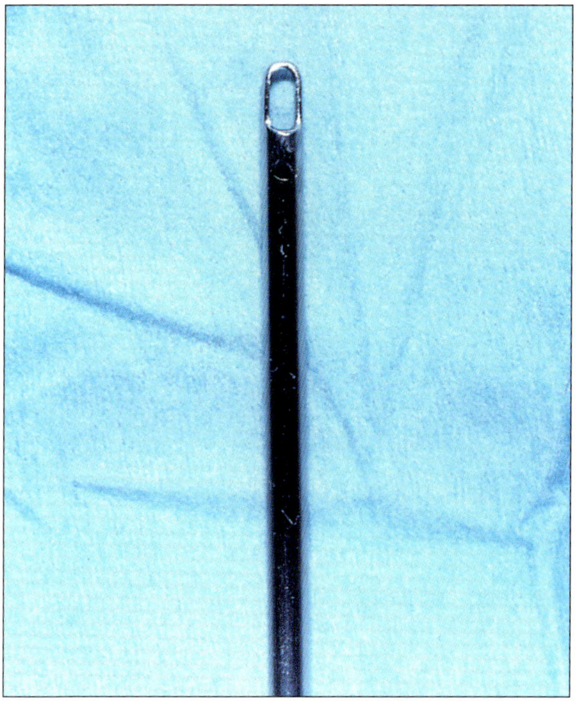

Fig. 5.14 Open tipped extraction cannula (Byron, Tuczon, AZ, USA)

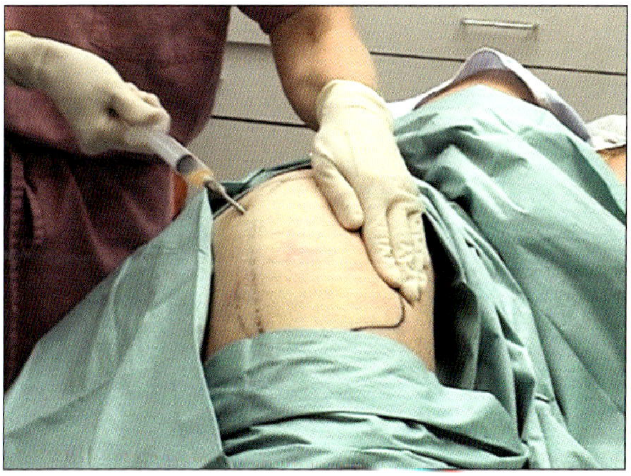

Fig. 5.15 Fat extraction

Facial anesthesia

The patient's comfort is paramount to a successful procedure. Facial anesthesia should be carried out

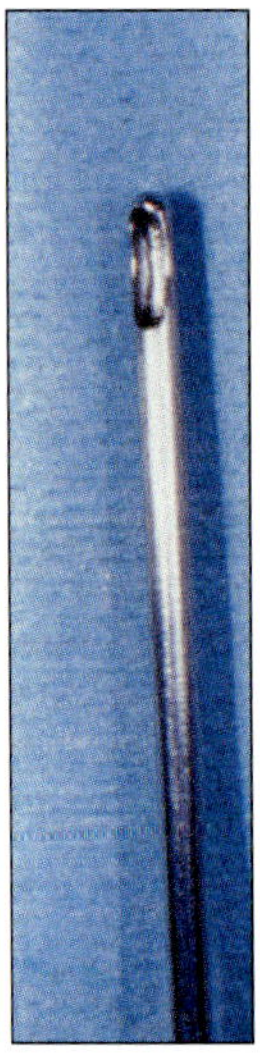

Fig. 5.16 Blunt infiltration cannula

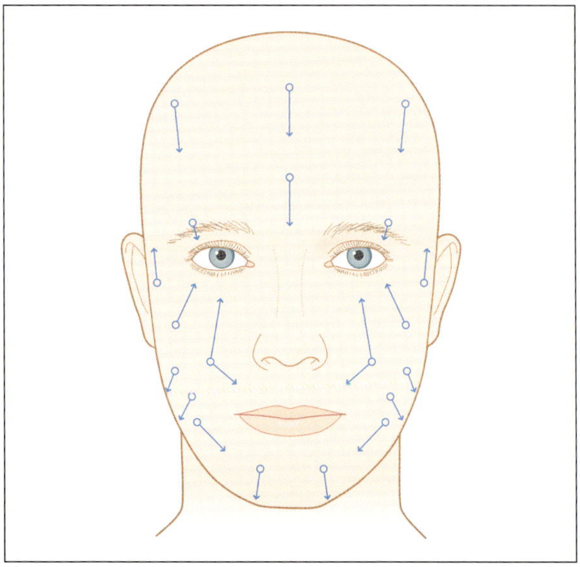

Fig. 5.17 Recommended entry sites and direction of infiltration

slowly while verbally soothing and distracting the patient. Patients are encouraged to bring headphones or a favorite CD to make the experience less unpleasant. Facial blocks with 1% xylocaine are used when appropriate in the infraorbital, mental, supraorbital and supratrochlear areas. The majority of the anesthesia takes place via local infiltration of 0.5% lidocaine (lignocaine) 4:1 with sodium bicarbonate. 30 gauge 1 inch needles are used to infiltrate broadly. Injections are kept in the deep fat to minimize ecchymosis, especially in the lateral orbit and temple. In the perioral area an intraoral route of anesthesia is less uncomfortable than the percutaneous route. In this area it is only necessary to fill the superior and inferior labial vestibule superficially to achieve adequate lip anesthesia.

General technique

All infiltration of fat is with blunt 17–18 gauge cannulas attached to 1 mL syringes of fat (Fig. 5.16). This not only offers superb control over the placement of minute droplets of fat, but also keeps the procedure safe by minimizing injection pressures and the risk of canalizing vessels. Blunt instrument infiltration allows the recipient tissues to 'spread' apart, thus anchoring the fat, rather than 'coring' out a tunnel as is the possibility with a sharp large bore needle. It also allows the dermasurgeon the freedom of placement in the periorbital area where sharp instruments run a high risk of perforation of the orbital septum or periocular vessels. Entry sites are made at various locations on the face to allow for easy access with an 18 gauge Nokor needle (Becton Dickinson, Franklin Lakes, NJ, USA) (Fig. 5.17). The dermasurgeon enters, bevel down on the cannula, weaving the cannula in a back and forth motion depositing approximately 0.05 mL of fat per stroke. Therefore, it should take 20 passes to empty a 1 mL syringe. All injection of fat takes place retrograde. Holding the 1 mL syringe with attached cannula in the dominant hand, the dermasurgeon uses the thenar eminance of this hand to push in the plunger in 'spurts' on the withdrawal phase of the movement through the tissue. Unless otherwise specified below, infiltration of fat occurs in all levels of subcutaneous tissue, starting deeply adjacent to mucosa or bone and working up through muscle and subcutaneous fat taking advantage of multiple entry sites and weaving fat in a crosshatched three dimensional lattice.

Forehead augmentation

The goals of forehead augmentation are to project the skin of the forehead anteriorly, thus achieving a lifting of the brow, and to form an interface subcutaneously to attenuate the pull of the frontalis muscle on the skin. All forehead infiltration is perpendicular to the brow, i.e. parallel to the fibers

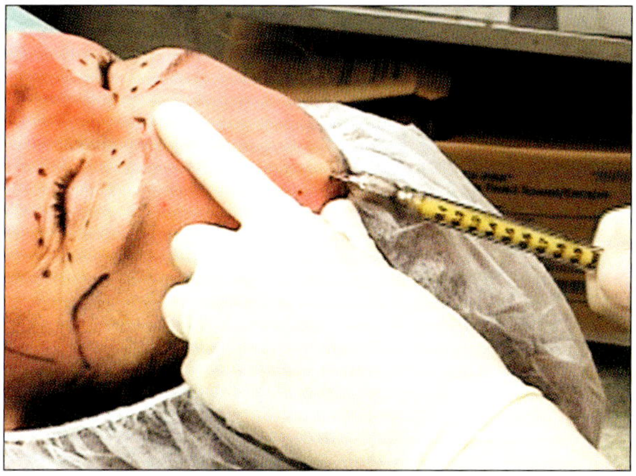

Fig. 5.18 Forehead infiltration

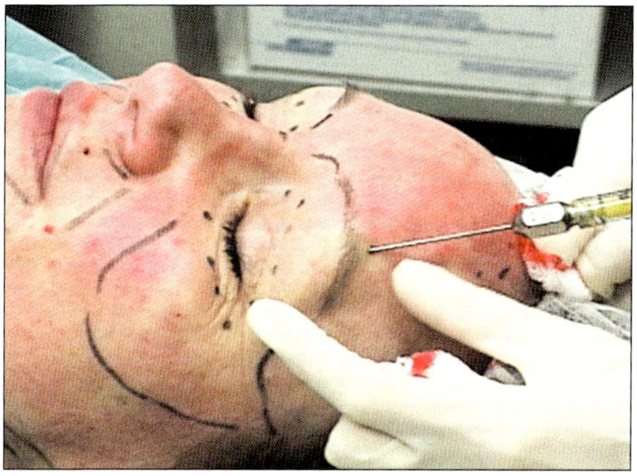

Fig. 5.19 Brow augmentation

of the frontalis muscle. Incisions are best made at multiple places in the hairline. The temple and glabella as well as the brow/lid complex can all be addressed through these incisions. Fat is deposited subcutaneously in the supragaleal plane anterior to as well as in and under the frontalis muscle. Visible ridging is common, especially in the temple, and requires smoothing out with firm pressure in all directions. Typically the forehead can hold 6–12 mL of fat, and the temples 1–3 mL each (Fig. 5.18).

Brow augmentation

As described above, brow filling can take place via an entry site at the hairline or from one just above the eyebrow. Fat is placed in 'droplets' depositing the base of the drop at the newly marked supratarsal crease and then pulling the 'tail' of the drop superiorly. Augmenting this area serves to advance the brow forward, filling up skin redundancy by applying an internal tenting force on the skin. The brow can take a total of 1–2 mL of fat and should be tapered to blend seamlessly with the neighboring temple and forehead (Fig. 5.19).

Suborbital augmentation

The plan for augmentation of the suborbital area depends on whether the patient displays the atrophic or the hypertrophic variant of aging in this area or whether augmentation is being performed to correct an overaggressive blepharoplasty. In the case of atrophic aging an incision is made at a point midway between the midpupillary line and the lateral canthus 2 cm out from the orbital rim. Fat is placed in linear threads throughout the suborbital area maintaining a perpendicular alignment to the lid margin. Fat is placed *under* the orbicularis oculi muscle in smaller than 0.05 mL aliquots using only blunt cannulas (Fig. 5.20). Fingers of the nondominant hand protect the globe at all times. Often it is necessary to make a second incision just lateral to the nasolabial fold with which to access the medial portion of the suborbital area, again in a plane under the orbicularis muscle (Fig. 5.21). This is the preferred incision site for bolstering the arcus marginalus with fat to support the lower lid and eliminate scleral show from blepharoplasty. In the hands of highly experienced fat transplant dermasurgeons an incison at the lateral margin of the orbit can be used to place fat directly subcuta-

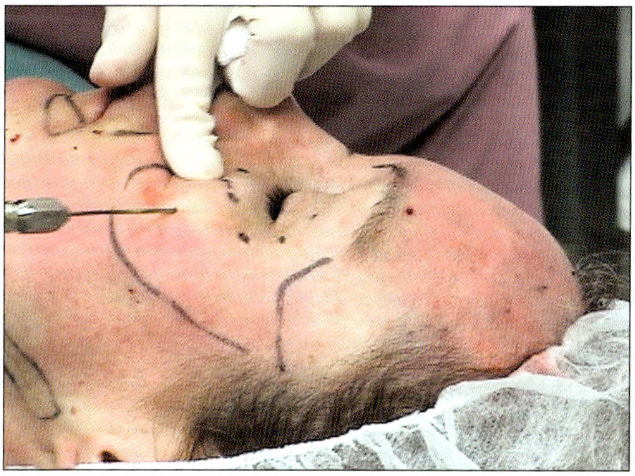

Fig. 5.20 Suborbital augmentation

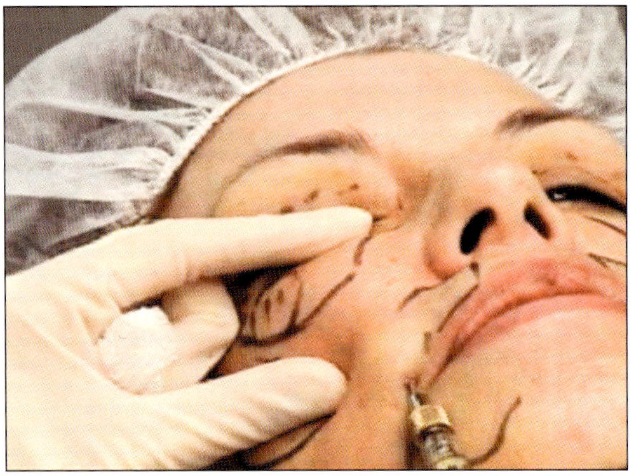

Fig. 5.21 Suborbital augmentation

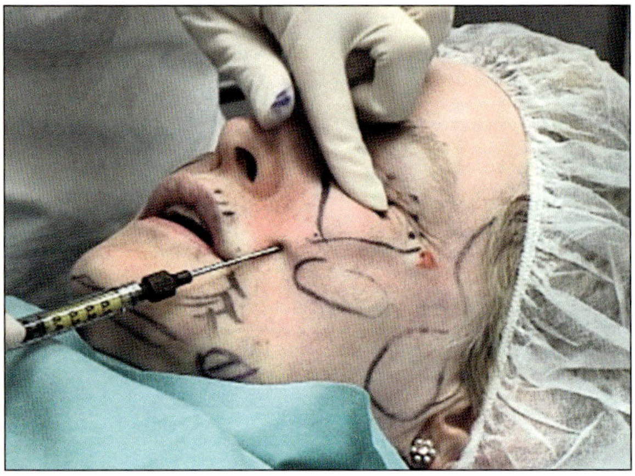

Fig. 5.23 Central malar augmentation

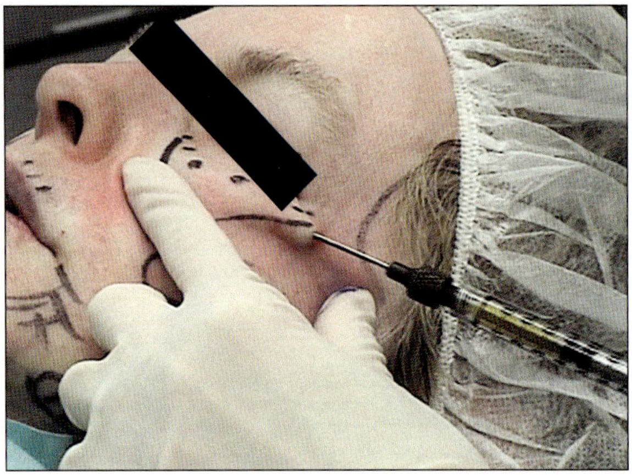

Fig. 5.22 Suborbital augmentation, lateral approach

neously above the orbicularis muscle (Fig. 5.22). In this scenario, fat is threaded in minuscule amounts with multiple passes required to deposit even 0.1 mL. This technique carries a high risk of textural irregularities, but is necessary if the dermasurgeon wishes to give the appearance of a prominent lower lid, or to fill close to the lashline. Hypertrophic suborbital aging requires filling of the cheek and will be discussed below.

Cheek augmentation

Certainly the most dramatic changes achievable by fat transfer are simply by restoring the profile arc of the midface to an aging individual. Not only does this small change return a critical point of highlight to the 'apple' of the cheek, but also it serves to tent out the skin of the midface, in essence lifting skin inferior to it. In the case of hypertrophic suborbital aging, the goal is to advance the cheek to the level of the suborbital protuberance or beyond, so that the orbital area appears to recede. From an incision in the base of the nasolabial fold, or just lateral to it, fat is placed diffusely in the central cheek superiorly to the level of the tear trough, fanning out laterally (Fig. 5.23). Then from an incision inferior and lateral to the zygomatic arch, fat is deposited parallel to the arch and perpendicular to the previous placement. Fat is placed in multiple layers starting underneath the zygomaticus muscles, coming up through the muscles, then subcutaneously. Finally, the area of the buccal fat pad is restored to its youthful fullness by either one of the above incisions or one inferior to the buccal hollow (Fig. 5.24). Placement amounts vary, but it is very common to place 7–15 mL in these areas to re-establish anterior projection of the midface.

Perioral augmentation

Involution in the perioral area with resultant collapse, shriveling and lengthening of the upper lip is a common manifestation of both fat atrophy and bony reabsorption secondary to chronologic aging. Fat replacement pushes the cutaneous portion of the lip forward, so that it appears shorter. It also interrupts the skin–muscle interaction that leads to a contracted pursed look. Fat replacement in the chin can soften or even alleviate the dimpling secondary to aging in patients with a past history of

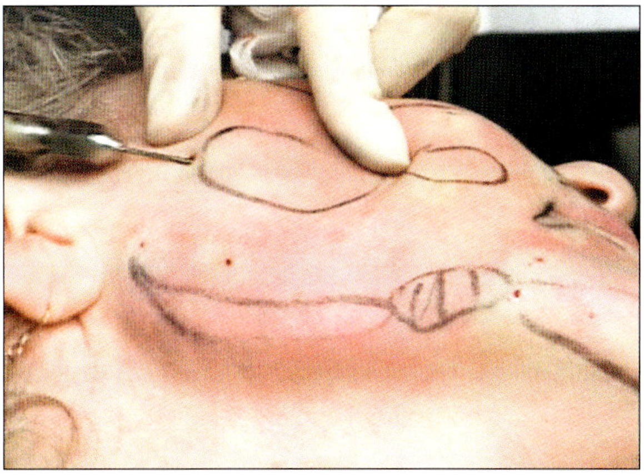

Fig. 5.24 Buccal augmentation

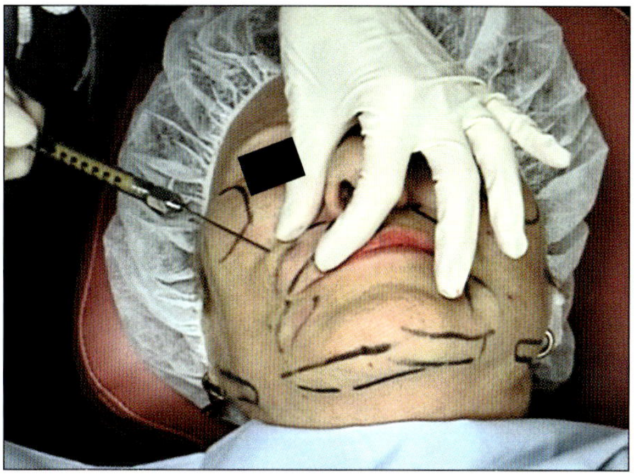

Fig. 5.26 Nasolabial fold augmentation

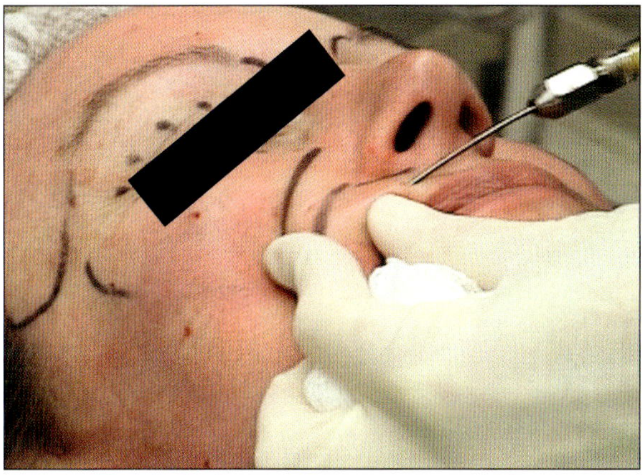

Fig. 5.25 Cutaneous upper lip augmentation

acne in this area. The cutaneous portion of the upper and lower lip can be reached by a medial incision in the philtral columns, an incision in or lateral to the nasolabial and labiomental crease, or from an incision at the angle of the mouth. The direction of infiltration is parallel to the border of the lip, extending from the upper vermilion to the subnasal area and lower vermilion down to the chin (Fig. 5.25). Infiltration amounts of 1–2 mL of fat per side upper and lower for a total of 4–8 mL in the entire cutaneous perioral area is normally required. If desired the mucosal portion of the lip can be augmented with 2–4 mL either with a 20 gauge sharp needle into the vermilion border or bluntly with an 18 gauge cannula depositing fine threads of fat into the body of the lip.

Nasolabial and labiomental crease augmentation

Often amelioration of the nasolabial fold is achieved by the anterior projection achieved through filling of the central cheek area, and the advancement of the cutaneous portion of the lip that makes up the medial nasolabial fold. However if additional augmentation into this fold is desired, an incision site lateral to the fold through which 1–2 mL of fat is placed perpendicularly is preferable to fat placement parallel in the fold (Fig. 5.26). The same holds true for the labiomental crease, where filling of the lateral cheek and buccal area redistributes the skin redundancy that forms this fold. When additional filling is desired, as it often is in this area, 1–2 mL of fat can be placed through an incision lateral to the fold, being careful to pull the tail of the fat droplet across the fold so as not to accentuate the insertion of the retaining ligament in this area (Fig. 5.27).

Jawline augmentation

To restore the 'rounded angularity' characteristic of a young jawline, 8–20 mL of fat is placed in the submandibular area. Incision sites are perpendicular to the arc of the jawline so that the fat is placed in droplets wrapping around the inferior surface of the mandible (Fig. 5.28). The level of placement is superficial at the level of investment of the platysma muscle. Care must be taken to place the fat evenly. If it appears to be forming clumps then an approach though a parallel incision to smooth out the area may be necessary. Enhancement of the chin can

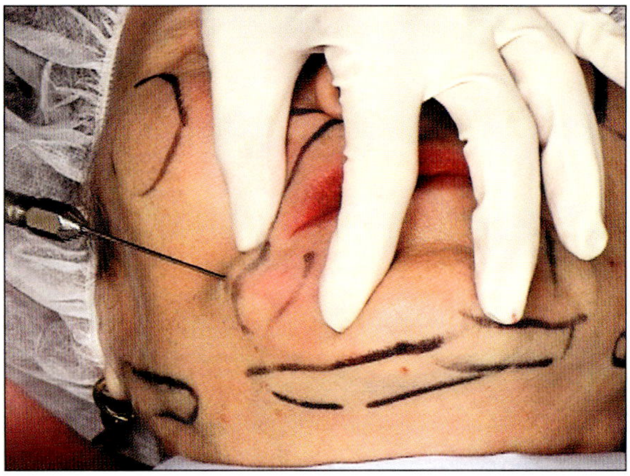

Fig. 5.27 Labiomental crease augmentation

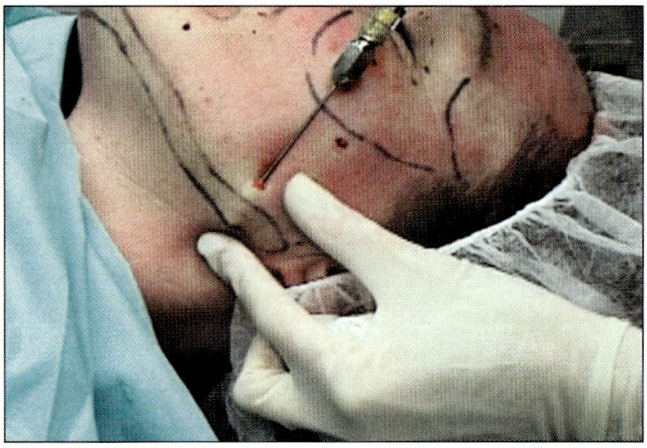

Fig. 5.28 Mandibular augmentation

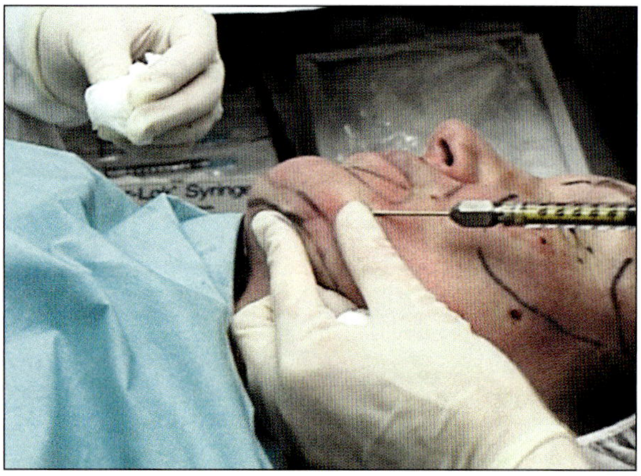

Fig. 5.29 Chin augmentation

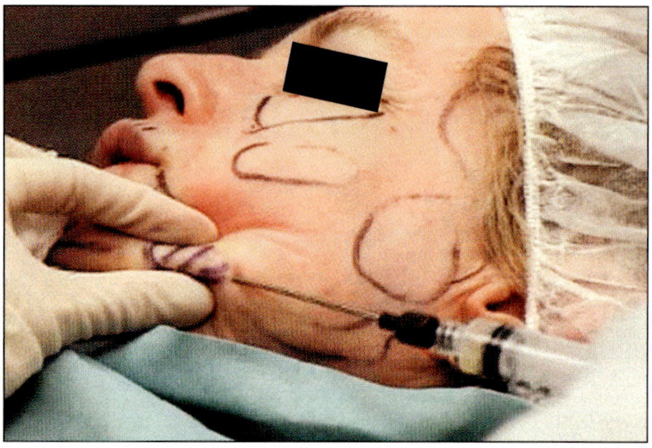

Fig. 5.30 Microliposuction of jowl fat

also be accomplished through one of the anterior incisions, approaching this area laterally (Fig. 5.29). Placement of 1–2 mL of fat in this area is usually sufficient, but difficult due to the tough fibrous tissue present subcutaneously.

Microliposuction

As discussed above, in certain patients with adequate skin tone, it may be desirable to microliposuction the hypertrophic fat deposits of the lower face to achieve true fat rebalancing. This can be accomplished with the same 17 gauge cannulas used to place the fat by attaching a 10 mL syringe and withdrawing the plunger to create negative pressure. This technique can be used in the areas lateral to the nasolabial fold, lateral to the labiomental crease, and in the jowl (Fig. 5.30). It is prudent to undercorrect staying in a deep plane. Typically 0.5–1 mL only of fat is removed from each area, and so repeat suction is required. In addition to erring on the side of caution, staging the suction procedures allows time for the skin to recontract to smaller insults.

Pearls for successful fat rebalancing

The number one mistake made by fat transfer dermasurgeons is underestimation of the amount of fat it takes to affect a volume change and tissue shift. It is helpful therefore to think in elliptical terms like teaspoon and tablespoon measurements to visualize the volume of fat it would take to cause projection in the desired plane. It is common for an atrophic cheek to require upwards of 15 mL (i.e. 1 tablespoon) of fat placed in one or multiple sessions to recapture the anterior projection reminiscent of

Common pitfalls of fat transplantation

- Underestimating the amount of fat it will take to cause volume change and tissue shifting
- Assuming that the change early on is due to fat and not edema
- Transplanting too much fat in one session
- Using sharp instruments
- Filling only the folds

Box 5.3 Common pitfalls of fat transplantation

youth. Since the blunt trauma incurred by the fat transfer cannulas causes prolonged edema, it is also common to assume that the change in volume early on is due to the transplanted fat. This leads to a false assumption, and once the edema subsides, the supposition that the fat has been absorbed. The other common mistake made with fat transfers is to fill only the folds. A good test as to whether this would indeed correct the problem is ask the patient to lie down, and examine the fold from this angle. If it is flattened, then only redraping of neighboring tissues will ameliorate this fold and not direct filling. Once the dermasurgeon starts thinking spatially in three dimensions this comes as second nature and panfacial fat rebalancing becomes the treatment of choice. Common pitfalls of fat transplantation are summarized in Box 5.3.

Side effects, complications, and alternative approaches

The most common sequelae of panfacial fat rebalancing are edema and ecchymosis lasting 2–14 days. Patients seem to have more down-time from the first procedure than from subsequent touch up procedures. Small nodules or tracts of fat or edema can persist in the periorbital area and often require feathering via perpendicular cannula passes on a follow up visit. Persistent uncorrectable irregularities are uncommon with judicious placement in experienced hands. Hard persistent nodules representative of sterile fat cysts require dilute steroid injections, or even incision to resolve. Postinflammatory pigmentation or hemosiderin pigmentation is occasionally encountered and can be treated with time or laser light sources. The author has encountered two patients who complained of prolonged pain in the temple and lateral zygomatic area following fat transfer in a deep structural plane, and one patient with muscular fasciculations of the lip levator that resolved after 3 months. Other rarely noted side effects are infection, eruption of herpetic lesions periorally, and submandibular lymph node enlargement. A review of the literature reveals such serious and disconcerting side effects as middle cerebral artery infarction, blindness, and abscess formation. The etiology of these events is unclear, but appears to be related to high pressure injections of fat through a large syringe or sharp needle with retrograde flow into the internal carotid system. It is imperative therefore that fat be transferred with only blunt instruments using 1 mL syringes during the withdrawal stroke of the movement.

Retention rates are variable in the literature and appear to be site specific and operator dependent. Long term retention of fat has been documented by many authors using a multilayer transplantation technique. Poorest retention is seen in the lips and perioral area probably due to the multiple dynamic and intrinsic muscular forces that contribute to folds in this area. The periorbital area and cheek have the best retention followed by the lateral jawline, forehead, and buccal area. Patients desiring further correction in low retention areas are often encouraged to augment with hyaluronic acid fillers, however these small volume fillers are not capable of the dramatic tissue shifts achievable with fat rebalancing in the structural plane (Figs 5.31–5.33).

Postoperative course and follow up

Intramuscular or oral steroids are recommended immediately postoperatively to minimize postoperative edema. Ice packs should be applied to the face frequently, for the first and second postoperative day. The harvest sites are covered with absorbable dressings to wick off the tumescent drainage and then a compression elastic garment such as a girdle or Lycra biking shorts applied. Structural fat rebalancing is most successful when done in repeated stages. Touch up procedures can be scheduled at 1 to 3 month intervals until the desired correction is achieved. These touch up sessions may be accomplished with either fresh fat harvested in the manner above, or previously frozen fat (Fig. 5.34). The use of frozen fat is highly controversial. It remains uncertain at this time whether frozen fat has the potential for long term augmentation but many surgeons who routinely augment with previously frozen fat comment on its ability for long

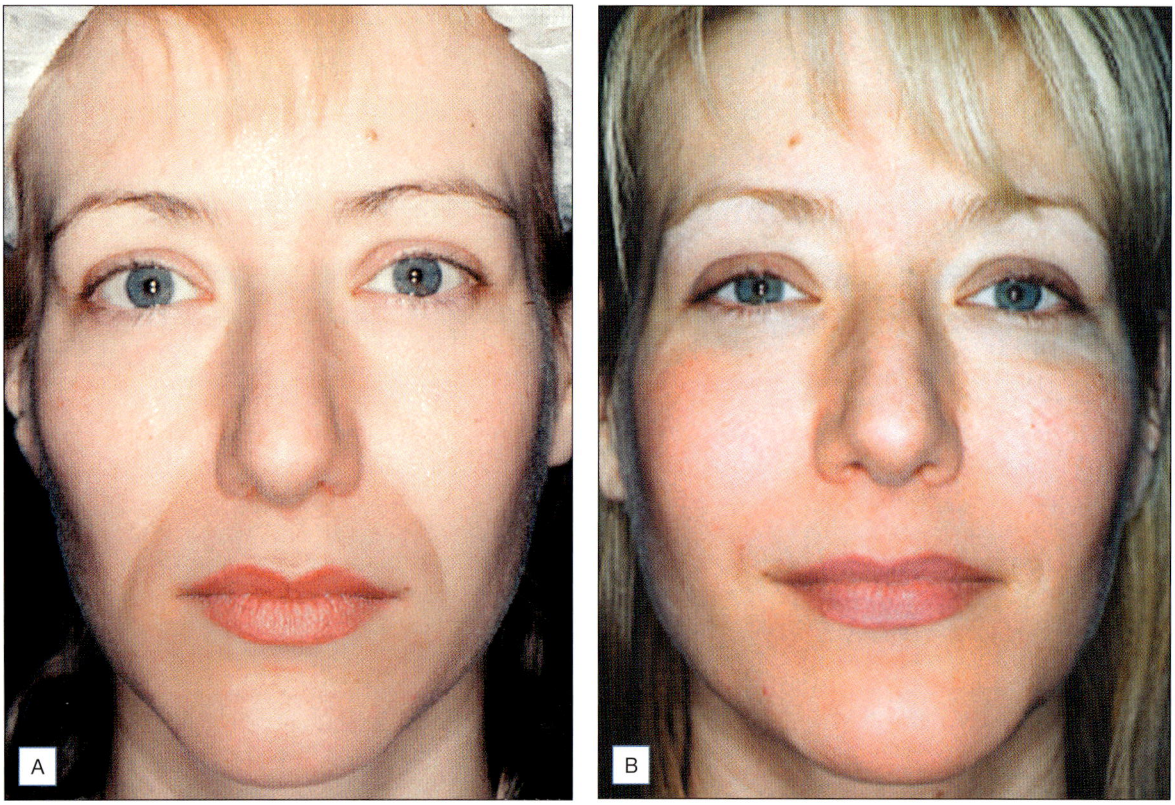

Fig. 5.31 (**A**) Age 32. (**B**) Age 37, at 2½ year follow up after fat rebalancing series

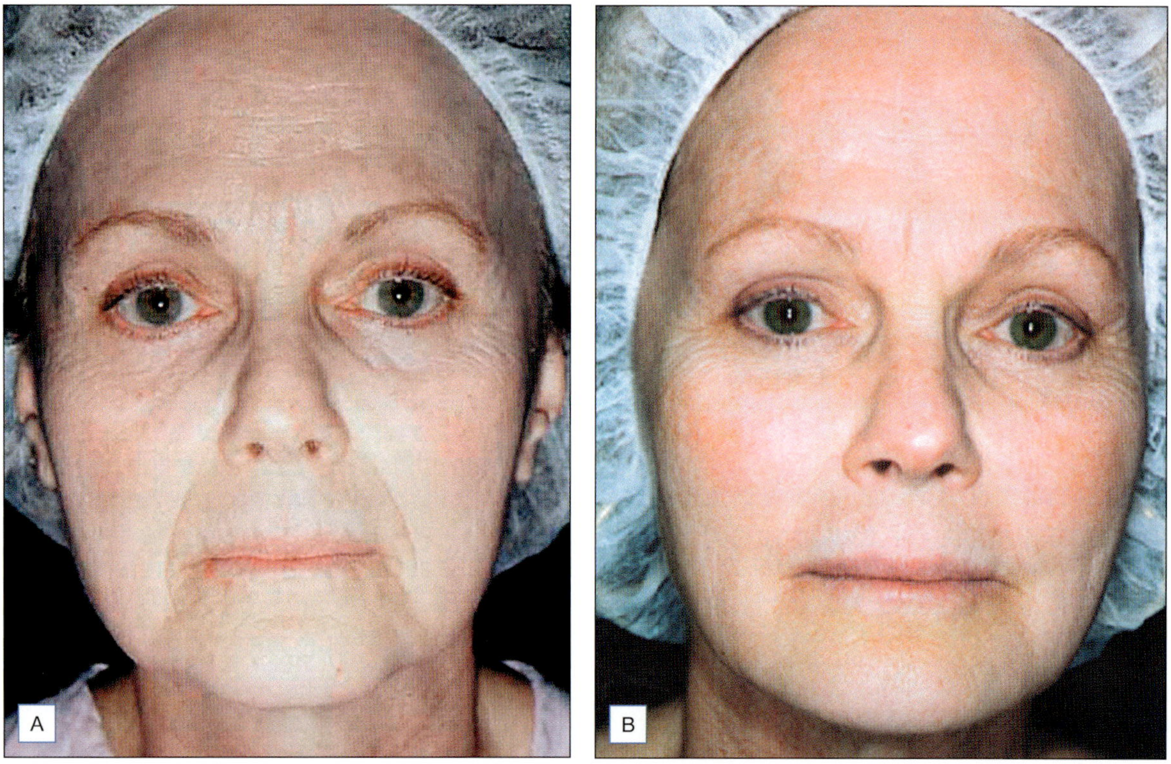

Fig. 5.32 (**A**) Age 53. (**B**) Age 56, at 1½ year follow up after fat rebalancing series

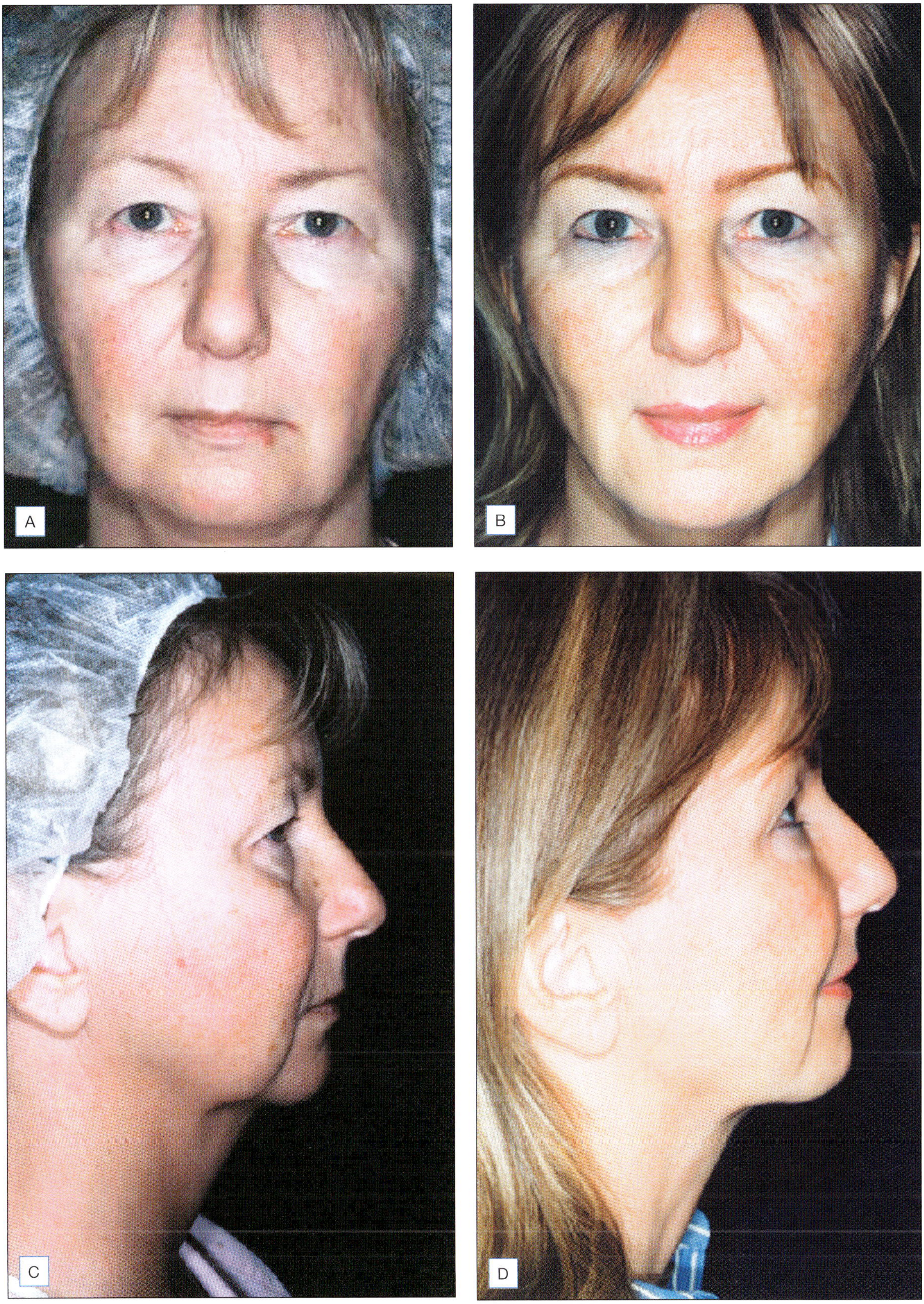

Fig. 5.33 (**A,C**) Age 50. (**B,D**) Age 55, at 2 year follow up after fat rebalancing series

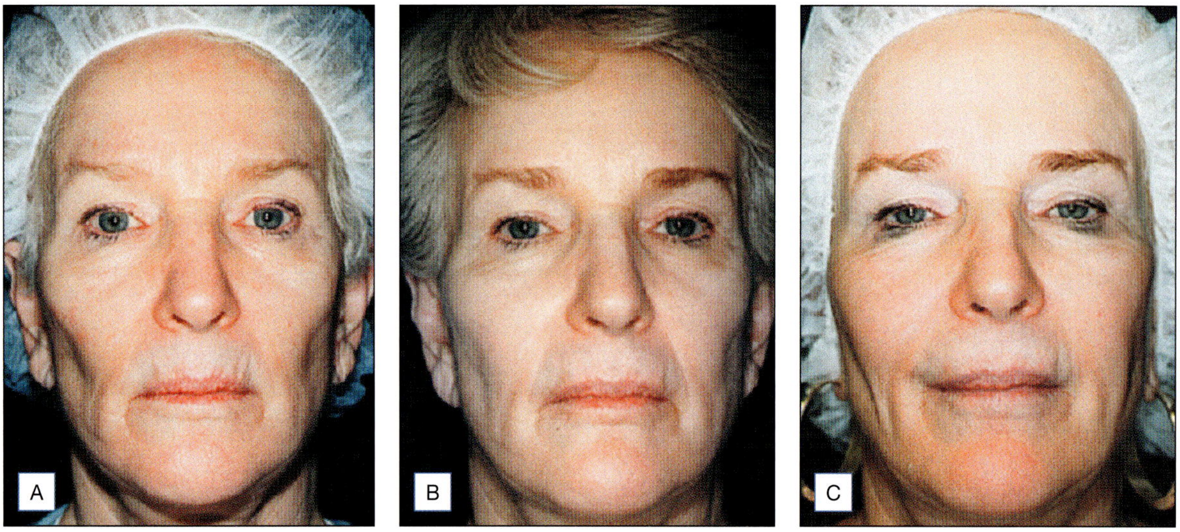

Fig. 5.34 (**A**) Age 50. (**B**) After first fat rebalancing session with fresh fat. (**C**) After two more sessions using only frozen fat, at 1 year follow up

term correction. If fat is to be frozen for future use, the fat should be frozen in 10 mL syringes after decanting infranate, but with triglycerides intact, meticulously labeled with patient's name, date of procedure, and social security number. Fat should be slowly frozen by placing it at −20°C, moved to temperature monitored and alarmed freezers for long term storage at −20 to −30°C, and then rapidly thawed when ready to use. Long term sterility of frozen fat has been shown for up to 2 years.

Further Reading

Bertossi D, Kharouf S, d'Agostino A, et al 2000 Facial localized cosmetic filling by multiple injections of fat stored at −30°C. Techniques, clinical follow-up of 99 patients and histological examination of 10 patients. Annales de Chirurgie Plastique et Esthétique 45:548–555

Carraway JH, Mellow CG 1990 Syringe aspiration and fat concentration; a simple technique for autologous fat injection. Annals of Plastic Surgery 24:293–296

Carruthers A, Carruthers J 1998 Clinical indications and injection technique for the cosmetic use of botulinum A exotoxin. Dermatologic Surgery 24:1189–1194

Carruthers A, Carruthers J, Cohen J 2003 A prospective, double-blind, randomized, parallel-group, dose-ranging study of botulinum toxin type A in female subjects with horizontal forehead rhytides. Dermatologic Surgery 29:462–467

Coleman SR 1995 Long term results of fat transplants: controlled demonstrations. Aesthetic Plastic Surgery 19:421–425

Coleman SR 1997 Facial recontouring with liposculpture. Clinics in Plastic Surgery 24:347–367

Coleman SR 2001 Structural fat grafts: the ideal filler? Clinics in Plastic Surgery 28:111–119

Danesh-Meyer HV, Savino PJ, Sergott RC 2001 Case reports and a small case series; ocular and cerebral ischemia following facial injection of autologous fat. Archives of Ophthalmology 119: 777–778

De Ugarte DA, Ashjian PH, Elbarbary A, Hendrick MH 2003 Future of fat as raw material for tissue regeneration. Annals of Plastic Surgery 50:215–219

Donofrio LM 2000 Structural lipoaugmentation: a pan-facial technique. Dermatologic Surgery 26:1129–1134

Donofrio LM 2003 The technique of periorbital lipoaugmentation. Dermatologic Surgery 29:92–98

Dreizen NG, Framm L 1989 Sudden unilateral visual loss after autologous fat injection into the glabellar area. American Journal of Ophthalmology 107:85–87

Egido JA, Arroyo R, Marcos A, Jimenez-Alfaro I 1993 Middle cerebral artery embolism and unilateral visual loss after autologous fat injection into the glabellar area. Stroke 24:615–616

Feinendegen DL, Baumgartner RW, Schroth G, Mattle HP, Tschopp H 1988 Middle cerebral artery occlusion and ocular fat embolism after autologous fat injection in the face. Journal of Neurology 245:53–54

Feinendegen DL, Baumgartner RW, Vaudens P, et al 1998 Autologus fat injections for soft tissue augmentation in the face; a safe procedure? Aesthetic Plastic Surgery 22:163–167

Flynn TC, Narins RS 1999 Preoperative evaluation of the liposuction patient. Dermatologic Clinics 17:729–734

Fulton J, Suarez M, Silverton K, Barnes T 1998 Small volume fat transfer. Journal of Dermatologic Surgery and Oncology 24:857–865

Goldman MP, Marchell N, Fitzpatrick RE 2002 Laser skin resurfacing of the face with a combined CO_2/Er : YAG laser. Dermatologic Surgery 26:102–104

Gosain AK, Amarante MT, Hyde JS, Yousif NJ 1996 A dynamic analysis of changes in the nasolabial fold using magnetic resonance imaging:implications for facial rejuvenation and facial animation surgery. Plastic and Reconstructive Surgery 98:622–636

Hanke CW 2001 The tumescent facial block: tumescent local anesthesia and nerve block anesthesia for full-face laser resurfacing. Dermatologic Surgery 27:1003–1005

Hudson DA, Lambert EV, Bloch CE 1990 Site selection for autotransplantation: some observations. Aesthetic Plastic Surgery 14:195–197

Jackson RF. 1997 Frozen fat—does it work? American Journal of Cosmetic Surgery 14:339–343

Klein JA 1990 The tumescent technique; anesthesia and modified liposuction technique. Dermatologic Clinics 8:425–437

Lawrence N 2000 New and emerging treatments for photoaging. Dermatologic Clinics 18:99–112

Lee DH, Yang HN, Kim JC, Shyn KH 1996 Sudden unilateral visual loss and brain infarction after autologous fat injection into the nasolabial groove. British Journal of Ophthalmology 80:1026–1027

Lilleth H, Boberg J 1978 The lipoprotein-lipase activity of adipose tissue from different sites in obese women and relationship to cell size. International Journal of Obesity 2:47–52

Markey AC, Glogau RG 2000 Autologous fat grafting: comparison of techniques. Dermatologic Surgery 26:1135–1139

Moore JH, Kolaczynski JW, Morales LM, et al 1995 Viability of fat obtained by syringe suction lipectomy: effects of local anesthesia with lidocaine. Aesthetic Plastic Surgery 19:335–339

Narins RS, Brandt F, Leyden J, Lorenc ZP, Rubin M, Smith S 2003 A randomized, double-blind, multicenter comparison of the efficacy and tolerability of Restylane versus Zyplast for the correction of nasolabial folds. Dermatologic Surgery 29:588–595

Nguyen A, Pasyk KA, Bouvier TN, Hassett CA, Argenta LC 1990 Comparative study of survival of autologous adipose tissue taken and transplanted by different techniques. Plastic and Reconstructive Surgery 85:378–386

Niechajev I, Sevcuk O 1994 Long term results of fat transplantation: clinical and histologic studies. Plastic and Reconstructive Surgery 94:496–506

Ostad A, Kageyama N, Moy RL 1996 Tumescent anesthesia with a lidocaine dose of 55 mg/kg is safe for liposuction. Dermatologic Surgery 22:921–927

Pessa JE, Zadoo VP, Mutimer KL, et al 1998 Relative maxillary retrusion as a natural consequence of aging combining skeletal and soft-tissue changes into an integrated model of midfacial aging. Plastic and Reconstructive Surgery 102:205–212

Pessa JE, Zadoo VP, Yuan C, et al 1999 Concertina effect and facial aging: nonlinear aspects of youthfulness and skeletal remodeling, and why, perhaps, infants have jowls. Plastic and Reconstructive Surgery 103:635–644

Schiffman MA, Mirrafati S 2001 Fat transfer techniques: the effect of harvest and transfer methods on adipocyte viability and review of the literature. Dermatologic Surgery 27:819–826

Shoshani O, Ullman Y, Shupak A, et al 2001 The role of frozen storage in preserving adipose tissue obtained by suction-assisted lipectomy for repeated fat injection procedures. Dermatologic Surgery 27:645–647

Sommer B, Sattler G 2000 Current concepts of fat graft survival: histology of aspirated adipose tissue and review of the literature. Dermatologic Surgery 26:1159–1166

Teimourian B 1988 Blindness following fat injections. Plastic and Reconstructive Surgery 82:361

6 Liquid Injectable Silicone

David S. Orentreich, Derek H. Jones

Introduction

Liquid injectable silicone (LIS) is a 'permanent' soft tissue augmenting agent that may be employed for a variety of cutaneous and subcutaneous atrophies. The term 'permanent' must be qualified. Although the material stays permanently in the skin with no significant loss through degradation, permanent **results** are usually not possible in areas subject to further volume loss, mimetic motion and the forces of gravity.

While there is a wide variety of excellent soft tissue augmenting agents on the market, LIS stands out with regard to superiority of routinely obtainable corrections and persistence of results. However, it is one of the most technique-dependent and least forgiving of fillers, and therefore should be used only by those with extensive training and experience.

LIS is also unique in its versatility. No other currently available filler can remedy such a wide variety of indications from the smallest of defects to major tissue loss. When properly administered, patients may expect permanent correction of scars, permanent lip and facial contour augmentation, and longlasting correction of wrinkles and depressions. It is also particularly advantageous from a cost–benefit perspective.

Patients benefiting from this treatment are those seeking improvement of cutaneous atrophies, especially those desiring longlasting correction. Patients with unclear treatment goals are better advised to choose temporary fillers. LIS is not the filler of choice for those needing immediate correction, as augmentation proceeds gradually over multiple treatments spaced out over 3–9 months. LIS is inappropriate for those seeking 'trial' augmentation (such as lip enhancement) prior to making a decision on permanent enhancement.

History of Liquid Injectable Silicone

The term 'silicone' refers to man-made polymers containing elemental silicon (Si). These polymers are not a single substance, but a family of compounds with varying chemical and physical properties, purity, sterility, and biocompatibility.

Silicone may exist as a solid, gel or liquid. Of the large and diverse family of silicones, this chapter will focus only on LIS or polydimethylsiloxane (see Fig. 6.1), which is the product used for soft tissue augmentation. It consists of repeating units of dimethylsiloxane terminated with trimethylsiloxane ends, as represented in Figure 6.1.

'Centistoke' (cs) refers to the viscosity of silicone oil, and is directly related to the chain length of repeating dimethylsiloxane units. Oils containing longer chains are thicker and more viscous. While a 1 cs product is equivalent in viscosity to water, 350 cs products are oils similar in consistency to mineral oils, and a 1000 cs product is similar in consistency to honey.

In the 1940s, Dow Corning (DC) introduced its first silicone product, a greasy material that was used to waterproof electrical systems of bomber planes and permit flight at higher altitudes.

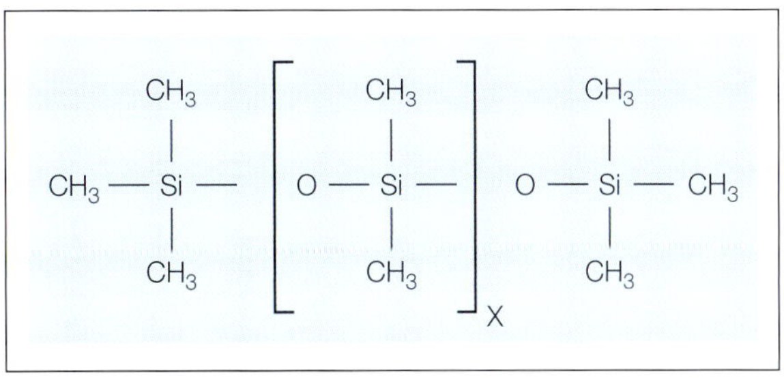

Fig. 6.1 Linear molecular structure of polydimethylsiloxane. There are trimethylsiloxane units at each end and repetitive dimethylsiloxane units in between

During this time, it was noted that various silicones appeared biologically and chemically inert and had a variety of medical applications, including use as a bio-implant. Subsequently, in the 1950s, both physicians, and unfortunately, nonphysicians had begun injecting silicone oil for human soft tissue augmentation. However, silicone oil injected in a large bolus tended to migrate along tissue planes to other parts of the body. It was believed that injecting silicone combined with known irritants such as vegetable fatty acids (e.g. the Sakurai formula, silicone containing 1% olive oil) might produce a more robust fibrous tissue reaction, thus limiting silicone migration. However, these adulterants contributed to frequent granulomatous reactions (nodules, plaques, ulceration) at the site of implantation.

In the early 1960s, DC introduced a purified, nonsterile silicone oil named DC 360 Medical Fluid. This 350 cs silicone (which today is still manufactured for its original purpose) was intended for use by the medical industry as a lubricant for needles and syringes, or as a coating for medicinal or blood containers. It was not intended to be injected into the human body for soft tissue augmentation. However, unauthorized injections for soft tissue augmentation were frequent among physicians and nonphysicians alike. The material was likely injected in large volumes using a variety of injection techniques. Reports of inflammatory reactions or migration were common, leading the FDA to declare DC 360 Medical Fluid a 'new drug' subject to regulation.

Based on anecdotal reports of initial success injecting DC 360 Medical Fluid utilizing small volumes over several injection sessions, DC sought and gained FDA approval in 1965 to investigate a more pure liquid silicone oil for cosmetic soft tissue augmentation. Its new product, named DC MDX 4-4011, was a 350 cs oil sterilized and purified to remove heavy metals and volatile low chain-length polymers. A total of 1300 patients were treated for a variety of conditions. DC stated that the study supported safety and efficacy of MDX 4-4011, with only one report of a 'severe' complication (migration of silicone in the leg of a polio patient treated 'off-protocol' with a large single injection volume). However, many specific aspects of the study protocol were apparently uncontrolled and left to investigators' judgment, including eligibility criteria, treatment technique, average volume per treatment, total volume injected, and interval between treatments. Dow dropped further study in 1976, citing poor study control and in anticipation of its inability to 'prevent misuse of the product.' In the meantime, unauthorized injection of noninvestigational and noninjectable grade silicone oil continued. Negative publicity surrounding adverse events led to the passage of a 1975 law criminalizing its use in the state of Nevada.

In 1978, DC initiated a new study (IND 2702) with MDX 4-4011 for treatment of severe atrophic deformities such as Romberg's disease, trauma, branchial arch syndrome, lipodystrophy and scleroderma. In this study, 128 subjects were treated by 26 investigators. Again, treatment technique was not controlled and varied from investigator to investigator. The various injection techniques employed included the fanning, tattooing and microdroplet serial puncture techniques. The average total volume of silicone injected per patient was 21 cc. The average total volume, per treatment volume, interval between treatments and total number of treatments per patient was uncontrolled and unknown. The study was completed and a final report was filed to the FDA in 1990. In 126 of 128 cases, either the subject or global panel rated treatment outcomes as good or excellent. Device-related anticipated adverse events were reported for 23 subjects, who had treatment outcomes judged to be good to excellent. Many (16/36) of these complications were transient and characteristic of normal responses to needle insertions (edema, pain and erythema). Needle size ranged from 22–25 gauge. Severe complications were reported in two patients who experienced edema unresponsive to conservative therapy and eventually requiring surgical correction.

The 1980s saw an increase in silicone oil injections of unknown purity for soft tissue augmentation. Both physicians and nonphysicians performed these procedures, and a number of reports linking injectable silicone to adverse reactions appeared, generating considerable negative publicity. Practitioners obtained silicone from multiple sources, including noncommercial and clandestine sources, with the injected substance often termed 'medical grade silicone.' However, there was no standardized regulation of purification or sterilization of these products. A compositional analysis of six purported 'medical grade' silicone oils commonly used during this period showed six **different** products, all of different viscosity. All products contained large amounts of elemental impurities (including one sample with large amounts of chlorine, a highly toxic catalytic remnant of chemical processing), and excessive amounts of low-molecular-weight components. Such impurities are known to unfavorably affect biocompatibility, and may lead to toxic and foreign-body reactions. In conclusion, impurities most likely present in the majority of these silicone oils must necessarily throw into question any adverse clinical reports regarding 'medical grade' injectable silicone oil used during this era.

By the 1990s, medical opinion on liquid injectable silicone had become polarized, with both critics and advocates relying on anecdotal data to argue their positions. The controversy continues today. On one side, physicians with substantial experience rely on a wealth of anecdotal data to argue that purified silicone oil injected correctly is safe and effective, and that complications are a result of impure substance or incorrect injection technique. Advocates argue that complications can be avoided by strict adherence to the following rules: (1) use only pure medical grade silicone intended for injection into the human body, (2) inject limited volumes at monthly or longer treatment intervals, and (3) limit injection technique to the micro-droplet serial puncture technique (~ 0.01 ml microdroplets injected at 2–4 mm intervals into the subdermal plane). The theory behind the purported success of the microdroplet technique lies in the observation that large volumes of silicone oil injected in bulk tend to track along tissue planes, migrating sometimes to distant sites of the body. However, a given volume injected in many tiny droplets (0.01 cc or less) provides a larger total surface area for contact with the patient's tissues than would the same volume injected into fewer but larger globules. The resulting fibroplasia that ensues around microdroplets within several days to weeks creates a collagenous capsule that serves to anchor the microdroplets in place, thus eliminating the potential for drift.

Critics, however, argue that injectable silicone is inherently unpredictable, with adverse events appearing sometimes years after injection and despite use of appropriate technique and substance. In one report by Rapaport et al, problems related to 'medical grade' silicone are described in 54 patients seen between 1974 and 1995. Problems included chronic cellulitis, nodules, foreign-body reactions, and migration to other parts of the body. However, variables that may support the etiology of complications (such as the purity of silicone injected, injection technique and volume of silicone oil injected) are not presented.

In 1992, on the backdrop of this controversy, the FDA restricted use of all silicone due to concerns related to possible toxicities with silicone breast implants. The FDA clarified its position on liquid injectable silicone: 'The FDA has not approved the marketing of liquid silicone for injection for any cosmetic purpose, including the treatment of facial defects or wrinkles. The adverse effects of liquid silicone injections have included movement of silicone to other parts of the body, inflammation and discoloration of surrounding tissue, and the formation of granulomas.' In 1992, the FDA issued a press release stating that 'Physicians will no longer be allowed to use liquid injectable silicone for cosmetic treatment unless the product is approved by the FDA either for marketing or for investigational studies.'

In 1994, a 5000 cs liquid injectable silicone, AdatoSil 5000 (Bausch and Lomb, Tampa, FL), was approved as an injectable intraocular tamponade to treat complicated retinal detachment. Silikon 1000 (Alcon, Fort Worth, TX), a less viscous 1000 cs silicone oil, was approved for intraocular use in 1997. Under the US FDA Modernization Act of 1997, which afforded physicians the right to use medical devices under the same off-label provisions previously applicable only to drugs, US physicians could, for the first time, legally employ standardized silicone oils of exceptionally high purity for soft tissue augmentation. The FDA has clarified that, under the new guidelines, off-label injection of FDA-approved liquid silicone for soft tissue augmentation is legal, as long as the physician does not advertise for such use and bases such treatment on the unique needs of individual patients.

Advocates and critics alike must not lose sight of the fact that prior to 1994, there was no standardized, injectable fluid silicone on the market for any indication. The silicone manufactured as a lubricant for needles and syringes, which arguably was and is standardized, was not available for physician use. Therefore, reports referring to local or systemic complications resulting from 'medical grade silicone' or 'unadulterated pure silicone' are impossible to verify. A true analysis of long-term postinjection efficacy and sequelae can only be made with standardized materials available after 1994.

In 2001, the FDA approved a clinical study of SilSkin (Richard-James, Inc., Peabody, MA), a highly purified 1000 cs oil, for the treatment of nasolabial folds (NLFs), marionette lines, and mid-malar depressions. In 2003, the FDA also approved SilSkin for investigational treatment of human immunodeficiency virus (HIV) associated lipoatrophy. It is hoped the data from these ongoing studies will clarify some of the differences of opinion regarding liquid injectable silicone.

Patient Selection

Indications for LIS include facial rhytids such as NLFs and marionette lines, facial contour depressions, nonbound-down depressed scars, and facial lipoatrophy related to HIV, trauma, normal aging or the spectrum of hemi-facial atrophy conditions. It is also useful in restoring lost volume to the aging face and hands. In addition, silicone may be used for soft tissue enhancement in the lip and cheekbone areas, as well as correction of postsurgical defects and depressions.

The exclusion criteria for LIS administration include:

1. Patients seeking augmentation of the breast, eyelids, bound-down scars, or injection into an actively inflamed or infected site.
2. Those seeking immediate correction, temporary correction, or those who are uncertain about facial enhancement (such as lip augmentation) are better treated with temporary fillers.
3. While there is no reason to believe that LIS administration would be injurious to pregnant or nursing women, the elective nature of this procedure and the absence of controlled studies make it inadvisable.

The ideal patient is one with a realistic attitude regarding achievable results, in good physical health and compliant with sun protection recommendations. Further, while LIS can improve many cutaneous defects, it is not a replacement for surgical re-draping (facelift, brow lift, blepharoplasty), resurfacing to correct solar dyschromia, or 'relaxing' with botulinum toxin to correct dynamic rhytids.

Expected Benefits

Prevention of rhytids

A remarkable quality of LIS is its use as a preventative rhytid treatment (see Figs 6.2A, 6.2B and 6.3).

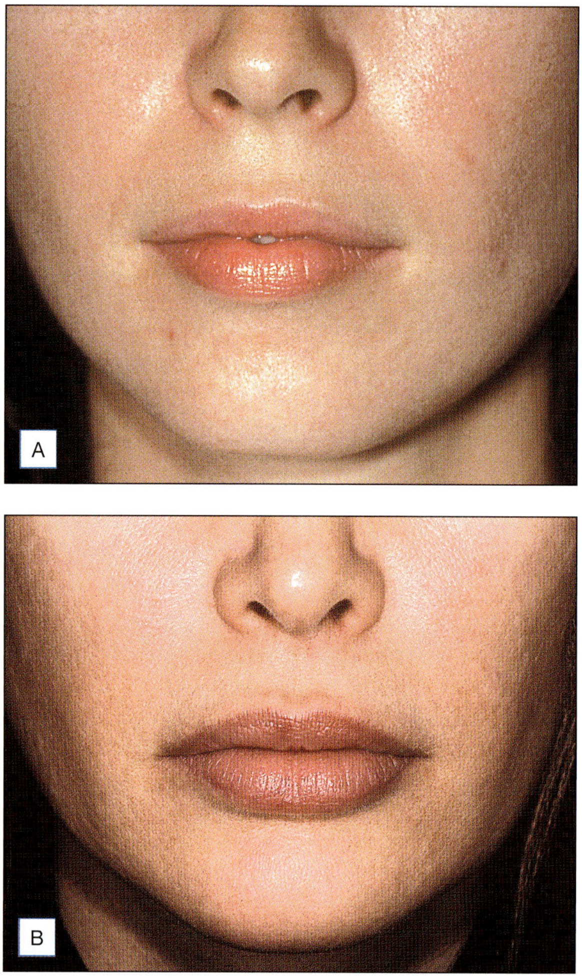

Fig. 6.2 (**A**) Patient pre-treatment 1990. Patient was seen at 28 years of age with the earliest stages of NLFs. (**B**) Patient post-treatment (maintenance) 2004. Fourteen years later, NLF formation is absent at age 42. Improvement in both NLFs and lips has been maintained

Patients are typically seen annually or bi-annually for maintenance.

Correction/improvement

An improvement of 30–90% may be expected, depending on the depth of the original depression (see Fig. 6.4). Hands are also amenable to treatment with LIS (see Fig. 6.5) as are lips (see Fig. 6.6).

Pain or discomfort

Injection of LIS is somewhat less painful in that the material itself has neutral pH and does not cause a

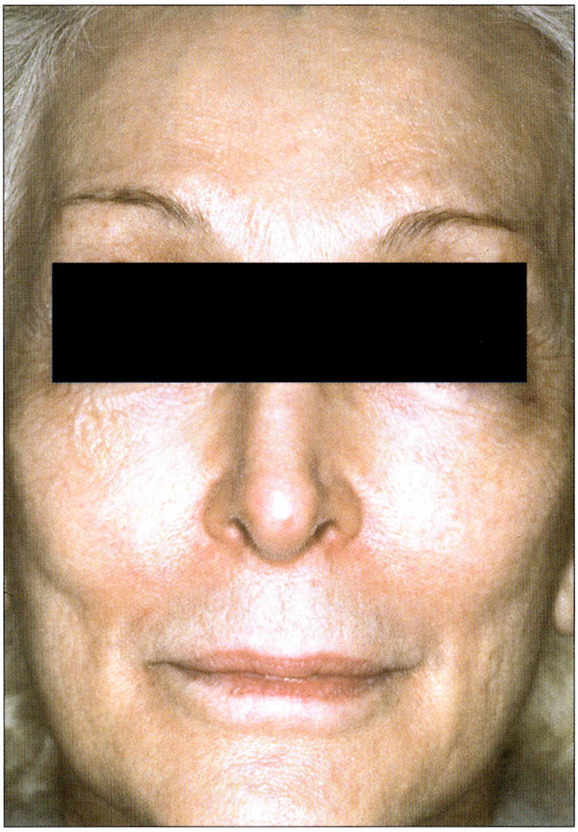

Fig. 6.3 Patient began receiving LIS injections 34 years ago, at age 38. While visible manifestations of aging are present, this 72-year-old woman's results are clearly evident. Additional treatments include dermabrasion, blepharoplasty and botulinum toxin injections

stinging sensation upon entering the tissue. However, it may be somewhat more painful due to the high number of needle punctures required. A large bore, 30 gauge needle (RJ Maxflo needles, Richard James, Inc., Peabody, MA) is used to decrease patient discomfort. Areas notably sensitive even with the application of topical anesthetics include the lips, corners of nose, hands, and malar groove. Other areas are relatively less painful to inject, either with or without having applied topical anesthetic. Depending on the patient, the physician may elect to use an intra-oral block on the lips and a radial, median nerve or ulnar block on the hands.

Cost

The cost of LIS is substantially less than any other filler marketed in the USA. The fluid volume required per patient visit varies widely, as does the number of visits needed. Regardless of the total volume, the benefit-to-cost ratio for the patient is significant compared to other currently available fillers.

However, for the physician, the benefit-to-cost ratio is more complex. Learning to use this material safely and effectively takes longer than the learning process with other injectable fillers. LIS is one of the least forgiving injectables. New practitioners should train with a colleague with extensive experience in LIS administration. After training, they may wish to confine themselves to treating less visible areas (e.g. acne scars on the back) until confidence in their ability to administer this filler properly has developed. When beginning facial injections, the cheek and NLFs are preferable areas to start with, progressing to forehead lines and lips (both more technically difficult areas) as more experience is gained.

In addition, as LIS is not approved by the US FDA for use as a soft tissue augmenting agent, not only an informed consent is required, but also a careful explanation of off-label use. Malpractice carriers should be consulted regarding coverage of off-label use of medical devices and the legal position regarding injecting LIS ascertained (for example its use has been illegal in Nevada since 1975).

Therefore, in terms of provider training, experience, and patient education, LIS may have less of a benefit-to-cost ratio for the physician. Nevertheless, the benefit in terms of lasting results and patient satisfaction is substantial.

HIV-associated Lipoatrophy

Among HIV-infected individuals, facial lipoatrophy has become epidemic. Those affected are stigmatized, leading to psychological distress, social and career impediments, and impaired compliance to HIV medications. Temporary treatment options, including bovine collagen (Zyplast), cadaveric collagen (Cymetra, Fascian), bioengineered human collagen (Cosmoplast), and fat transfer are limited by excessive cost, necessity of frequent treatments, and/or lack of a natural look or feel beneath the skin. Sculptra (polylactic acid) has recently been approved by the FDA panel for the temporary correction of HIV facial lipoatrophy [ASDS White Paper Sculptra™ (poly-L-lactic Acid)]. However, its use is also limited by temporary tissue residence, and formation of nodules and foreign-body reactions at implantation sites. Radiance (calcium hydroxylapatite) is another filler currently being used to treat

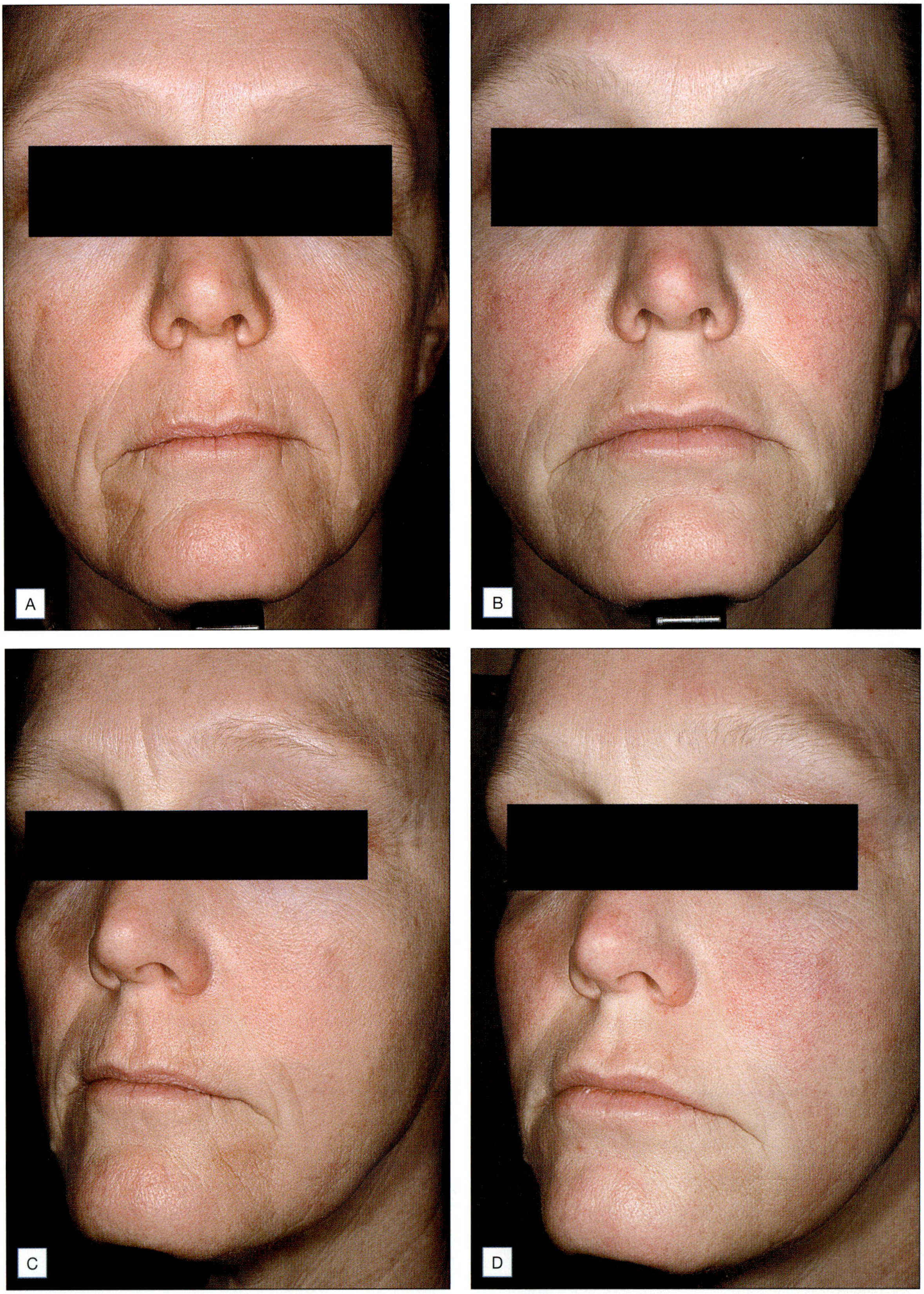

Fig. 6.4 Treatment for rhytids. (**A**) Frontal pre-treatment. (**B**) Frontal mid-treatment. (**C**) Oblique pre-treatment. (**D**) Oblique mid-treatment. Patient continues to undergo treatment

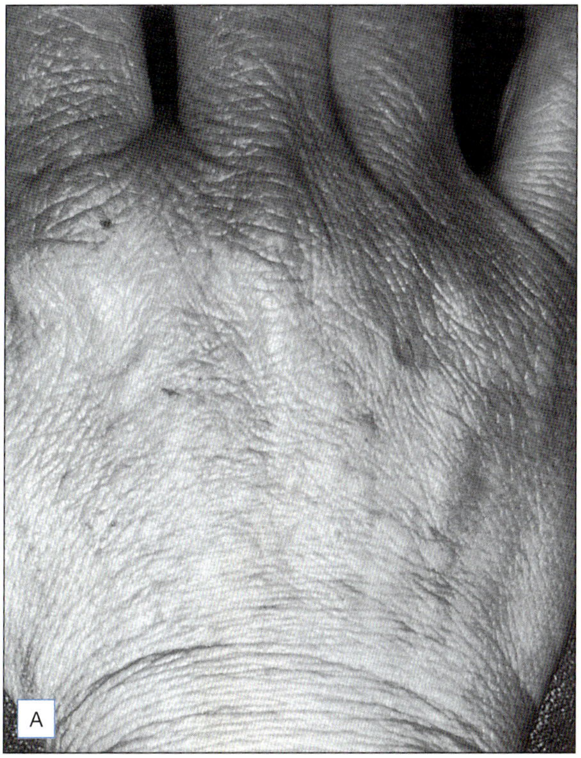

Fig. 6.5 (**A**) Immediately after initial treatment. (**B**) 6 months post-treatment LIS and cryotherapy

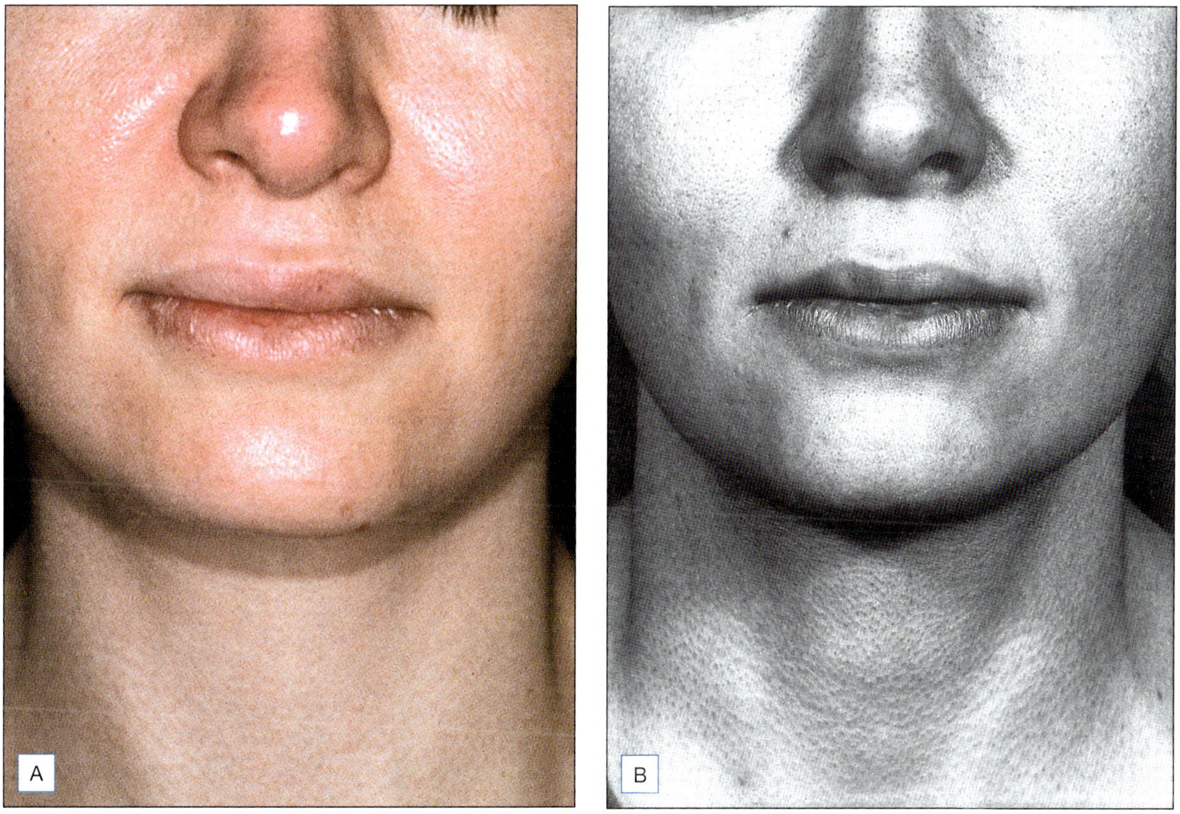

Fig. 6.6 Treatment of lips and NL folds. (**A**) Patient pre-treatment. (**B**) Patient post-treatment

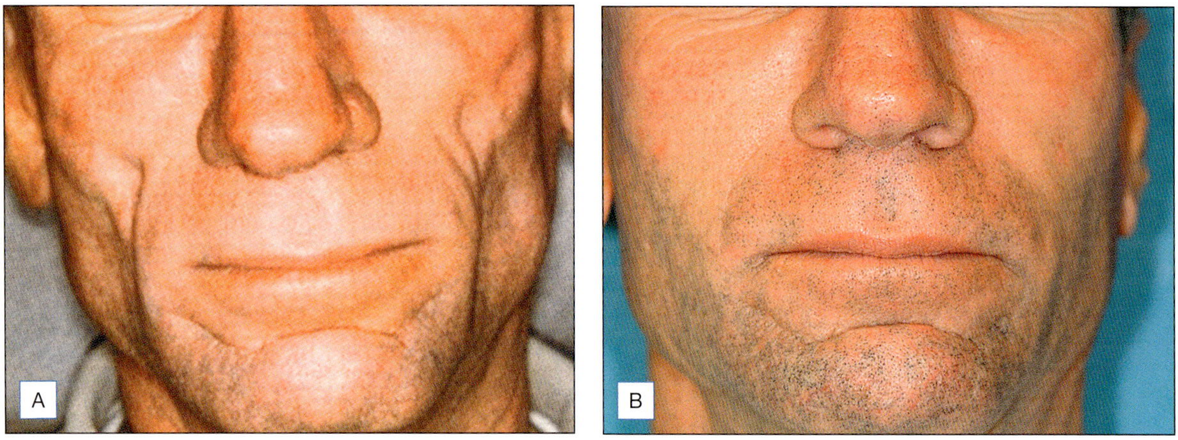

Fig. 6.7 HIV-associated lipoatrophy stage 3. (**A**) Patient pre-treatment. (**B**) Patient post-treatment

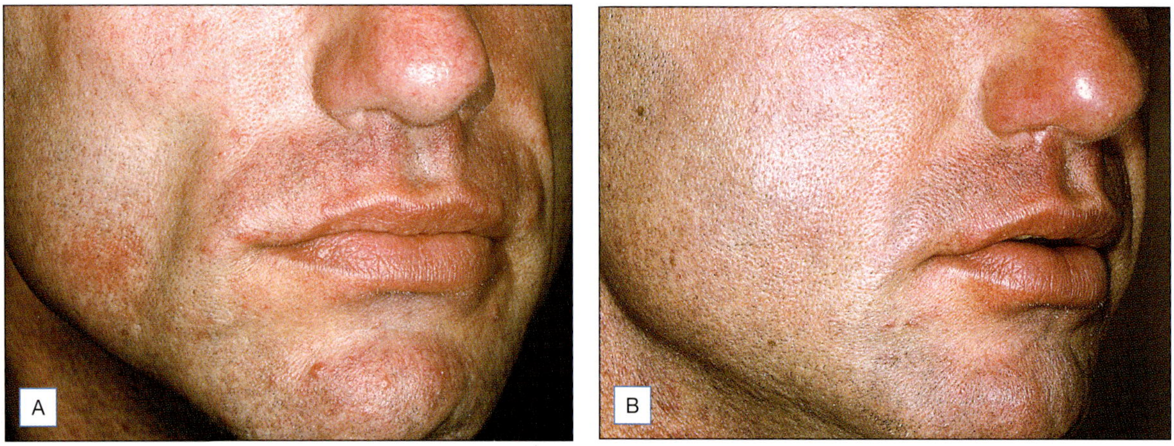

Fig. 6.8 HIV-associated lipoatrophy stage 3. (**A**) Patient pre-treatment. (**B**) Patient post-treatment (13 mL)

HIV-associated lipoatrophy. Radiesse™ is a radio-opaque implant approved for radiological and otolaryngology indications. Studies regarding safety, efficacy and longevity are lacking. Rhytidectomy and surgical implantation of rigid cheek implants offer unsatisfactory correction. Affected patients require more natural, persistent, affordable, safe and effective treatment options.

The authors are currently evaluating the safety and efficacy of highly purified 1000 cs silicone oil (Silikon 1000) for the treatment of HIV-associated lipoatrophy. To date, hundreds of patients with HIV facial lipoatrophy are being treated utilizing an average of 2 cc of Silikon 1000 injected at monthly intervals with the microdroplet serial puncture technique. Recently, data on 77 patients with a complete correction were analyzed to determine the number of treatments, amount of silicone, and time required to reach complete correction, relative to initial severity. The volume of silicone, number of treatments, and time required to reach complete correction were directly related to initial severity of lipoatrophy ($P < 0.0001$). Supple, even facial contours were routinely restored (see Figs 6.7 and 6.8), with all patients tolerating treatments well. No adverse events were noted. Although we have demonstrated that highly purified 1000 cs silicone oil is a safe and effective treatment option for HIV facial lipoatrophy, longer term safety and efficacy in HIV patients remain to be proven.

Instrumentation

In the USA, the most appropriate liquid injectable silicone for soft tissue augmentation is Silikon 1000 (Alcon, Fort Worth, TX). AdatoSil 5000 is too

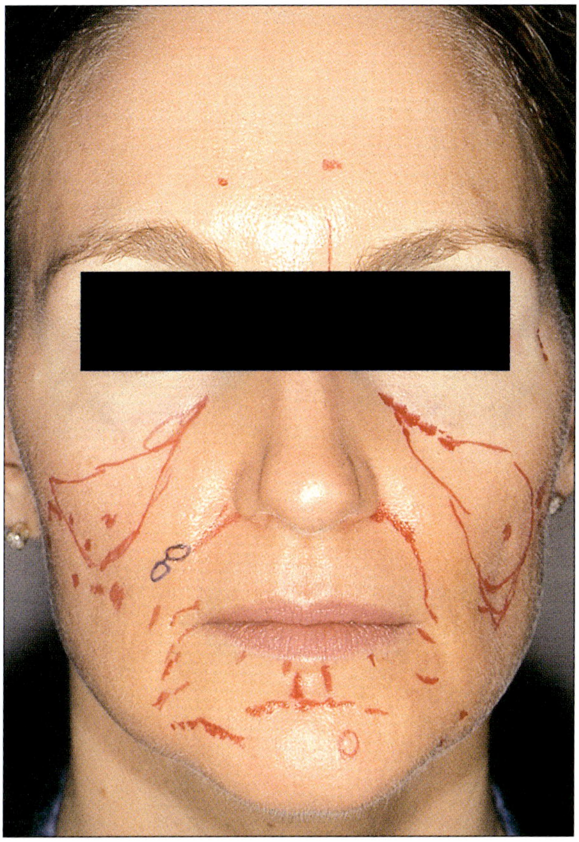

Fig. 6.9 Typical pre-injection markings for patient with rhytids, depressions, and scarring

viscous to be injected in a timely fashion through the 30 gauge needles recommended for injecting LIS. Using standard sterile technique, the silicone oil is drawn through a 16 gauge Nokor needle into a BD 1 cc Luer-Lok syringe immediately prior to use. The syringe is filled to the 0.5 cc mark to allow better control of the plunger. Silicone for injection is not to be stored for longer periods in the syringe, as contaminants in the rubber stopper of the plunger may possibly leak into the LIS and contribute to a foreign-body reaction. The liquid silicone is more easily injected through the wider internal bore 30 gauge RJ MaxFlo Needle (RJ Development, Peabody, MA). Rubber electrical bushings, with an inner diameter of 0.5 in (obtainable through most hardware stores) may be autoclaved and placed over the barrel of the Luer-Lok syringe to provide a cushion for the physician's second and third fingers during injection. Alternatively, the Becton Dickinson (Franklin Lakes, NJ) 3/10 cc insulin syringe can be used to inject (note that the insulin syringe must be back-loaded). Each method has a different 'feel.' Injecting with both syringes allows a useful comparison.

Patient Preparation

The skin is thoroughly cleansed with antibacterial cleanser. If a patient wears make-up, special attention is taken to ensure all traces of make-up are removed prior to injecting, as it is theoretically possible to 'tattoo' components of make-up, including silica, a common make-up ingredient, into the skin, resulting in a potential foreign-body reaction. The patient is seated with overhead lighting adjusted to delineate areas to be treated. Areas to be injected are outlined with a fine Sharpie pen or other marker (Fig. 6.9). Careful and precise marking is of utmost importance to obtain precise correction.

Marked areas are usually anesthetized with topical anesthetic under plastic occlusion for 30 minutes. Care is taken not to disturb the markings when removing the topical anesthetic. A facial tissue is pressed gently against the skin to absorb the anesthetic cream, and slowly and carefully lifted off, repeating until all anesthetic has been removed.

The patient may be injected in a seated or recumbent position, depending on the physician's preference. However, marking should be done with the patient in the seated or standing position.

Method of Injection

The only method used by the authors is the Orentreich microdroplet serial puncture technique (MDT), developed by Norman Orentreich in 1952, and perfected in 1955. In the authors' opinion, the MDT is the method of injection that consistently yields the best results, while minimizing the risk of unwanted effects. Other techniques, even in experienced hands, are more likely to create undesirable effects such as tendency to produce pooling or beading of the silicone in the injection tract.

Using the MDT, the needle is inserted into the skin at intervals of 2 mm to 5 mm at the appropriate angle for optimal penetration and deposition. A microdroplet of LIS is defined as a volume of 0.005–0.01 mL. It is deposited at the appropriate depth on each insertion of the needle. It is not necessary to aspirate prior to injection. When incidentally injected into a blood vessel, the LIS simply flows through and does not block the vessel, but is excreted in the urine.

Injection concepts

The angle of insertion varies: more oblique (approaching perpendicular) for areas of greater depth, such as when injecting skin in the lip or cheek area. A relatively acute (approaching parallel to the skin) angle for more superficial deposition or more acute (approaching parallel to the skin) for superficial deposition. A relatively acute angle of injection is indicated when treating skin that overlies bony, vital, and vascular structures.

Assiduously avoiding finger pressure on the plunger of the syringe while the needle is entering or exiting the skin ensures that the LIS is deposited at the appropriate depth, and the possibility of unintentional superficial deposition and potential beading is minimized.

Unlike many temporary fillers, the intentional production of any overcorrection immediately after injection of LIS is to be avoided. With LIS, the defect is deliberately under-corrected, with gradual augmentation achieved over several sessions. A useful analogy is 'planting seeds' under the depressed area to stimulate collagen growth.

Direct manual pressure suffices to stop any minor bleeding that can occur, and to prevent or minimize ecchymosis. Firm pressure also can help to lessen any minor escape of LIS through the skin surface through the needle track. Attempting to further disperse LIS after injection by means of massage or other modality is of unproven value and can unnecessarily traumatize facial tissues. The injection of a microdroplet at each puncture site obviates the need for dispersion by imprecise techniques.

Depositing LIS at different depths in the skin can produce either desirable or undesirable effects. Superficial intradermal injection of LIS into skin of normal thickness can produce a 'beading' effect, particularly when skin overlies bone (i.e. on the forehead). Certain scars and rhytids lack dermal thickness however; in these circumstances, controlled superficial intradermal injection is intentional and produces the desired augmentation. A suboptimal correction usually results if LIS were to be injected at the deeper dermal subcutaneous interface under these same defects.

The total amount of LIS injected is dictated by the level of correction desired. When the microdroplet serial puncture technique is used, each needle puncture and injection deposits between 0.005–0.01 mL of LIS. The average single treatment session for a middle-aged patient with facial rhytids requires a total of 0.25–0.75 mL of LIS. Injections of this volume can entail as few as 25–50 (or as many as 75–150) individual needle punctures, and usually suffices to treat the neck, labial commissure grooves, nasolabial creases, malar grooves, crow's feet, frown lines, and forehead lines. The total number of punctures depends on the size of the microdroplets and the total volume of LIS used.

When treating facial lipodystrophy or hemifacial atrophy, a larger total volume (always administered in microdroplets), approaching 2 mL per session, is used. In areas of deeper depression, the physician should avoid during any one injection session, an immediate 'second pass' over areas that have just been treated. Doing so may cause microdroplets to coalesce into large droplets and increase the risk of drift. In an experienced practitioner's hands, a second pass may be undertaken 5 mm or more deeper to the first pass in order to build volume more quickly. As the endpoint of treatment approaches, the volume injected per visit diminishes and the time interval between treatments lengthens until the final result is achieved.

Although large cumulative volumes are required for larger defects, use of the microdroplet technique is still essential. Because fibroplasia and resultant augmentation occur at the surface of LIS droplets, the amount of new collagen formed is directly proportional to the total surface area of the injected silicone microdroplet 'implant' (the implant comprising hundreds of microdroplets). A given volume of LIS dispersed into many small droplets provides a larger total surface area for collagen deposition than would the same volume divided into fewer, large drops (see Fig. 6.10). The microdroplet injection also effectively eliminates migration by stimulating a collagen capsule that holds the microdroplets at the site of implantation. The surface tension surrounding a microdroplet is sufficient to hold it in place. The same surface tension is not adequate to hold a macrodroplet ($\geq$ 0.01 mL) in place.

Treatment protocol

Intervals between sessions are usually 1 month in the early stages of treatment. Intervals longer than

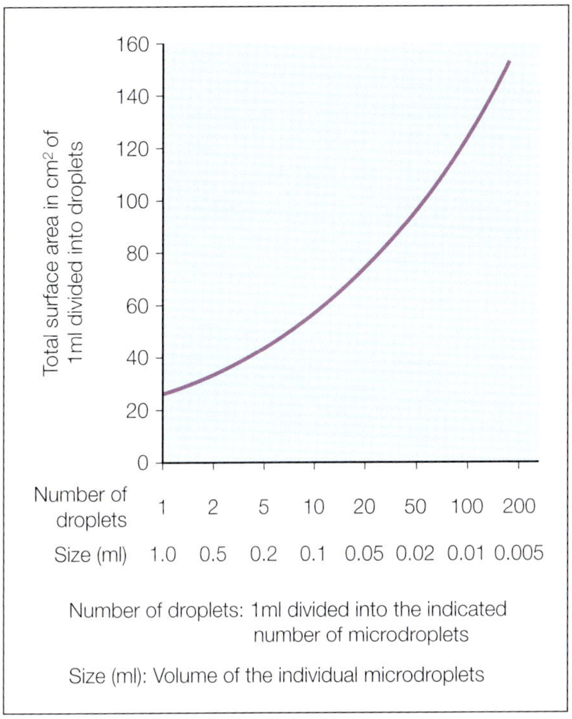

Fig. 6.10 Cumulative surface area (vs. volume) for 1 mL LIS divided into microdroplets

Technique pearls for different esthetic regions

Premise: The mechanism of action of LIS as an augmenting agent is wholly different from that of most other fillers. Those accustomed to using temporary fillers may initially find the MDT counterintuitive and cumbersome. Comfort with the MDT will come with strict adherence to the technique and with time

1. Exercise particular care in marking. NL folds are marked, usually wider at the nose, and injected in a random zigzag pattern to avoid repeating the same injection sites on future visits. Employ random placement of needle punctures while adhering to the 2–4 mm rule
2. Carefully blot topical anesthetic off skin to preserve original markings
3. Skin may be stretched to facilitate needle entry, or pinched to hold it away from underlying structures
4. Lips are usually injected at the 'wet line.' Finger pressure on the skin adjacent to the vermilion border will evert the wet line. Needle is perpendicular to lip surface
5. Be aware of bevel orientation, particularly when angle of injection is acute
6. Neck – stretch skin to facilitate needle entry. Bevel down, 45° angle (md ≤ 0.005 mL)
7. Periorbital lines (crow's feet) – very acute angle (~30°). Only the lightest touch on the plunger, i.e. md ≤ 0.005 mL

Box 6.1 Technique pearls for different esthetic regions

1 month pose no problem; however both physician and patient must be aware that augmentation will proceed at a slower rate, and a final result will take proportionately longer to achieve. As the defects improve, longer intervals of 2–6 months or more are appropriate to avoid overcorrection. Treatments given less than 1 month apart are permissible if different areas are treated.

'Pearls'

(See Box 6.1).

Side effects and complications

Adverse reactions and precautions

Edema

Edema can result from the trauma of needle insertion and usually resolves within several hours to days. Because the edema itself can produce temporary correction of defects, judgment of cosmetic improvement cannot be made until the edema resolves and collagen deposition takes place. Edema with LIS is usually slight compared to edema provoked by other fillers.

Ecchymosis

If ecchymosis occurs, it is usually mild and related to needle puncture, needle gauge, vascularity of underlying tissue, and the surface anticoagulant property of LIS. Bruising is more prominent in areas with a dense vascular network. It is advisable but not essential for patients to avoid the use of anticoagulants (especially aspirin or ibuprofen) prior to treatment. When anticoagulant therapy cannot be discontinued, prolonged manual pressure is advised. The application of firm pressure reduces the incidence and extent of ecchymosis. Patients are permitted to apply make-up to camouflage bruising immediately after treatment.

Erythema

Slight to moderate transient erythema sometimes appears immediately after injection. The triple response of Lewis ('weal and flare') reaction can be more pronounced in patients with dermatographism and a tendency towards contact or pressure urticaria. It typically persists for a few hours and can be masked with make-up. Rarely, persistent erythema of an injected area can result if the injection of LIS has been made too superficially or with impure materials. Persistent erythema can be diminished by topical application of anti-inflammatory corticosteroid preparations or intradermal injection of triamcinolone acetonide 1–2.5 mg/mL in 0.05–0.10 mL aliquots. Rare persistent cases of erythema respond to pulse-dye laser.

Dyschromia

On rare occasions, the injection of silicone has been reported to cause a brownish yellow discoloration of the skin. Dyschromia is avoidable and is usually the result of either very superficial deposition or injection of impure material. A bluish tinge can result from superficial deposition of LIS into very thin, translucent skin, such as striae and atrophic scars, from light passing through skin infiltrated with a clear material. Carefully documenting pre-existing pigmentation in the form of written records and photographs is useful.

Texture and sensation

The texture of soft tissue augmented with evenly dispersed microdroplets of LIS is quite natural. The patient does not experience any unnatural sensation or sensitivity to touch in such locations. Larger cumulative amounts of LIS, as is sometimes required to correct hemifacial atrophy and lipodystrophy, can impart a slightly firmer consistency on palpation. In the context of overall cosmetic improvement, this texture is usually acceptable to the patient; it occasionally reverts to a near-normal texture given time. Injection of LIS in greatly excessive amounts or, purportedly, too superficially in the dermis has been known to cause distention of the skin and blockage of lymphatics; fullness or a *peau d'orange* texture can result.

Overcorrection

Overcorrection at a particular site of LIS implantation can occur if an excessive quantity is injected at one time or cumulatively over several sessions. Attempting to satisfy a patient's desire for instant gratification by injecting large volumes violates a fundamental principle of LIS-MDT therapy.

Overcorrection of deeper tissues while attempting contour elevation is very uncommon when the MDT is used with intervals of 1 month or more between treatment sessions. When it occurs, it usually takes the form of a diffuse enlargement of the treated area.

The term **beading** (Fig. 6.11) is used to describe small (1–5 mm), firm papules that form at individual sites of needle insertion. They are usually skin colored but can be slightly erythematous or brownish yellow. These papules are the result of collagen deposition around superficially implanted microdroplets; they are not granulomas. They can occur when attempting either surface remodeling or contour elevation. A few patients develop beading at augmentation sites even after precautions have been followed. In some cases, the effect is temporary and the problem subsides spontaneously during the ensuing months.

Beading and overcorrection are amenable to intralesional injections of anti-inflammatory corticosteroids, usually triamcinolone acetonide (1.0–5.0 mg/mL, with approximately 0.05–0.10 mL injected per cm^3 of elevated tissue). Improvement can be temporary, with the return of overcorrection after the effects of the corticosteroid have dissipated. This treatment can be repeated. Micro-electrodesiccation, punch excision, dermabrasion, or tangential shave excision surgery can provide permanent resolution.

Although experience is limited, the use of suction-assisted lipectomy to treat tissues excessively augmented with unknown fluid implant materials, impure silicone, or even LIS can be worthwhile in selected cases. When improvement is achieved by liposuction it is probably because of the removal of adipose tissue and not LIS.

Common skin lesions that can be mistaken for LIS beading include benign nevi, milia, eccrine hidrocystoma, and sebaceous hyperplasia. Some patients

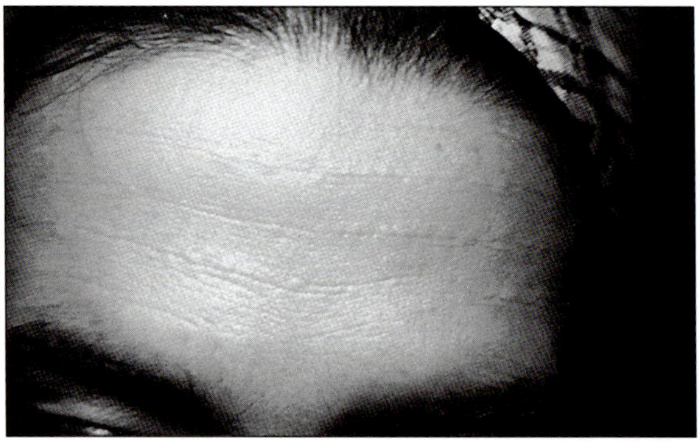

Fig. 6.11 Beading secondary to superficial intradermal injection

present with sebaceous hyperplasia in areas previously injected by LIS. Sebaceous hyperplasia is characterized by yellowish papules measuring 1–5 mm with central umbilication. Each of these lesions can be treated by electrodesiccation.

Embolism

As with any injection of an augmenting material, care must be taken to avoid intravascular injection of LIS. The authors have not observed or encountered any reports of ophthalmic symptoms after microdroplet LIS injection into facial skin. The absence of amaurosis after LIS injections is likely the result of LIS's fluid nature and anti-coagulant surface property.

Granulomatous reactions

Granulomatous inflammatory reactions to injected purported 'silicone' have been called **siliconomas**, a misnomer because silicone itself cannot become a tumor (**-oma**). Furthermore, cells that phagocytose silicone (macrophages) do not multiply in a tumorous fashion. Critical scrutiny of reports of granulomatous reactions to purported silicone reveal that these cases fall into several causal categories: cases of overinjection, injecting into contraindicated sites, injection of impure silicone, and injection of substances of unknown chemical composition.

There are reports in the literature of 'silicone' granuloma reactions responding favorably to a variety of modalities, including Imiquimod 5%, high-potency topical steroids, and antibiotic treatment with satisfactory responses. While it is important to note the success of these treatments, it is equally important to note that in the cases referenced, the presence of LIS was never conclusively established.

Idiosyncratic reactions to liquid injectable silicone

Very rarely, instances of local, isolated reactions of an inflammatory nature have occurred in the author's practice, with an approximate incidence of 1:5000 to 1:10 000 treatment sessions. These reactions, characterized by a well-demarcated area of moderate swelling with or without erythema, can appear months or years after injection or involve one, or rarely several, of the many areas treated. They frequently are preceded by an infection at a distant site such as acute sinusitis, furuncle, otitis media, or dental abscess. If a biopsy is performed, the histopathology is consistent with a nonspecific chronic inflammatory reaction. An intradermal skin test to LIS performed on the volar forearm is invariably negative. The reactions respond within days or weeks to intralesional corticosteroid injections and broad-spectrum oral antibiotics; treatment is repeated as needed until resolution of symptoms is complete. After the negative intradermal skin test and resolution of the idiosyncratic reaction, one of the authors (DO) has performed further LIS augmentation on some of these patients without incident.

One theoretical explanation for these idiosyncratic reactions is that rarely, an inert material such as LIS tissues implanted into normal tissues may act as a nidus for infection. Infectious organisms can come in contact with the surface of the microdroplets by local extension or via the circulation. Although LIS does not support the growth of microorganisms, the relatively reduced perfusion in the microenvironment at the surface of any inert implant may allow the proliferation of bacteria.

Drift

Drift is defined by movement of a soft tissue augmenting agent to a site distant from where it was originally injected. Drifting of LIS (or other injectable implant for that matter) can occur when a large volume (many times greater than a microdroplet) is injected into a single site during a single treatment session. Distant migration of silicone gel from ruptured breast implants has also been reported. These large volumes, which were not contained by the receiving tissues, migrated by gravity, muscle action, and external pressure along tissue planes of least resistance.

The microdroplet injection technique effectively eliminates drift by stimulating a collagenous capsule that holds the LIS at the site of implantation. Only the most fibrotic bound-down tissues are not distensible enough to retain microdroplets of LIS.

Areas of naturally occurring age-related ptosis of facial tissue, which can develop concomitantly with or subsequent to LIS administrated over many years, have been erroneously blamed on drifting LIS. These areas correspond to typical bulges seen with chronologic and photo aging, such as NLFs, cheek pouches, the jawline jowls, and 'dewlaps'. In some instances, these bulges existed prior to LIS treatment but were noticed by neither the patient nor the physician. Increased attention to appearance leads to close scrutiny of the face by both patient and physician. General dissatisfaction with an aged appearance causes the patient and occasionally the physician to attribute responsibility for the facial sagging on LIS drift. Examination of pretreatment photographs usually dispels this misconception and underscores the importance of obtaining pretreatment photo documentation.

Gravity exerts its effects on the soft tissues of the face equally. When ptosis of facial tissues inevitably occurs, areas augmented with LIS sag in concert with all other areas of the face. The authors have seen no independent drift of LIS injected with the MDT.

Finally, gravitational movement of LIS has been putatively reported months to years after injection. Such drift is difficult to reconcile with the laws of physics because the specific gravity of LIS is less than that of water, and thus LIS floats on water. Because the specific gravity of human soft tissue is even greater than that of water, LIS would migrate or drift upward in a cephalad direction, which it does not. The authors have never observed the presence of LIS in relatively cephalad locations, years or decades after it was injected using the MDT, nor are they aware of any published reports of such occurrences.

Connective tissue disease

The occurrence of connective tissue disease, including human adjuvant disease, has been reported after augmentation mammoplasty by the injection of foreign substances such as paraffin, processed petrolatum, impure silicone, or mixtures of these. Scleroderma has been reported in women after silicone gel bag augmentation mammoplasty; however, no cause-and-effect relationship was established. The incidence of scleroderma in women with breast augmentation has been calculated to be the same as that for nonbreast-augmented women. To the authors' knowledge, there is no cause-and-effect relationship between connective tissue disease and LIS therapy.

Troubleshooting

(See Table 6.1).

Acknowledgment

The authors would like to thank Anna-Sophia Leone for her assistance in the preparation of this manuscript.

Troubleshooting	
Problem	**Possible causes**
Treatment progressing slowly	Injecting too deeply? Inadequate total volume/treatment?
Patient claims LIS is 'drifting'	Assuming use of MDT, point out facial redundancies prior to treatment to ensure that pre-existing redundancies are not erroneously attributed to LIS migration
Beading	Injection too superficially, or check if thumb is on plunger while inserting or withdrawing plunger. Treat with electrodesiccation
Dyschromia	Very superficial injection, usually into atrophic scars, which lack adnexal structures
Ecchymosis	Apply finger pressure to skin immediately after withdrawing syringe, discontinue use of anticoagulants prior to treatment when possible
Transient edema	Expected. Resolves over the course of several days

Table 6.1 Troubleshooting

Further Reading

Alani RM, Busam K 2001 Acupuncture granulomas. Journal of the American Academy of Dermatology 45(6 suppl):5225–5226

Ashley FL, Thompson DP, Henderson T 1973 Augmentation of surface contour by subcutaneous injections of silicone fluid. Plastic and Reconstructive Surgery 51:8

Baumann L, Halem M 2003 Lip silicone granulomatous foreign body reaction treated with Aldara (imiquimod 5%). Dermatologic Surgery 29(4):429–432

Benedetto AV, Lewis AT 2003 Injecting 1000 centistoke liquid silicone with ease and precision. Dermatologic Surgery 29(3):211–214

Blocksma R, Braley S 1973 Implantation materials. In: Grabb WC, Smith JW (eds) Plastic Surgery. 2nd edn. Little, Brown, Boston, pp 131

Bondurant S, Ernster V, Herdman R 2000 Committee on the Safety of Breast Implants, Washington, DC; Institute of Medicine, Safety of Silicone Breast Implants. National Academy Press

Coleman S 2001 Injectable silicone returns to the United States. Aesthetic Surgery Journal 21:576–578

Delage C, Shane JJ, Johnson FB 1973 Mammary silicone granuloma: Migration of silicone fluid to abdominal wall and inguinal region. Archives of Dermatology 108:104

Dow Corning 1990 IDE Number L002702 Limited Applications for Silicone Injections Using Dow Corning MDX4-4011, final report to the FDA

Duffy DM 1998 Injectable liquid silicone: New perspectives. In: Klein AW (ed.) Tissue Augmentation in Clinical Practice: Procedures and Techniques. Marcel Dekker, New York, pp 237–267

Duffy DM 2002 The silicone conundrum: a battle of anecdotes. Dermatologic Surgery 28:590–594

Durst S, Johnson BS, Amplatz K 1974 The effect of silicone coatings on thrombogenicity. American Journal of Roentgenology Radical Therapy in Nuclear Medicine 20:904

Ellenbogen R, Rubin L 1975 Injectable fluid silicone therapy: Human morbidity and mortality. Journal of the American Medical Association 234:308 http://ww.fda.gov/cder/guidance/105-155.htm

Jaques LB, Fidlar E, Feldsted ET et al 1946 Silicones and blood coagulation. Canadian Medical Association Journal 55:26

Jones D, Carruthers A, Orentreich D, Brody H et al 2004 Highly purified 1000-cst silicone oil for treatment of human immunodeficiency virus-associated facial lipoatrophy: an open pilot trial. Dermatologic Surgery 30:1279–1286

Jones D 2004 Treatment options for HIV facial lipoatrophy. Dermatologic Surgery 2004 (in press)

Kagan HD 1963 Sakurai injectable silicone formula. Archives of Otolaryngology 78:663–668

Kozeny GA, Barbato AL, Vertuno LL et al 1984 Hypercalcemia associated with silicone-induced granulomas. New England Journal of Medicine 311:1103–1105

Latish E 1999 From Eric Latish, Chief Dental, ENT, and Ophthalmic Devices Branch, Division of Enforcement II, Office of Compliance, Center for Radiologic Health, US Food and Drug Administration (letter)

McDowell F 1978 Complications with silicones—what grade of silicone? How do we know it was silicone? (editorial). Plastic and Reconstructive Surgery 61(6):892–895

Milojevic B 1982 Complications after silicone injection therapy in aesthetic plastic surgery. Aesthetic Plastic Surgery 6:203

Orentreich D, Leone AS 2004 A case of HIV-associated lipoatrophy treated with 1000-cs liquid injectable silicone. Dermatologic Surgery 30:548–551

Orentreich DS 2000 Liquid injectable silicone: techniques for soft tissue augmentation. Clinical Plastic Surgery 27(4):595–612

Orentreich N, Durr NP 1985 The four R's of skin rehabilitation. In: Graham JAG, Kligman AM (eds) The Psychology of Cosmetic Treatments. Praeger, New York, pp 227

Parel JM, Villain F 1994 Silicone oils: Physicochemical properties. In: Ryan SJ, Glaser BM (eds) Retina. Mosby, St Louis, pp 2131–2149

Pearl RM, Laub DR, Kaplan EN 1978 Complications following silicone injections for augmentation of the contours of the face. Plastic and Reconstructive Surgery 61(6):888–891

Rapaport MJ, Vinnik C, Zarem H 1996 Injectable silicone: cause of facial nodules, cellulitis, ulceration, and migration. Aesthetic Plastic Surgery 20(3):267–276

Selmanowitz VJ, Orentreich N 1974 Cutaneous corticosteroid injection and amaurosis. Analysis for cause and prevention. Archives in Dermatology 110(5):729–734

Selmanowitz VJ, Orentreich N 1977 Medical grade fluid silicone: A monographic review. Journal of Dermatological Surgery and Oncology 3:597

Sperber PA 1964 Chemexfoliation and silicone infiltration in the treatment of aging skin and dermal defects. Journal of the American Geriatric Society 12:594

Wilkie TF 1977 Late development of granuloma after liquid silicone injections. Plastic and Reconstructive Surgery 60:179

Winer LH, Sternberg TH, Lehman R et al 1964 Tissue reactions to injected silicone liquids: A report of three cases. Archives of Dermatology 90:588

Wolff K, Tappeiner G 1993 Mycobacterial diseases: Tuberculosis and atypical mycobacterial infections. In: Fitzpatrick TB, Eisen AZ, Wolff K et al (eds) Dermatology in General Medicine. 3rd edn. McGraw-Hill, New York, pp 2370–2395

Zandi I 1985 Use of suction to treat soft tissue injected with liquid silicone. Plastic and Reconstructive Surgery 76:307

7 Combination Materials

Hayes B. Gladstone, Peggy Wu, Alastair Carruthers

Introduction

Since fat was first used to fill defects in the 19th century, the search for useful materials has included both biodegradable materials such as collagen and hyaluronic acid and nonbiodegradable materials such as silicone oil. The current authors' patients desire both a safe product and long-term correction. One way to produce a longer lasting material is to combine a permanent or extended life material with another material which is essentially a vehicle. The vehicle disappears relatively rapidly, leaving the longer lasting material to produce the long-term correction. Examples include polymethylmethacrylate (PMMA) beads in a bovine collagen vehicle (Artecoll, Artefill, Artes Inc., San Diego, CA) and calcium hydroxylapatite beads in a methylcellulose vehicle (Radiesse FN, Franksville, WI, USA).

The challenges have been to make these combination fillers into a material that is easily injectable, that is at least semi-permanent, and that does not cause intense inflammatory reactions that will lead for example to granulomas. To date these fillers have been moderately successful in achieving these stated goals. For the appropriate patient, they may be more effective than currently other Food and Drug Administration (FDA)-approved fillers. Most of the fillers discussed in this chapter are not yet (Fall 2004) approved in the USA by the FDA for cosmetic indications, though several have undergone extensive use in Canada, Europe and Asia. Nonetheless, it is important for the dermatologist to be familiar with them, since it is anticipated that they will shortly enter the US market. This chapter is not meant to be an exhaustive compilation of all fillers, but rather to discuss in depth some of the representative new generation of combination fillers so that the practitioner will become more knowledgeable about them.

Artecoll/Artefill

Background

Artecoll is a permanent, injectable soft tissue filler consisting of PMMA microspheres 30–42 μ in diameter suspended in a 3.5% partially denatured bovine collagen solution. This product has been used in Europe since 1994 and Canada since 1998, primarily for the treatment of facial wrinkles. It is currently pending FDA approval for use in the USA under the trade name Artefill.

The allure of Artecoll/Artefill is its permanence. Though the bovine collagen, which serves as a vehicle for the PMMA beads, degrades after 1–3 months, the microspheres themselves are made of a nonresorbable synthetic material. These beads induce a long term foreign body reaction and become encapsulated in fibrous connective tissue, producing long-lasting augmentation.

History

Since its appearance on the market in 1994, Artecoll has been used worldwide (with the exception of the USA and Japan) in an estimated 200 000 patients. Patient satisfaction was reported at 91% while the overall complication rate was estimated at 3%.

Development of this product began in 1985 by German plastic surgeon Gottfried Lemperle, beginning with animal studies and resulting in a PMMA suspension in gelatin for use in humans dubbed Arteplast. Unfortunately, this material induced granuloma formation in a significant number of the individuals who were injected. Lemperle determined that this was due to the presence of smaller particles which could be ingested by macrophages as well as the rough surface of the beads. Subsequent iterations improved the surface, size and uniformity of the beads and changed the liquid phase of the material to collagen. A few preliminary studies on Artecoll have addressed patient satisfaction and complications within approximately 2 years of injection; other published literature on the subject consists of reviews and case reports.

Structure

Artecoll is biphasic in nature: it consists of a solid phase of PMMA microspheres suspended in a liquid phase collagen vehicle in a ratio of 1:4. Artefill is identical to Artecoll. The microspheres are made of PMMA, a plastic (also known as Plexiglas or Lucite) used in bone cement, dentures and hard contact lenses. The collagen component is a 3.5% solution of denatured bovine atelocollagen; without the telopeptide immunogenic ends, the collagen molecule is less antigenic. Artecoll/Artefill also contains 0.3% lidocaine hydrochloride to reduce pain after implantation.

PMMA has been shown to be biocompatible, nonallergenic and chemically inert in its use in the past 40 years as bone cement and in hip and dental implants. The collagen in Artecoll/Artefill is also known to be biocompatible and nontoxic, although it is more likely than PMMA to induce an allergic response. The current production process of bovine collagen minimizes the chance for contamination with infectious agents such as bovine spongiform encephalopathy (BSE) and has an allergy rate of 0.08%. Because of the possibility of a hypersensitivity reaction to collagen, skin testing is required with a single intradermal test injection of Artecoll/Artefill collagen at least 4 weeks before the planned implantation.

The PMMA particles in Artecoll range from 30–42 microns in diameter, are round and have polymerized, smooth surfaces (Rofil Medical International, Breda, Holland). At this size they are large enough to avoid phagocytosis and are small enough to promote optimal connective tissue encapsulation. Because irregularity in the shape of the spheres is correlated to granuloma formation, care is taken to smooth out the surfaces and remove any dust or charge by a complex washing and straining procedure and ultrasound technology.

Artecoll is supplied as approximately 0.5 mL of product in a 1.0 mL syringe with a Luer–Lok. Also supplied with the syringe is a 26 (preferred) or 27 gauge 0.5 in needle. Another option is the RJ Maxflo 30 gauge needle with an internal diameter similar to the 27 gauge needle. This needle tends to be more comfortable to the injectee but may occasionally become blocked. Although the PMMA–collagen gel state suspension is stable at room temperature, it should be kept in the refrigerator prior to use. Heating the syringes under warm water prior to use will reduce the viscosity of the suspension. However at 40°C the collagen gel melts and the two phases will separate, leaving the PMMA microspheres to sink to the bottom. This phenomenon can result in reduced efficacy if during implantation only the collagen fluid is injected as it pushes through the microspheres, which remain in the syringe and block the needle. To regain the gel suspension the solution can be run under cold water but neither procedure is recommended. With good technique, the material can be satisfactorily used straight from the refrigerator.

Mechanism of action

Upon implantation, Artecoll, which is placed at the border of the dermis and subcutaneous fat, fills the wrinkle or skin defect with volume. Gradually in the next 1–3 months, the 80% collagen component of Artecoll/Artefill is degraded. Meanwhile the 30–42 μm PMMA spheres are nonbiodegradable and too large for phagocytosis by macrophages and giant cells. They become a scaffold promoting connective tissue deposition and are eventually encapsulated by fibroblasts and collagen. The body's fibrous connective tissue response replaces the collagen carrier volume during the first 1–4 months. Nevertheless, to avoid overcorrection and for desired results, two to four injection sessions are usually needed with an interval of at least 2 months.

Indications

Artecoll/Artefill is a long-lasting filler substance with uses ranging from facial wrinkles and folds, acne scars, augmentation and similarly sized soft tissue contour defects in the face and other areas. It is best used in areas of thicker skin (i.e. not crows' feet) so that the implant is not visible or palpable. The physician should be prepared for a slight learning curve, as the implant is more viscous in consistency than collagen, and it may take some practice to learn the correct injection pressure.

Contraindications include individuals with a known allergy to collagen or lidocaine, a positive skin test (recommended 4 weeks before planned implantation), susceptibility to keloids, atrophic skin diseases, autoimmune disease, and immunosuppression.

Duration of action

Artcoll/Artefill is a permanent filler. Although the collagen component is degraded over months, the PMMA beads are not broken down by the body and remain encapsulated within the body's fibrous connective tissue for long-lasting subdermal augmentation. The manufacturer, Artes Medical Inc., describes the correction as 'long-term' to account for the continuous aging process and as 10 years is the longest clinical experience thus far with Artecoll.

Patient selection

The permanent nature of this implant warrants careful selection of patients. Patients should be overall healthy and not pregnant. Previous reactions to other injections or prior surgeries or trauma to the area are relative contraindications.

Ideal patients are those with well-defined wrinkle lines and folds with little excess skin. These are often patients between the ages of 40–50 without surplus skin that would indicate a need for a facelift. Those with thin and flaccid skin, sebaceous skin and large pores would not be good candidates as the filler may be palpable or visible, or shine through the skin of such patients. Also, younger patients have a greater tendency towards scar formation. A good candidate should fully understand the possibility of permanence with an Artecoll/Artefill implant, and may therefore be someone who has used more temporary fillers and wishes longer-term augmentation.

Most importantly, there should be a mutual understanding of expectations between the physician and patient. In particular, the patient should be aware that s/he may need more than one injection to achieve correction, and that especially over the course of the first 6 months the implant will be changing before the final result is apparent. Ideally, two to four injection sessions at least 1 month apart will be necessary. It is essential to avoid injecting Artecoll in too large a volume at a single visit since this is more likely to cause problems.

Technique

About 4 weeks prior to implantation, an injection should be given either behind the ear or in the forearm to test sensitivity to Artecoll/Artefill collagen (Fig. 7.1). For injection into the perioral or perinasal area, local nerve block with 1% or 2% lidocaine solution or at least a topical anesthetic such as LMX 5 or Betacaine applied 30–60 minutes before the procedure is usually indicated.

In general, Artecoll/Artefill is injected just below the border of the dermis into subcutaneous fat with a 26 gauge, 0.5 in needle. Before injecting, one should check that the needle is not blocked by gently squeezing some of the filler out of the tip. The physician should insert the needle horizontally beneath the wrinkle (tunneling technique) and, while maintaining a constant pressure on the syringe plunger and continuous movement of the needle, fill the channel as the needle is withdrawn. Because it is three times more viscous than collagen, Artecoll/Artefill requires a higher and more constant pressure applied throughout the injection. There will also be some resistance in the correct layer of skin, although the material should flow smoothly into the tissues. If greater pressure is required, stop injecting and remove the needle. Check product flow as a blocked needle is the most likely cause of needing more injection pressure. If the filler is injected too superficially, i.e. in the papillary dermis, an undesirable

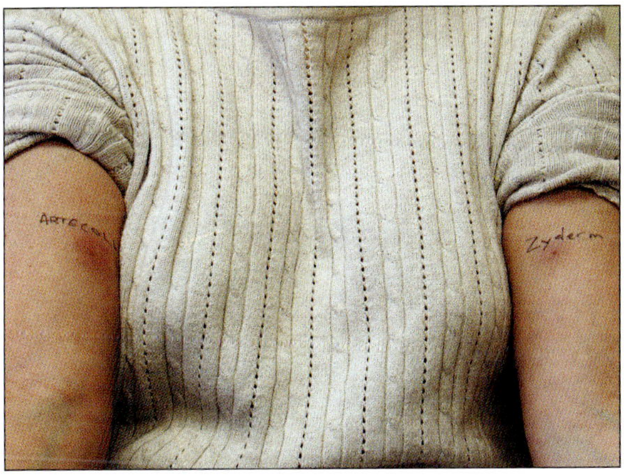

Fig. 7.1 Positive skin test to both Zyderm and Artecoll

blanching effect will be seen. Should this occur, the needle should be withdrawn and implantation resumed one needle diameter (0.4 mm) deeper. The outline but not the gray of the needle should always be seen under the skin. After injection, the implant should be massaged with the fingertip to smooth out any lumps and assure an even distribution. The patient should avoid strong mimic muscle movement in the site the first few days following implantation; immobility can be promoted with taping of the implant site or botulinum toxin injection.

First implantation of up to 0.5 mL Artecoll/Artefill is usually sufficient to correct one of the following: both glabellar frown lines, one nasolabial fold (NLF), one upper or lower lip, one corner of the mouth. Some patients may wish for more correction than can be safely attempted with Artecoll in the first session. In these cases one can overlay the Artecoll with Restylane or Perlane, and as these substances dissipate, the volume can be supplemented by further Artecoll injections.

Lip enhancement

Injection of Artecoll in the lips is a procedure commonly performed in Canada. However when the FDA panel met in February 2003 to evaluate its safety in this site, their recommendation was for it to be considered a contraindication due to reports of lumpiness in the lips (Fig. 7.2). Nevertheless, injection into the lips is possible, with some precautions. Ideally the orbicularis oris should be relaxed with botulinum toxin prior to injection to prevent filler migration and aggregation with movement of the lips. Also, it is important not to inject too much Artecoll into the lips (never more than one syringe, if not much less). If more volume is required, overlay with a temporary filler, such as a hyaluronan, can be carried out. Artecoll correction of the lips should take place over two to four treatments with conservative amounts each session and long intervals in between. The patient should always be warned prior to injection that minor lumpiness is the rule rather than the exception, and these usually resolve without treatment over 6 months. Treatment, if necessary, consists of making a small incision on the surface of the lip to remove the unwanted matter, most often a foreign-body granuloma. This complication is thought more to be due to limitations of technique and product rather than an immunological response.

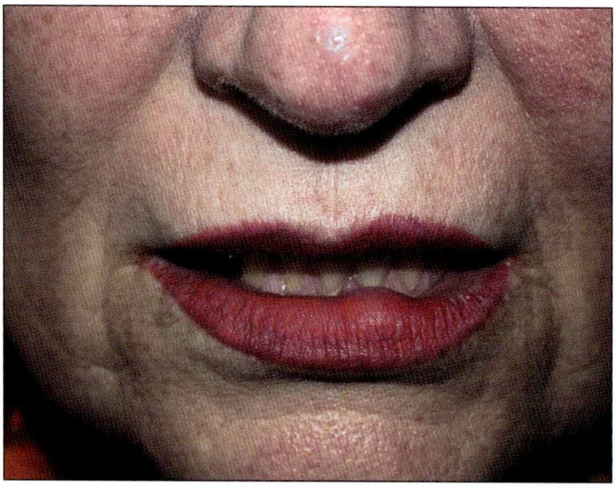

Fig. 7.2 Lip lumpiness after Artecoll injection

Other cosmetic subunits and indications that are appropriate for Artecoll injection are: glabellar frown lines, horizontal forehead lines, single crow's feet, irregularities of the nose, NLFs, perioral lip lines, marionette lines, horizontal chin folds, horizontal neck folds, and acne scars (Fig. 7.3 A–D).

Complications and treatment

The overall complication rate of Artecoll used in wrinkles was estimated at 3% in 1994. Common acute side effects include redness, swelling and moderate pain in the first 2 days after implantation. Bruising rarely occurs but can last up to 1 week, and patients may describe itching at the implantation site within the first few months. If the injection is done too superficially, it can cause long term itching and redness; this can be treated with corticosteroid creams or injections. Other technical side effects include uneven distribution, an over-deep implantation of the filler or accidental dislodgement through pronounced facial expression. The first two side effects can be corrected with another injection of Artecoll and the last prevented by keeping the site as immobile as possible with tape for approximately 3 days.

Allergic reactions to the collagen component in Artecoll are rare (three in more than 4280 patients), but possible. These can be treated with intralesional triamcinolone injections. Telangiectasias can occur at the implantation site of patients with thin skin but they usually disappear within 6 months; if they do not completely resolve, they may be treated with lasers. Hypertrophic scarring has also been reported

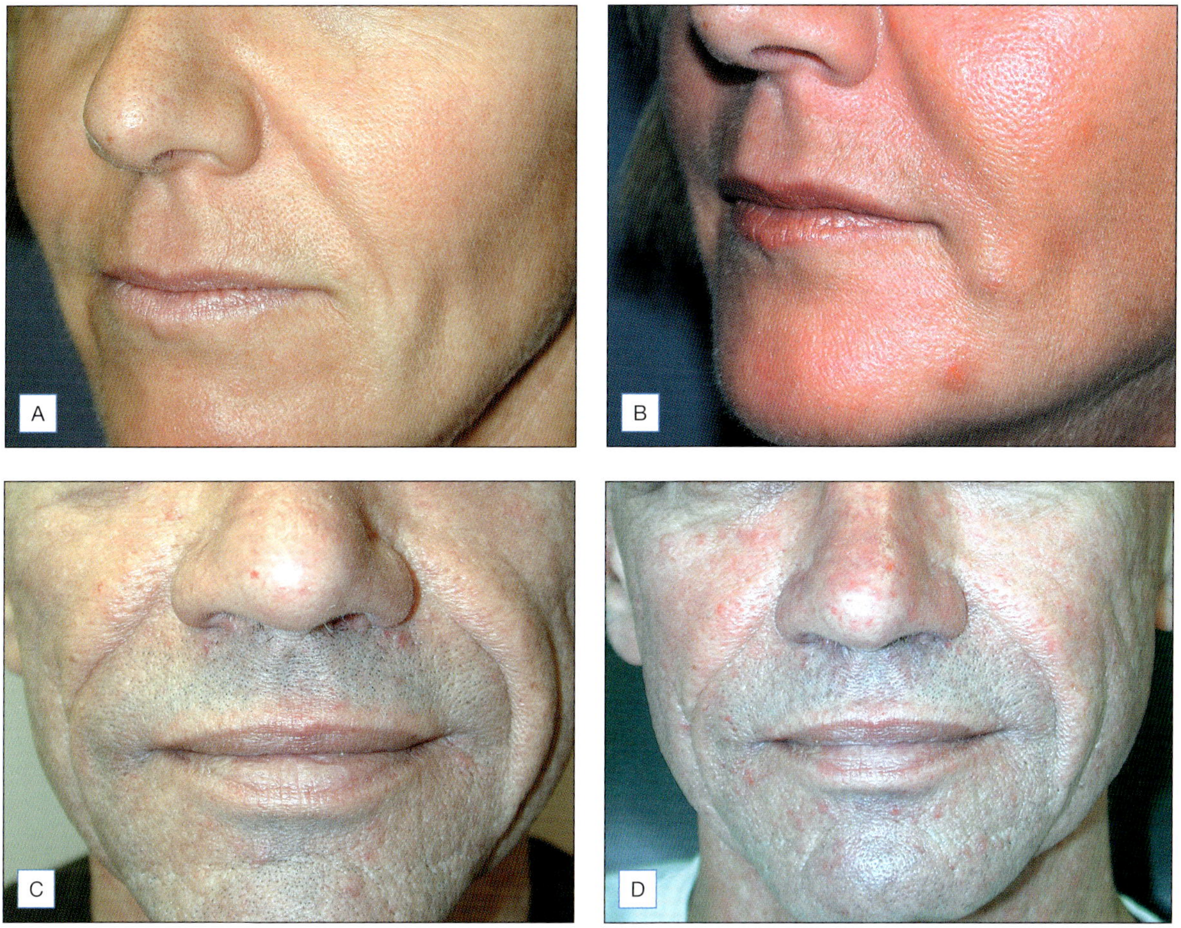

Fig. 7.3 (**A**) Pre-Artecoll treatment of cheeks producing softening of NLFs. (**B**) Post-Artecoll treatment of cheeks producing softening of NLFs. (**C**) Pre-Artecoll treatment of NLFs. (**D**) Post-Aretcoll treatment of NLFs

due to an overzealous version of the normal fibrous connective tissue response and can be treated with intralesional triamcinolone injections.

Finally, granuloma formation, though much feared and highly publicized, is rare and occurs in less than 0.01% of patients. No granulomas were reported in 251 patients in eight centers across the USA in clinical trials for FDA approval, although follow up was discontinued at 1 year. Granulomas typically appear 6–24 months after Artecoll treatment (Fig. 7.4) and differ histologically from the expected foreign-body reaction in that there is a wide distance between the microspheres filled with macrophages, giant cells, fibroblasts and broad bands of collagen fibers. The treatment of choice is a series of intralesional injections of corticosteroids. Local steroids work by inhibiting fibroblast and macrophage activity, thereby preventing collagen deposition, giant

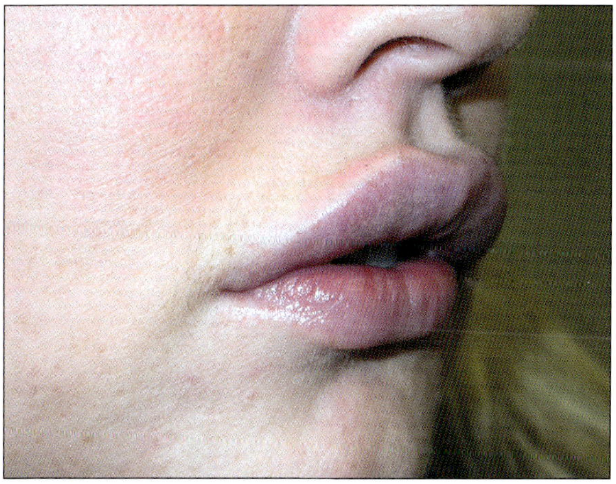

Fig. 7.4 Artecoll granuloma of the upper lip occurring 2 years after the third injection

cell formation and associated swelling, itching or pain. Up to 20 mg lidocaine and triamcinolone in a 1:1 mixture or 5 g betamethasone can be injected through a 1 mL syringe and 30 gauge needle into the offending nodule. Two to five injections in 3-week intervals may be necessary. Excision is also an option to remove unwanted nodules in the worst cases of granulomas, hypertrophic scars or dislodgement.

Radiesse

Background

Radiesse is a product made from calcium hydroxylapatite. Presently, it is approved in the USA for use in laryngoplasty and craniofacial defects. It has also been used in imaging procedures due to its radio-opaque nature. Its use for soft tissue augmentation is an off-label indication.

The product has gained popularity among some cosmetic surgeons because it offers the potential to serve as a long term soft tissue filler. Calcium hydroxylapatite is the matrix material found in both bone and tissue. The bioengineered product serves as a scaffold for native cells including osteoblasts and fibroblasts to form a permanent soft tissue correction.

History

Calcium hydroxylapatite has been used in urology as well as otorhinolaryngology over the past decade. When injected into the bladder neck or vocal cords, the material was found to be stable for years. In addition, no significant inflammatory reaction was noted.

In 2002, the material was used in Italy for cosmetic indications, and after the data was presented, Radiesse use in the USA began in earnest. Several plastic surgeons and dermatologists in the USA began to use this product as a facial cosmetic filler. Currently Radiesse FN is used off-label for cosmetic uses. In the summer of 2004, the name of this product changed to Radiesse in the USA.

Structure

Radiesse is comprised of two components: a gel carrier and the matrix particle. The aqueous gel contains glycerin, sodium carboxymethylcellulose and water. Not only are the vehicle components nonallergenic and nontoxic but the calcium hydroxylapatite is inert. These qualities are especially advantageous when compared with other semi-permanent or permanent fillers such as Artecoll/Artefill or silicone. Since all of the ingredients are nonallergenic, skin testing is not required prior to use. According to the FDA, all of the ingredients are classified as 'Generally Recognized as Safe'.

Each bioceramic sphere of hydroxylapatite ranges in size from 25–125 μ. During the manufacturing process, the spheres are washed free of any dust particles or nonuniform spheres. Molecular calcium hydroxylapatite is identical to the scaffolding of human bone and this material has a history of biocompatible usage in maxillofacial surgery and urology. According to Bioform, there has been 'no reaction from or rejection of the implant' to date.

The material comes in sterile 1 cc syringes and is a milky white suspension. Placement in the mid or superficial dermis (especially in light or thin-skinned patients) will result in visible material. Because of its viscosity, Radiesse has flow dynamics that are similar to hyaluronic acid when injected with a 25 or 26 gauge needle.

One other structural property unique to this filler is its radio-opacity. This is important when injecting around the mouth or other areas where surgery or radiologic evaluation is planned. Migration risk is minimized with this material since the structure allows for native tissue ingrowth once the carrier gel is absorbed. Prior to this ingrowth, migration is possible and care should be taken to minimize this risk when injecting, and in the immediate post-procedure period.

Mechanism of action

Once injected into the subcutaneous space, the gel is absorbed. What remains is a matrix of material that will take on characteristics of the cells that populate it. As the cells from the surrounding tissue grow into the scaffolding of the biomatrix they produce their respective materials. When injected into the subperiosteal space, the material stimulates production of bone. When injected into the soft tissue spaces, the fibroblasts produce collagen. This property of assuming characteristics of adjacent tissue requires precise placement of the filler in order for the permanent correction to occur – placement out of reach of fibroblastic ingrowth will mean that the permanent collagen will not be laid down or will be formed in the wrong location. Since the collagen produced is native and the material injected is inert, the filler formed has the potential to be stable and permanent.

Indications

Radiesse should be used for patients who have had good experience with other, long-lived soft tissue augmentation products. It should be used by physicians experienced with soft tissue augmentation using a variety of products including collagen, hyaluronans and fat.

Aside from allergy, which would be rare, there are no absolute contraindications. Caution should be used for first-time patients who may benefit from a material that has a shorter duration of effect, and is more forgiving.

While this is an off-label use of Radiesse, there are several specific indications. These include depressed scars including acne scars, deep NLFs, marionette lines, lips, and glabellar folds (Fig. 7.5A,B). Other less common areas include use for cheek and chin augmentation.

Duration of correction

There is not enough data to suggest that the material will be permanent. In one study evaluating the efficacy of Radiesse on NLFs, at 6 months patients rated their improvement as 2.53 (on a scale of 1–4, with 4 being the greatest improvement) while an independent physician evaluator rated the improvement as 2.87. This study suggests that there is still significant effacement of the NLFs, but that patients may require another treatment between 6–9 months to maintain the effect.

Patient selection

Given the potential for long term issues, patient selection is very important when injecting Radiesse.

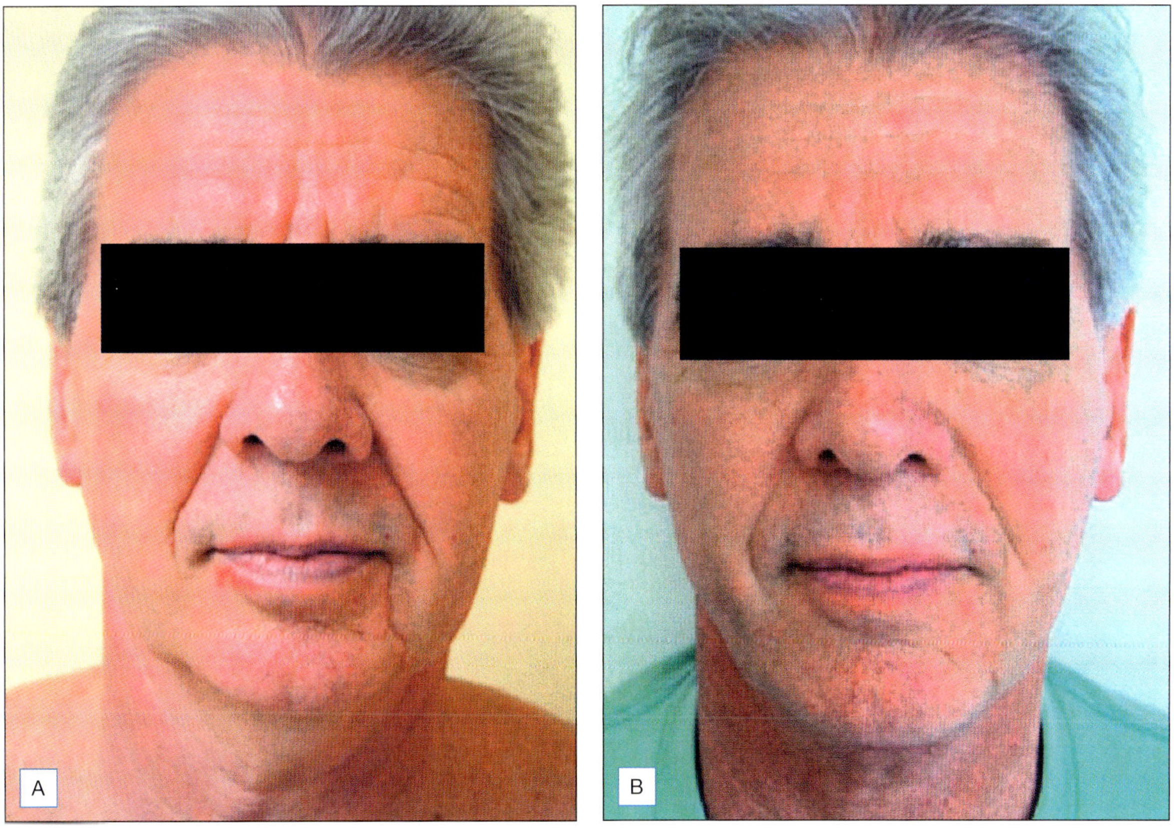

Fig. 7.5 (**A**) Pre-calcium hydroxylapatite treatment of glabellar furrow, NLFs and left mental scar. (Photo courtesy of Dr Greg S. Morganroth). (**B**) Post-calcium hydroxylapatite treatment (1 cc) of glabellar furrow, NLFs and left mental scar. (Photo courtesy of Dr Greg S. Morganroth)

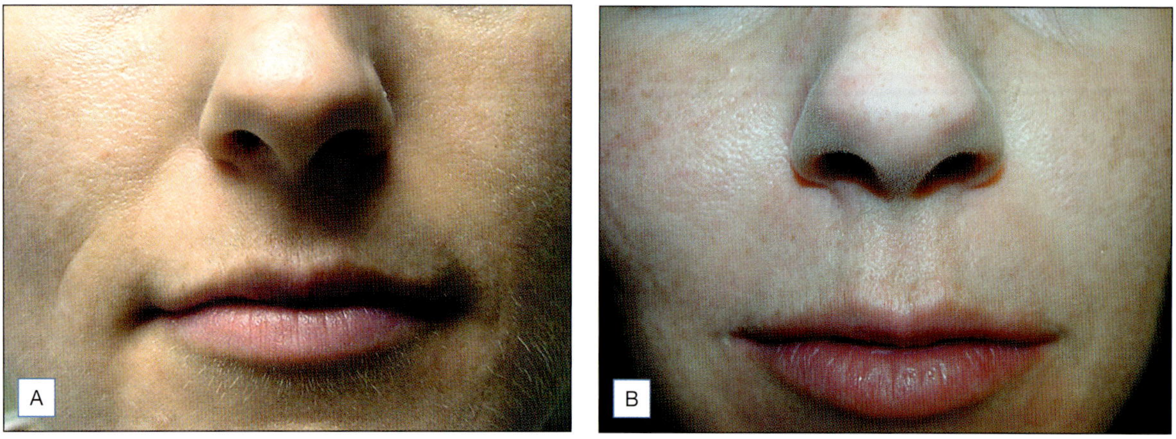

Fig. 7.6 (A) Pre-calcium hydroxylapatite treatment of NLFs. (B) 6 months' post-calcium hydroxylapatite treatment of NLFs

Specifically, patients should be in good health and not be pregnant. Prior surgery or trauma of the areas as well as prior injections with silicone are relative contraindications.

The most important selection criterion is realistic patient expectations and understanding of the limitations of the procedures. Patients who are going to be miserable if they can palpate the implant are poor candidates for the procedure, as are patients who expect a one-time injection resulting in a perfect and permanent correction.

An ideal patient for this procedure is someone who has had experience with other fillers, and due to its off-label use has had a previous relationship with the practitioner. This patient should have the ability to follow up should there be adverse effects.

Technique

When injecting Radiesse, a 27 gauge needle should be used to obtain even flow with low resistance. Alternatively, the RJ MaxFlow needle may be used. Prior to injection, LMX 5% should be applied over the site; a nerve block can be performed or local anesthetic can be infiltrated into the area to be injected. The advantage of the latter technique is that there will be less bruising due to direct constriction of the blood vessels. Because of the localized swelling and mild distortion, it is important to wait 15–20 minutes before injecting the Radiesse.

Nasolabial folds

Radiesse provides excellent results in NLFs (Fig. 7.6 A,B). Injections of Radiesse should be made using serial punctures with material deposited at the deep dermal–subcutaneous junction. Each injection should be made with about 0.05 cc of material. Injections are made as the needle is withdrawn and not as it is advanced. Typical quantities used for a moderately deep nasolabial crease would be about 0.5–1 cc. Obviously, deeper rhytides will require more material. Threading can also be used with Radiesse, though technically it is more difficult due to the importance of precision in injecting this material. Repeated treatment sessions should be planned for moderate or deep rhytides, with each session spaced about 6 weeks apart.

Marionette lines

Isolated marionette lines are also areas that respond well to treatment with Radiesse (Fig. 7.7A,B). Multiple 'rippled' marionette lines secondary to skin laxity may make placement more challenging. Injections of Radiesse should be at the dermal–subcutaneous junction. A serial puncture technique depositing approximately 0.05 cc per puncture is used to deposit the material. When injecting the marionette lines, care must be taken to support the corners of the mouth. A small amount of material (0.05 cc) may be placed in the lateral aspect of the lower lip to help support the area. The total amount of material required to treat moderately deep marionette lines is about 0.5 cc per side. Multiple treatment sessions approximately 6 weeks apart are used for optimal outcomes.

Lip

Radiesse should be used with great caution for lip augmentation and correction of both the upper and

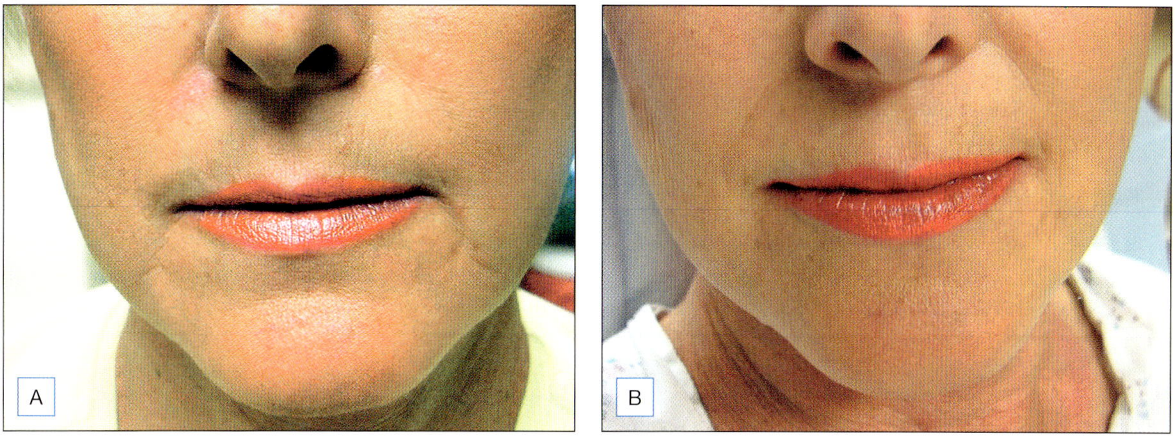

Fig. 7.7 (**A**) Pre-calcium hydroxylapatite treatment of marionette lines. (**B**) 6 months post-calcium hydroxylapatite treatment of marionette lines

lower lips. The constant motion of the mouth tends to cause migration of the filler. Additional potential problems include lumps and bumps that can occur in this area with frequency.

When injecting the lips, anesthesia may be obtained with a mucosal block using lidocaine with epinephrine. Dental gel applied to the mucosa as well as buffering of the injection will make the injections more comfortable.

The areas to be treated should be cleansed with surgical cleanser suitable for this area (dental preparation works well for lips). Consideration should be given to antibiotic coverage when injecting the mouth given the microbial content of the mouth and the permanent nature of the filler. For upper lip rhytides, a 27 gauge needle should be inserted, oriented away from the mouth. While withdrawing the needle, slowly fill each rhytide with material. Great care should be taken to avoid overcorrection. In addition, placement too superficially will cause visible bumps while deep placement runs the risk of being posterior to the orbicularis muscle.

Lip augmentation with Radiesse should be done gradually and with caution. Experience with other fillers such as the hyalurons and collagen is imperative for injecting Radiesse into the lips. To increase lip volume or definition, a serial puncture technique is recommended. Small injections utilizing about 0.01 cc of material are used to deposit material. The injections should be made along the vermilion border and placement should be above the orbicularis and in the dermal–subcutaneous junction. Most patients will require no more than 0.5 cc of Radiesse to treat both the upper and lower lips. Unlike other fillers, Radiesse does not require overcorrection.

As with other materials, the shape and anatomy of the lip need to be respected and the material should not be injected in a straight line across the lip. This type of injection (irrespective of the material) will make the lips look large but not natural.

Chin

Chin furrows and atrophic chins are good candidates for treatment with Radiesse. Preparation of the area is as described previously and anesthesia is obtained with local anesthetic. To fill a transverse furrow, serial punctures should be made with each depositing about 0.1 cc of material. To treat a moderately deep chin furrow about 0.3–0.5 cc of material is used. Treatment of an atrophic chin may utilize from 0.5–1 cc of material. For chin augmentation, the material is injected and gently molded with the fingers to form a symmetric chin.

A technique that works nicely in conjunction with Radiesse treatment of the chin is to use 2–3 units of botulinim toxin (Botox) injected into the mentalis. This additional injection will minimize the risk of migration of material.

Glabellar rhytides

Given the particle size and viscosity, great care should be exercised when using Radiesse in the glabella area if it is used there at all. Very minute amounts of material (0.05 cc) should be deposited in each serial puncture. The material should be injected as the needle is withdrawn and the correction should be to full correction but not overcorrected. When treating the glabellar region, it is recommended that Botox be used as adjunctive treatment to minimize the movement of the treated area and thereby decrease the risk of migration. The amount of material used for glabellar rhytides is about 0.25 cc for moderate rhytides.

Complications and treatment

There is remarkably little data on the complication rate of Radiesse when used for cosmetic indications. Most of the information regarding antigenicity and granuloma formation has been inferred from experience in other fields. To date, no antibody formation has occurred and there are no reports of hypersensitivity. Complications that occur vary by the area treated. For all areas, bruising and swelling are common (more than half of the patients will have mild or moderate bruising that is self-limited). Pain associated with the injection is also mild and can be treated with acetaminophen in most cases. In one series of 35 patients, there were no reported complications including infection or granulomas after injecting into the NLFs. There was mild bruising, and in several patients there was a mild erythema along the injection site that resolved spontaneously in 48–72 hours (Fig. 7.8).

The complications that are the most troubling to patients are persistence of palpable areas in the skin and nodule formation. Nodule formation that is mild and self-limited occurs in about one-third of patients injected. About 10% of patients will have nodules that require treatment with either intralesional steroids or incision and drainage using a number 11 needle. These complications should be considered when injecting Radiesse into the lips.

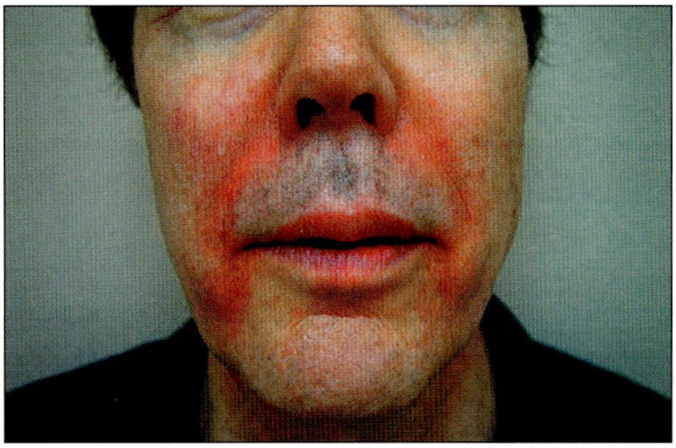

Fig. 7.8 Transient erythema 24 hours after injection of calcium hydroxylapatite. (Photo courtesy of Dr Greg S. Morganroth)

No reports of embolism or arterial occlusion have occurred yet in this application but these can be expected given the characteristics of the implant.

Dermalive/Dermadeep

Background

Dermalive and Dermadeep are semi-permanent soft tissue implants composed of acrylic hydrogel in a hyaluronic acid vehicle. Both products are essentially the same in constitution, however the acrylic hydrogel particles are larger in Dermadeep and used for pronounced tissue defects while Dermalive consists of smaller acrylic hydrogel particles and is injected less deeply into the tissue. Since 1998, Dermalive/Dermadeep has been marketed in France and the rest of Europe primarily for long term correction of facial lines and creating volume. It is currently not FDA approved for cosmetic use in the USA.

Dermalive/Dermadeep is a good alternative for bioresorbable materials such as pure hyaluronic acid or collagen because its effects are longer lasting. While the body absorbs the hyaluronic gel vehicle within 3–4 months, the nonbiodegradable acrylic hydrogel component reportedly remains for in excess of 12 months. The acrylic hydrogel and the tissue response to the implant, account for its long term effects.

History

Dermalive/Dermadeep (Euromedical Systems Ltd.), a by-product of the manufacture of intraocular lenses, has been used in over 150 000 patients in Europe and other parts of the world since its appearance on the market in 1998. In the only published clinical study focused on Dermalive/Dermadeep, 88% of 455 patients with an average of two injections per patient were satisfied after 3 years.

Structure

As previously stated, Dermalive/Dermadeep consists of two phases: a fluid carrier and a solid phase in 60% and 40% volumes, respectively. Both components are nonanimal in origin and therefore less likely to cause allergy. The fluid vector is hyaluronic acid, a linear polysaccharide of repeating disaccharide units, which is produced by *Streptococcus equi* in bacterial fermentation and subsequently purified for use. Hyaluronic acid is nonallergenic and is FDA approved and used in synovial fluid and wrinkle implants.

The solid phase of the implant, acrylic hydrogel, is a copolymer of hydroxymethylmethacrylate (HEMA) and ethylmethacrylate (EMA). HEMA and EMA have been widely used and well tolerated in other medical applications such as intraocular lenses and burn dressings. The acrylic hydrogel solids are polygonal, translucent and intentionally irregular in shape with smooth walls. The sizes of the particles range from 45–65 μm for Dermalive and 80–110 μm for Dermadeep — too large for phagocytosis. Extensive sifting and purification is done to obtain the specified geometry of the acrylic hydrogel fragments.

Dermalive/Dermadeep is packaged in sterile unit-dose pre-filled syringes in different quantities: 0.8 mL syringes with a 27.5 gauge needle for Dermalive and 1.2 mL syringes with a 26.5 gauge needle for Dermadeep. Its viscous consistency makes it easy to control and inject.

Mechanism of action

Dermalive/Dermadeep is a semi-permanent biphasic implant. Most of the hyaluronic acid fluid vector, accounting for 60% of its volume, is resorbed in the first 3 months following injection. The other 40% is nonresorbable acrylic hydrogel. The hydrogel particles are nonspherical in shape, preventing long-range migration and concentric fibroses, and are smooth-walled, promoting integration of the product into the body by acting as a scaffold for collagen fibers to form in a loose network around the particles. It is the laxity of these fibers that produces natural-looking results. In practice, approximately 50% of the implant remains after resorption, due to the development of new collagen around the acrylic hydrogel particles. This fibrotic reaction takes about 3 months, which is the recommended interval between injections. More than one injection of Dermalive/Dermadeep is often needed, with 3–4 injection sessions at maximum.

Indications

Dermalive and Dermadeep are semi-permanent filler substances best used in the long-term correction of natural or acquired skin depressions due to aging or trauma, or in the creation of volume. Dermalive should be used primarily to fill medium to deep skin depressions, such as the NLFs, glabellar lines, marionette lines, facial scars, and to enhance the borders of the lips and to correct skin adherence after rhinoplasty. Use of Dermadeep, meanwhile, is indicated only in the reduction of pronounced NLFs and creation of volume in the cheeks, sunken malar eminences and the chin.

Contraindications for Dermalive/Dermadeep implantation come in two forms—the first related to site of injection and the second related to the patient. Sites that are contraindicated for Dermalive implantation include the mucus part of the lips, the periorbital zone, horizontal lines across the forehead and vertical wrinkles on the upper lip. Patients who should not receive Dermalive/Dermadeep injections are those with a history of hypertrophic scarring, immunotherapy, autoimmune or inflammatory diseases, multiple allergies, and (rarely) known allergy to sodium hyaluronate or hyaluronic acid.

Duration of action

Dermalive/Dermadeep is considered a semi-permanent implant; its effects should last at least 12 months. While the hyaluronic acid component is resorbed, the nonbiodegradable acrylic hydrogel particles are left behind and induce a tissue response to yield long-lasting results.

Patient selection

Given the long-lasting effects of Dermalive/Dermadeep, prudent patient selection is important. Patients should be in overall good health and not pregnant or breastfeeding. In addition to the contraindications listed earlier, sites with previous injections of long-term wrinkle reduction implants (such as silicone, Artecoll, Goretex, etc.) should be avoided.

Patients who are good candidates are those with obvious wrinkle lines and folds with little excess skin. Those with thin skin would not be ideal for Dermalive implantation, as the risk of complications such as overcorrection, whitening of treatment site, and visibility of the implant is increased in such patients. Age is also a consideration—younger patients have a greater tendency towards scar formation. Finally, someone who has used more temporary fillers and achieved desired augmentation effects may be more suitable for the potential permanence of Dermalive/Dermadeep.

As with many corrective and cosmetic procedures, good communication between physician and patient and a mutual agreement of expectations is of primary importance. For instance, both parties should understand that it may take more than one injection of Dermalive/Dermadeep to achieve the augmentation effects desired and that the implant will be changing over at least the first 3 months. Thus the ideal patient is probably someone who is familiar and has a good rapport with the physician — someone who has tried temporary fillers with good results and is looking for something more permanent.

Technique

Since Dermalive/Dermadeep has no elements of animal origin and is generally nonallergenic, no pretest is required. Prior to injection, local anesthesia in the form of a nerve block (especially for work in the perioral region, blocking the suborbital nerves and chin) is usually indicated and at the very least an anesthetizing cream such as LMX-5 should be used.

The retrograde threading infiltration technique for Dermalive/Dermadeep is preferred. Correct placement of Dermalive is at the dermal–subcutaneous border. This area can be located by first penetrating the subcutaneous with the needle and raising it into the deep dermis. It is important to be careful not to inject too superficially or use the multipuncture injection technique. If Dermalive is injected too superficially in the dermis, overcorrection or blanching of the treatment site can occur, resulting in visibility of the implant. Multipuncture injection can lead to the accumulation of the implant at one site.

Dermadeep, meanwhile, should be injected into subcutaneous layer. Injecting Dermalive/Dermadeep too deeply presents little danger of complication; the main consequence in such a case is insufficient wrinkle reduction. Patients will typically need 2–3 injections, spaced at least 3 months apart to allow the previous implant time to stabilize.

Complications and treatment

In 2001 the global complication rate of Dermalive/Dermadeep was estimated at 1.2 per 1000 patients. Sixty per cent of those cases were felt due to improper technique such as injection too close to the skin surface or use in the presence of contraindications (i.e. (i) injecting in areas with previous injections of silicone or Artecoll, (ii) use in multi-allergic patients or those with autoimmune or inflammatory disease, (iii) overfilling, or (iv) not waiting for long enough intervals between injections). Reported short-term side effects after injection of Dermalive/Dermadeep are pain following injection, itching, discoloration, tenderness, palpable lumpiness, redness and edema. Most patients will not experience those side effects. However, in the estimated 25% of patients who have had or may experience side effects such as moderate to pronounced edema or redness, those unwanted effects should self-resolve within 1–2 days after injection into the skin and within 1 week for lip injections.

Delayed hypersensitivity, which can manifest weeks to several months after injection, to hyaluronic acid has been documented and would contraindicate further use of such materials. Another potential long-term side effect is migration of the implant from the intended site. In a study of 455 patients injected with Dermalive/Dermadeep and followed up to 3 years, no cases of allergy or migration were observed. However, localized hypersensitivity reactions in the form of redness, tenderness and rarely acneform papules have been reported in an estimated one of 2000 patients.

Long-term side effects include nodules, swelling or redness at the point of injection appearing an average of 6 months after injection. Serious complications like granuloma, superficial necrosis and uticaria are estimated at less than one in 15 000 treatments. In approximately 12% of cases, undesirable effects emerged during or following upper respiratory infections or psychological shock. Ten per cent of these cases spontaneously resolved with no treatment. The remaining cases were most often treated with intralesional injections of betamethasone. At the first sign of a nodule or other complication, a series of corticosteriod injections with an interval of 1–3 weeks between each is usually effective. Surgical excision is a last resort and rarely necessary.

Bioplastique

Background

Bioplastique is a permanent, biphasic, soft tissue implant. It consists of solid silicone particles suspended in a polyvinylpyrrolidone gel. Since its development in 1987, applications of Bioplastique in Europe and other parts of the world have included soft tissue augmentation in the face as well as other parts of the body, such as the hands or chest and treatment of urological conditions, i.e. stress incontinence, etc. Bioplastique is not FDA approved for use in the USA.

Bioplastique is a longer lasting alternative to temporary fillers, and its uses are quite diverse, even among permanent fillers. Injection of Bioplastique promotes a low-grade inflammatory response. That phenomenon, in combination with the nonbiodegradable nature of the silicone solid, produces lasting effects.

History

Bioplastique (Uroplasty BV, the Netherlands), was invented in 1987 by Drs Robert Ersek and Arthur Beisang III. Its development was built on the pioneering work of Professor Jaime Planas of Barcelona, who cut pieces of solid silicone rubber into very small pieces and injected them to correct soft tissue defects in his patients. Silicone itself has been used in soft tissue augmentation for the past 40 years. Together Drs Ersek and Beisang have published a number of studies on animals and humans, including a 6-year report on the outcomes of 127 cases, describing applications and safety of Bioplastique. However, there have been no controlled clinical studies quantifying efficacy and safety to date.

Structure

Bioplastique consists of permanent polymer (silicone) particles and a gel (polyvinylpyrrolidone) carrier in a ratio of approximately 3:2. The non-animal origin of the implant materials renders an allergic reaction unlikely. The biocompatible gel vehicle polyvinylpyrrolidone (CHNO) is a water-soluble homopolymer with an average molecular weight of 13 600 Da. It belongs to a family of polymers that have been used as medication extenders and vehicles for the past 50 years. Polyvinylpyrrolidone is absorbed and transported through the tissue and finally excreted unchanged from the kidneys.

Meanwhile the solid phase of the implant, dimethyl siloxane, or silicone, is a similar rubber-like polymer to that used in heart valves, vascular shunts, pacemaker leads, and nose and chin prostheses since 1960. It is a nonbiodegradable, inert substance. The silicone particles are spheroid and range from 100–600 µm (average 150 µm) in size to prevent migration to lymph nodes or other parts of the body and phagocytosis by foreign body macrophages. At this size they are also too small to be perceived as surface irregularities on palpation. These polymer particles are fabricated with a textured surface to promote tissue ingrowth upon implantation, which in turn prevents micromotion. Further, using textured particles is thought to reduce the rigidity of scar tissue and contracture by enhancing the symmetry of collagen formation around the particle.

Bioplastique is packaged into 1 mL syringes with blunt-tipped 20 gauge needles, four in cannulae attached to a high-pressure leveraged gun. The blunt-tipped cannulas are specially designed to push aside important structures like nerves, arteries and veins. The ratcheted injection gun delivers precise amounts of gel mixture in a dependable, predictable manner.

Mechanism of action

The permanent nature of Bioplastique is derived from the nondegradable silicone particles and tissue response to the implant. The gel functions as lubrication during injection, to evenly suspend and maintain some distance between the silicone particles and to prevent movement after injection. Within about 4 days, most of the gel carrier is absorbed and replaced by fibrin in the first stage of the host's immune response. Meanwhile, the body continues to mount a reaction to the foreign bodies, a process necessary for Bioplastique's long-lasting augmentation effects. The fibrin serves as an intermediate spacer and matrix during the 3–4 weeks it takes for fibroblasts to form collagen and collagen to organize around the silicone. The textured surface of the implant is designed to enhance the fibrous response and strengthen connections to the host. In fact the host collagen replaces the gel vehicle in a volume slightly greater than 1:1 and tends to expand over time, unlike other temporary and permanent fillers. With that in mind, care should be taken to always undercorrect the defect. Bioplastique may be used in multiple sessions to avoid overcorrection. The minimal interval between injections is 6 weeks, as most of the tissue's fibrous response will have played out by this time.

Indications

Bioplastique is a permanent filler substance with a myriad of uses within soft tissue augmentation. Indications for facial use include lip, chin and cheek augmentation, depressed scars, filling in glabellar lines, rhinoplasty cases of saddle noses, and repairing cleft lip and nose. Not limited to facial applications, Bioplastique can also be used in cases of skull defects, correcting areas of lipoatrophy and lipotrops from liposuction, pectus escavatum and hand augmentation.

Use of Bioplastique would be contraindicated in a patient who has had a previous reaction to any silicone derivative. Since the kidneys excrete the gel phase, it would not be advisable for patients with kidney disease to receive injections. Generally patients with a history of hypertrophic scarring, bleeding disorder, immunotherapy, or autoimmune or inflammatory diseases should avoid implantation with Bioplastique. Although Bioplastique is non-animal in origin and no allergic reactions have been reported to date, allergy testing prior to use is an option but not required.

Duration of action

Bioplastique is a permanent implant. Its silicon particles remain and generate a fibrous tissue reaction resulting in long-lasting effects. Thus, it is important to augment incrementally and avoid overcorrection because the results are not as easy to correct as prevent.

Patient selection

It is important to find the appropriate patient for Bioplastique implantation. Its effects are permanent and thus not easily reversed. Overall patients should be healthy and not pregnant or breastfeeding. Patients who have had a reaction to silicone or silicone-derived implants in the past or who show severe inflammatory reaction upon allergy testing would not be good candidates.

Patients who are suitable candidates are those who would like to make permanent the results they have seen with temporary implants in the past. Given the greater than 1:1 ratio of augmentation effect to injection volume, a patient with a larger volume defect would be fitting. Patients with thin skin would be at higher risk of complications such as overcorrection, whitening of treatment site, and visibility or palpability of the implant with injection of Bioplastique. The patient may expect to return 1–2 times for additional injections of Bioplastique to achieve desired augmentation results.

Technique

Bioplastique has no elements of animal origin and though an option, no pretest is required. The area to be treated should first be outlined with a surgical marker and thoroughly infiltrated with 1% Xylocaine and 1:100 000 epinephrine to anesthetize and constrict blood vessels in the treatment site. Subcutaneous bleeding must be minimized so as not to compromise the placement of the implant. A regional nerve block may not sufficiently anesthetize the area.

The skin puncture should be approximately 1 cm distal to the treated area. If the defect is a scarred area, as in cleft lip, insert a pencil tip trocar through the puncture site to create channels in the tissue. This can be done by passing the trocar back and forth on many different planes. Bioplastique should be primarily placed subdermally, at the dermal–subcutaneous border; care must be taken not to inject too superficially. The cannula is then inserted through the puncture site and passed back and forth through the pre-tunneled channels. As the cannula is withdrawn, injection should be done slowly with gentle pressure on the injection gun. Approximately one 20 gauge wide line of material should be injected into each channel. Once enough Bioplastique has been delivered to the channels, pressure is applied to the area between the puncture site and defect, and pressure released from the gun. The cannula is then quickly withdrawn, the defect is rinsed with local anesthesia and elastic tape is applied over the defect and puncture site.

If the defect area is not scarred, such as the uninjured lip for augmentation, then no pre-tunneling is required and the cannula is passed back and forth along the length of the lip and about the middle of the muscle. Again the key is to inject slowly as the cannula is withdrawn; subsequent steps are similar.

Each click of the ratcheted, levered gun delivers 1 mL, which can make a line 30 cm in length. Typical implant volumes range from 0.2 mL for upper or lower lip and 1–2 mL for cleft lip deformity nose to 45.5 mL in pectus excavatum.

Complications and treatment

In the study with the longest follow up of Bioplastique patients (up to 6 years) to date, Ersek et al found that in eight out of 127 cases (5%), the material had to be removed, presumably due to overcorrection. Two out of 127 (1%) cases had suspected infection although cultures were negative. The eight cases were felt to be caused by too much material placed too close to the surface of the skin, especially in the lip area. There were no reported incidences of particle migration or loss of substance.

At least three cases of foreign-body granulomas from Bioplastique injection have been reported. These manifested clinically as nodules that appeared weeks to months after initial implantation and were excised and confirmed on histology. In the event of a complication, it is possible to remove Bioplastique using sharp cannulas or biopsy needles and standard needle biopsy. Direct surgical excision is a last resort but also a possibility.

Further Reading

Alcalay J, Alkalay R, Gat A, et al 2003 Late-onset granulomatous reaction to Artecoll. Dermatologic Surgery 29:859–862

Artecoll product information website. Available: http://artecoll.com

Bergeret-Galley C, Latouche X, Illouz Y-G 2001 The value of a new filler material in corrective and cosmetic surgery: DermaLive and DermaDeep. Aesthetic Plastic Surgery 25:249–255

Bioform Medical product website. Available: http://www.bioforminc.com/US/Products/Radiance.htm

Brown LH, Frank PJ 2003 What's new in fillers? Journal of Drugs in Dermatology 2:250–253

Carruthers A, Carruthers J 2004 Polymethylmethacrylate microspheres/collagen as a tissue augmenting agent. Dermatologic Surgery (in press)

Consumer information website. Available: http://www.consultingroom.com/Esthetics/Products/Product_Display.asp?ID=54

Damrose EJ, Berke GS 2003 Advances in the management of glottic insufficiency. Current Opinion in Otolaryngology Head and Neck Surgery 11(6):480–484

Ersek RA, Gregory SR, Salisbury AV 1997 Bioplastique at 6 years: clinical outcome studies. Plastic and Reconstructive Surgery 100(6):1570–1574

Euromedical Systems Limited product website. Available: http://www.euromedicalsystems.co.uk/dermalive_euromedical.htm

Gladstone HB, Morganroth GS 2003 Evaluating calcium hydroxylapatite for facial augmentation. Presented at the Annual American Society for Dermatologic Surgery Meeting. New Orleans, LA

Hoffman C, Schuller-Petrovic S, Soyer HP, et al 1999 Adverse reactions after cosmetic lip augmentation with permanent biological inert implant materials. Journal of the American Academy of Dermatologists 40(1):100–102

Hubbard W. Personal communication. Bioform Inc, Franksville, WI

Kubo M, Kuwayama N, Hirashima Y, Takaku A, Ogawa T, Endo S 2003 Hydroxylapatite ceramics as a particulate embolic material: report of the clinical experience. American Journal of Neuroradiology 24(8):1545–1547

Lemperle G, Hazan-Gauthier N, Lemperle M 1995 PMMA microspheres (Artecoll) for skin and soft-tissue augmentation. Part II: Clinical investigations. Plastic and Reconstructive Surgery 96(3):627–634

Lemperle G, Hazan-Gauthier N, Lemperle M 1998 PMMA-microspheres (Artecoll) for long-lasting correction of wrinkles: refinements and statistical results. Aesthetic Plastic Surgery 22:356–365

Lemperle G, Holmes R, Larson FG 2000 Granuloma formation and electrical surface charges after Bioplastique and Arteplast implantation. Aesthetic Plastic Surgery 24:74–75

Lemperle G, Morhenn V, Charrier U 2003 Human histology and persistence of various injectable filler substances for soft tissue augmentation. Aesthetic Plastic Surgery 27(5):354–366

Lemperle G, Ott H, Charrier U, Hecker J, Lemperle M 1991 PMMA microspheres for intradermal implantation I. Animal research. Annals of Plastic Surgery 26:57–63

Lemperle G, Romano JJ, Busso M 2003 Soft tissue augmentation with Artecoll: 10-year history, indications, techniques, and complications. Dermatologic Surgery 29(6):573–587

Lupton JR, Alster TS 2000 Cutaneous hypersensitivity reaction to injectable hyaluronic acid gel. Dermatologic Surgery 26:135–137

Mayer R, Lightfoot M, Jung I 2001 Preliminary evaluation of calcium hydroxylapatite as a transurethral bulking agent for stress urinary incontinence. Urology 57(3):434–438

McClelland M, Egbert B, Hanko V, et al 1997 Evaluation of Artecoll polymethylmethacrylate implant for soft-tissue augmentation: biocompatibility and chemical characterization. Plastic and Reconstructive Surgery 100(6):1466–1474

Olenius M 1998 The first clinical study using a new biodegradable implant for the treatment of lips, wrinkles and folds. Aesthetic Plastic Surgery 22:97–101

Ozyuvaci H, Bilgic B, Firatli E 2003 Radiologic and histomorphometric evaluation of maxillary sinus grafting with alloplastic graft materials. Journal of Periodontology 74(6):909–915

Piacquadio D, Jarcho M, Goltz R 1997 Evaluation of hylan b gel as a soft tissue augmentation implant material. Journal of the American Academy of Dermatology 36:544–549

Requena C, Izquierdo MJ, Navarro M, et al 2001 Adverse reactions to injectable aesthetic microimplants. American Journal of Dermatopathology 23(3):197–202

Rudolph CM, Soyer HP, Schuller-Petrovic S, et al 1999 Foreign body granulomas due to injectable aesthetic microimplants. American Journal of Surg Pathology 23(1):113–171

Sclafani AP, Jacono A 2002 Soft tissue implants. Emedicine. Online. Available: http://www.emedicine.com/ent/topic730.htm

Sklar JA, White SM, Radiance FN 2004 A new soft tissue filler. Dermatologic Surgery 30:764–768

Waris E, Pakkanen M, Lassila K, et al 2003 Alloplastic injectable biomaterials for soft tissue augmentation: a report on two cases with complications associated with a new material (DermaLive) and a review of the literature. European Journal of Plastic Surgery 26:350–355

8 Management of the Lips and Mouth Corners

Jean Carruthers, Vic A. Narurkar

Introduction

The perioral region is an extremely important area for esthetic enhancement. With the passage of time, hereditary factors, photodamage, and smoking contribute to the development of the typical features of perioral rhytides, decrease in vermilion lip fullness, and prominence of melolabial and melomental folds in the context of gravitational ptosis of the lower face (Fig. 8.1).

Successful rejuvenation of the perioral region requires sophistication in the application of multiple technologies. Injectable biodegradable biologic fillers include collagen implants (Zyderm/Zyplast, Cosmoderm/Cosmoplast), nonanimal stabilized hyaluronic acids (Restylane/Perlane, Juvederm), animal derived hyaluronic acids (Hylaform Plus), polylactic acid (Sculptra/Newfill), and autologous fat. More permanent fillers such as Artecoll and perhaps Radiance, ablative, fractional, nonablative resurfacing and BTX-A injections are also important components of the therapeutic armamentarium for perioral rejuvenation.

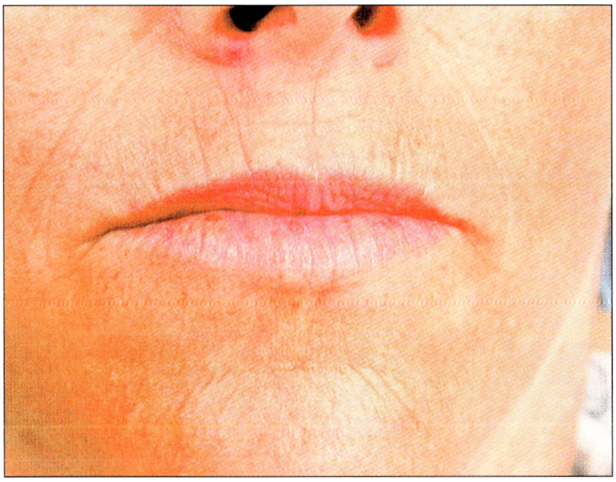

Fig. 8.1 Advanced perioral aging

The Glogau photoaging classification offers a rational approach to perioral rejuvenation. In general, the more advanced staging on the classification, the more common it will be to incorporate a plurality of treatments.

The problems being treated

The deflating vermilion lip is the most common concern for perioral rejuvenation. Photoaging, smoking and repetitive muscular pursing of the orbicularis oris combine with intrinsic aging to produce reduced show of the vermilion with superficial and deep lip rhytides (so called 'smokers' lines or 'lipstick lines').

Atrophic changes in the chin produce the 'apple dumpling' effect. Resorption of maxillary and mandibular bone as well as subcutaneous fat allows the mouth corner complex to descend, resulting in the 'mouth frown' and deep melomental folds, and hollowing of the chin behind the mentum and anterior to the jowls.

Patient selection

The selection of the appropriate patient for perioral rejuvenation is based on the extent of damage as described by the Glogau photoaging classification, the Fitzpatrick skin type of the patient, and the extent of associated bone and fat resorption. Semi-permanent fillers that do not require skin testing are usually suitable in all patients. In addition, subjects must disclose any tendency for herpes labialis and whether there are any other general health related issues, including allergy. Depending on the composition of the desired filler, skin testing may be necessary. Fillers containing bovine collagen such as Zyderm and Zyplast and Artecoll (Artefill) require skin testing, and approximately 3% of candidates have shown an allergic reaction to Zyderm. In addition, patients with known connective tissue disorders such as systemic lupus erythematosus are not suitable candidates for these implants. Nonanimal stabilized hyaluronic acid fillers do not require skin testing and show less than 1/10,000 incidence of delayed type hypersensitivity reactions. Semipermanent fillers such as Artecoll show overall complication rates of 3%. Patients with a known history of recurrent oral herpes simplex should be premedicated with systemic antiviral therapy such as valacyclovir prior to injection, particularly with deeper placed implants, as herpetic reactivation can produce epidermal compromise and atrophic and hypertrophic scarring. Individuals who are professional musicians or singers may need to consider the treatment and the initial effect it may have on oral expressive tone. There is no absolute contraindication for BTX-A injections for the perioral area but proper technique and conservative dosing is necessary to avoid asymmetry and unwanted facial paralysis. Lasers and light sources for photorejuvenation are highly dependent on Fitzpatrick skin type. Visible lasers and intense pulsed light with low cut-off filters (500–600 nm) should be used with caution in darker skin types for nonablative rejuvenation as there is significant overlap with melanin and this can lead to hypopigmentation and hyperpigmentation in darker skin types. Near infra-red lasers (1064, 1320, and 1540 nm) are the safest wavelengths for nonablative rejuvenation in darker skin but inadequate cooling may result in unwanted thermal injury leading to atrophic scars. Ablative laser resurfacing of perioral rhytides is not recommended in darker skin types and segmental ablative laser resurfacing carries the risk of post treatment unmatched pigmentation, even in lighter skin types, as the resurfaced region shows a difference in pigmentation (typically hypopigmentation) from the untreated skin.

Expected benefits

Table 8.1 summarizes expected benefits of the various approaches to perioral rejuvenation. Superficial rhytides are best addressed with BTX-A injections, nonablative rejuvenation, and superficially placed semipermanent fillers. The duration of these treatments is typically 3–4 months. These are ideally suitable in younger patients with limited damage. Moderate and deep perioral rhytides are best addressed with layering techniques of medium and deep placed longlasting fillers. Ablative laser resurfacing, manual dermabrasion/dermasanding, and chemical peeling is also a viable option but carries the risk of post treatment segmental pigmentary changes. Combination nonablative laser/light therapy and medium and deep fillers may be synergistic. The duration of these treatments is typically 4–9 months. The best approach to lip augmentation depends on the nature of the defect and the subject's esthetic desires. For genetically thin lips, structural augmentation with a deeper placed filler followed by volume correction with a superficial filler is ideal. For pure cosmetic enhancement of lips, a superficially placed filler with emphasis on the white roll and expansion of the vermilion is ideal.

The onset of benefits varies depending on the conditions being treated. Placement of fillers often produces an immediate result, although edema and bruising can temporarily mask the true correction. The onset of effect of botulinum toxin injections typically is evident at 2–10 days postinjection. Nonablative laser and light source rejuvenation shows a highly variable clinical outcome and multiple and repeated treatments may show clinical effects at varying intervals. Ablative resurfacing results in immediate epidermal and dermal injury which can take 4–6 weeks to resolve. The final results of ablative resurfacing may not be evident for up to 6 months following resurfacing.

Topical anesthesia (Ela-Max) is typically sufficient for most BTX-A injections, nonablative lasers and light sources, and selected fillers for lower melolabial fold augmentation. Infraorbital and mental nerve blocks and topical anesthetic are essential for most peroral fillers except collagen implants as

Approaches to perioral rejuvenation

Entity	Approach
Superficial rhytides	Botulinum A toxin injection Nonablative treatments Superficial fillers
Moderate rhytides	Medium and deep placed fillers
Deep rhytides	Ablative laser resurfacing and fillers
Lip augmentation—architecture	Medium placed fillers
Lip augmentation—volume	Superficial placed fillers

Table 8.1 Approaches to perioral rejuvenation

there is no anesthetic in the injectable material. For lip augmentation and lip rhytides, nerve blocks are essential. Ablative segmental resurfacing often requires sedation and/or general anesthesia if the entire face is also being treated.

Biologic fillers and BTX-A are the most gratifying in-office procedures as they produce consistent and reproducible results with little risk. The main disadvantange that patients express is the need for repeated treatments. Nonablative light and laser treatments are usually very safe and comfortable but in the perioral area have a lower patient satisfaction rate and are best performed as an adjunct to fillers and BTX-A. Ablative resurfacing produces more definitive and longer lasting results but the exaggerated healing time and risks make these procedures less popular.

The art of perioral rejuvenation involves careful patient selection, the use of the appropriate technology for the appropriate indication, and the use of combination therapies for a complete result. Often, combination of resurfacing, BTX-A and semipermanent fillers produces a more complete result. Thorough patient education with emphasis on realistic outcomes is essential for patient satisfaction.

Overview of Treatment Strategy

Treatment approach

An algorithm for perioral rejuvenation is presented in Table 8.2. Glogau photoaging classifications provide an excellent guideline to treatment strategies. Patients with Glogau type 1 photoaging typically have minimal damage in the perioral area. True rhytides are just discernible. Nonablative laser and pulsed light resurfacing may have some benefits for these patients, with the possible addition of BTX-A for very superficial vertical lip rhytides.

Patients with Glogau type 2 photoaging have mild to moderate vertical lip rhytides, early signs of vermilion atrophy, and some lower melolabial ptosis. Superficial and mid-dermal filler placements are appropriate for these patients with adjuvant laser and pulsed light nonablative treatments and BTX-A injections.

Patients with Glogau type 3 photoaging have more prominent vertical lip rhytides, further vermilion atrophy, and prominent melolabial ptosis. Mid-dermal and deep dermal filler placements, lip and chin BTX-A injections are essential with the possibility of lip augmentation with fillers. There is limited use of nonablative resurfacing.

Patients with Glogau type 4 photoaging have severe perioral rhytides, extreme lip atrophy, deep melolabial folds, and drooping and significant photodamage. The role of fillers and BTX-A are purely adjunctive in these patients. Ablative resurfacing, typically for the full face, is often warranted and surgical procedures are indicated prior to placement of fillers and BTX-A. These patients often require large volumes of fillers for complete correction of defects and therefore may not be suitable candidates for nonsurgical/ablative treatments as the primary modality for correction. Facelift may also be required.

Patient interviews

Careful patient selection and a detailed consultation are key factors for successful outcomes in any esthetic procedure. What the patient may desire may not be realistically possible and it is crucial to educate the patient about the realistic outcomes of perioral rejuvenation. Box 8.1 is a summary of a patient checklist and is a useful guide for consultation. An excellent approach during the patient screening process is to provide a mirror for the patient and

Algorithm for perioral rejuvenation						
Glogau type	**Nonablative technique**	**Botulinum toxin A injections**	**Superficial filler**	**Medium filler**	**Deep filler**	**Ablative resurfacing**
1	+	+	+/–	–	–	–
2	+	+	+	+	–	–
3	+/–	+	+/–	+	+	+/–
4	–	+/–	+/–	+	+	+

Table 8.2 Algorithm for perioral rejuvenation

Patient checklist for perioral rejuvenation

1. Synchronization of patient expectations and physician expectations
2. Detailed discussion of realistic outcomes of various modalities used in perioral rejuvenation
3. Detailed discussion of therapeutic options and their limitations
4. Detailed discussion of the time of onset, time of maximum benefit, and duration of treatments
5. Emphasis on repetitive nature of these procedures
6. Avoidance of the word 'permanent' correction
7. Education of ablative and surgical procedures when indicated
8. Discussion about maintenance treatments
9. Discussion of costs of procedures by a patient care coordinator in a discrete and private setting without the presence of the physician

Box 8.1 Patient checklist for perioral rejuvenation

elicit the patient's perspective of esthetic goals. This is particularly critical as the physician's perception of the esthetic goal may be different from the patient's perception. Once the therapeutic goals are established, a thorough explanation of treatment options is performed, with emphasis on the repetitive nature of these procedures. These include the onset of action of the various technologies, the duration of effect, and the appropriate intervals for treatments (Table 8.3). An atlas and diary of before and after pictures may be helpful but can often be misleading as they may convey only the optimal results. Patients seeking more 'permanent' options should be educated about the duration of these procedures, as surgical and ablative options for perioral rejuvenation also have their limits. We avoid using the word 'permanent' for any procedure. When there is hesitation about maintenance treatments, we emphasize how maintenance is part of any therapeutic goal, the same as for such as diet, exercise, and overall physical wellness. Once the consultation is complete, a patient care coordinator can discuss the costs and the patient signs a form which states they have been informed of the fees. A copy is given to the patient and the original form is placed in the chart. If the patient elects to schedule a procedure, an appropriate deposit is collected at the time of booking. It is critical for the physician to be removed from discussion of the fees and their collection and this entire process should be performed in a private and discrete setting with a patient care coordinator.

Treatment Techniques

We have outlined treatment techniques based on Glogau photoaging, which provides a useful guide to address the sequence and modalities of treatment. Table 8.4 outlines the Glogau photoaging classification and the treatment techniques suitable for the appropriate patient.

Glogau photoaging 1

This patient will typically present for cosmetic lip augmentation. The patient is advised to take arnica 2–3 days prior to the procedure to reduce ecchymoses and valaciclovir 2 g twice daily the day before the procedure if they have a history of recurrent oral herpes simplex. Anesthesia is first administered with topical anesthetic such as Elamax over the vermilion area. An infraorbital and mental block is then

Perioral rejuvenation summary

Approach	Onset of effects	Duration of effects	Potential risks
Botulinum toxin A	2–10 days	3–4 months	Asymmetry of lip
Nonablative treatments	6 weeks	Variable	Superficial blistering and potential for scars
Biodegradable fillers	Immediate	3–9 months	Edema, ecchymoses, allergic reaction, migration
Semipermanent fillers	Immediate	12–60 months	Similar to biodegradable fillers, granuloma formation
Ablative resurfacing	6 weeks to several months	3–5 years	Pigmentation change, erythema, infections, atrophic and hypertrophic scars

Table 8.3 Perioral rejuvenation summary

Glogau photoaging classification for perioral rejuvenation		
Glogau photoaging type	**Defect(s)**	**Treatment**
Any	Cosmetic lip enhancement	Superficial/medium depth fillers
I	Superficial vertical lip rhytides	Nonablative laser and pulsed light Botulinum toxin A
II	Superficial lip rhytides Lip atrophy Melomental folds	As above Medium depth fillers Medium depth fillers
III	Superficial lip rhytides Dyschromia/telangiectasias Moderate vertical lip rhytides Corner of mouth droop Advanced melolabial and melomental folds	As above Nonablative laser and pulsed light Medium depth fillers Medium depth fillers Deep fillers
IV	Deep rhytides	As above and ablative laser resurfacing (sequential and combination therapy)

Table 8.4 Glogau photoaging classification for perioral rejuvenation

performed with 1% lidocaine (plain or with epinephrine) (lignocaine) through the intraoral approach and a small amount is injected at the junction of the gum line and lip mucosa. It is critical not to distort the lip. Our approach is to utilize a medium depth filler such as Restylane for lip architecture. A 30 gauge needle bent at 45 degrees is utilized and a serial puncture technique is utilized (Fig. 8.2) inferior to the white roll in the vermilion border. For patients desiring additional volume, a more superficially placed filler such as Restylane fine lines or Cosmoderm is placed in the white roll with a 30 gauge needle bent at 45 degrees (Fig. 8.3). The philtrum and the angle recently identified as the Glogau–Klein point can be peaked for fullness. An ice pack is applied postoperatively. The patient is advised the volume of the lips may increase significantly and may not return to the expected size for 1 week. For patients who have an important event or social function and desire immediate lip augmentation, we limit the treatments to superficially placed fillers such as CosmoDerm and advise against placement of medium depth fillers. Prednisone 30 mg as a single dose after the injection, or possibly repeated once or twice, may be necessary in some individuals to reduce the swelling for the first few days.

Lip augmentation with fillers produces immediate results and has an outstanding patient satisfaction rate. It is critical to educate the patient about the degree of volume achieved by these procedures, as the immediate results are often disguised by edema. Some patients may experience anxiety over the nature of the edema and need to be informed

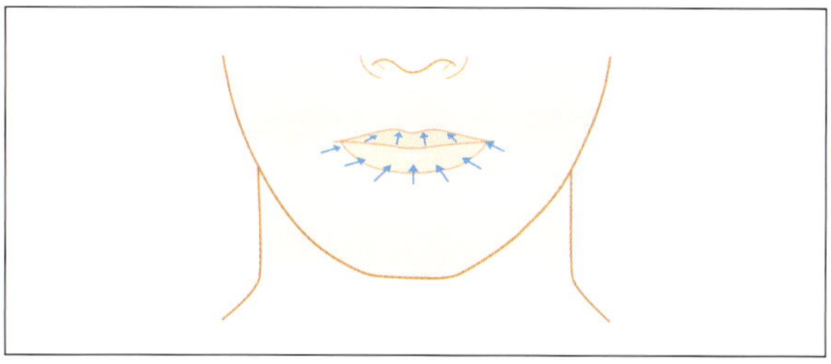

Fig. 8.2 Technique for lip augmentation for lip architecture. Placement of filler in the body of the lip using a serial threading technique

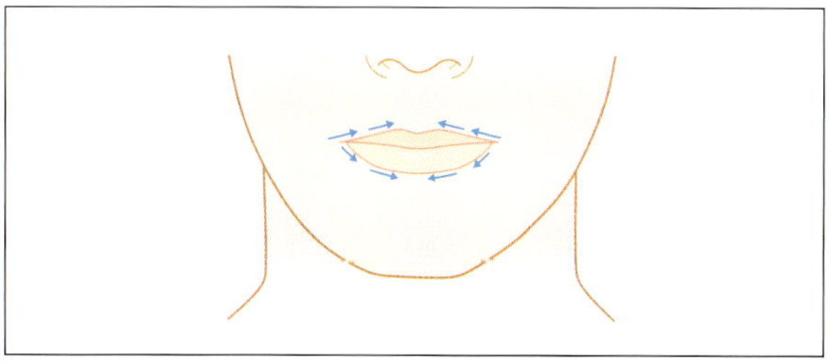

Fig. 8.3 Technique for lip augmentation for volume. Injection of filler in while roll (natural tunnel) at the junction of the vermilion border and the body of the lip

that this will subside in 24–48 hours. Our approach for lip augmentation is to be initially conservative and typically administer a single syringe of fillers for new patients and then reassess in 1 week if the patient desires additional augmentation. For patients with thinner lips, the layering technique is preferable, even in new patients, using vermilion placement of medium depth fillers and white roll placement of superficial fillers (Fig. 8.4).

Expected postoperative results of lip augmentation include edema and ecchymoses. Complications are exceedingly rare and include inadvertent intravascular injection resulting in immediate blanching of the site, exaggerated edema, hypersensitivity reaction to the filler, and herpetic reactivation. Careful technique can avoid intravascular injection, and if it does occur the lip with its superb collateral circulation is highly forgiving. Warm compresses, the use of Wydase for hyaluronic acid fillers, and close follow up is critical for favorable patient outcomes. Hypersensitivity reactions are also exceedingly rare and can be treated with intralesional steroids and pulsed dye/intense pulsed light treatments. Exaggerated edema can be prevented by postoperative ice, head elevation, and anti-inflammatory agents such as Celebrex. Herpetic reactivation can be prevented by preoperative treatment with valaciclovir.

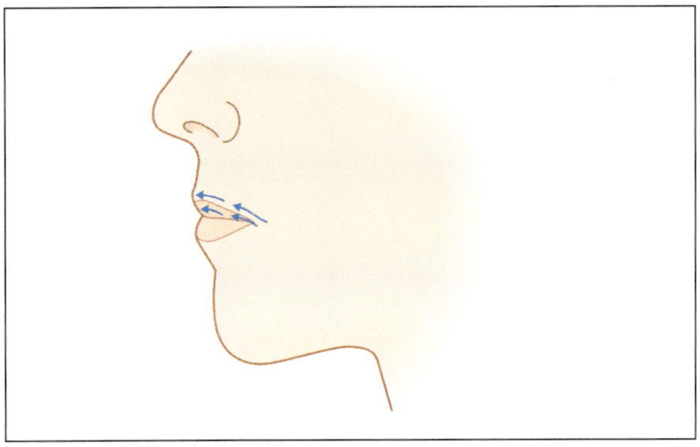

Fig. 8.4 Layering technique for lip augmentation. Superficial filler placed in white roll. Medium-depth filler serial threading into body of lip

Glogau photoaging 2

This patient typically presents with superficial vertical lip rhytides, some lip atrophy, and the appearance of lower melolabial fold drooping and superficial melolabial folds. The approach to lip augmentation is identical to Glogau photoaging type 1. In addition the vertical lip rhytides are more prominent. BTX-A injections will address early superficial lip rhytides. Topical anesthetic is administered with Elamax and 4–6 units of BTX-A are placed in the shoulders of the lip rhytides (Fig. 8.5) with a tuberculin or diabetic syringe. Often these patients may be undergoing nonablative photorejuvenation. BTX-A injections can be performed on the same day as nonablative rejuvenation. For more advanced vertical lip rhytides, placement of a filler is indicated and superficially placed fillers are ideal. Regional anesthesia is performed along with topical anesthesia and the fillers are placed with a bent 30 gauge needle directly into the groove of the

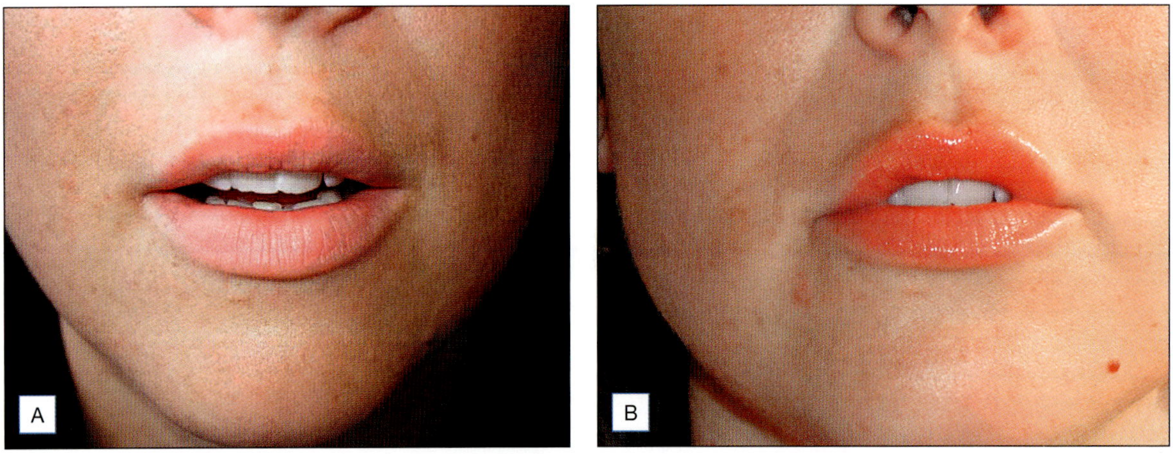

Fig. 8.5 Before (**A**) and after (**B**) photographs of Glogau type 1 photoaging for perioral rejuvenation

rhytide (Fig. 8.6). Overcorrection is not indicated. Simultaneous white roll enhancement and/or vermilion augmentation result in a more complete effect, as lip atrophy is often evident with the presence of vertical lip rhytides. Combination of BTX-A injections, direct filler injections into rhytides, and vermilion augmentation produce the most complete effect in these patients. The true efficacy of nonablative laser and pulsed light rejuvenation in this region remains controversial but may have synergistic effects when combined with the aforementioned techniques. The lower melolabial folds and chin drooping is addressed by injection of medium depth fillers and BTX-A into the depressor anguli oris (Fig. 8.7). Hyaluronic acid derivatives such as Restylane are ideal and the technique of fanning (Fig. 8.8) is performed to the corners of the mouth while a serial threading technique (Fig. 8.9) is ideal for placement of the filler in the lower melolabial folds. Both procedures utilize a bent 30 gauge needle which is directed medially. Gentle massaging of the material immediately after injection with a Q-tip for proper placement may be necessary for perfect results, but in general we aim to place the material in its final position rather than injecting and then massaging. Full correction of the region (Fig. 8.10) is an ideal postoperative result. The postoperative sequelae and care are identical to the treatment of lip augmentation.

The most common pitfall encountered in these patients is incomplete correction, thereby stressing the importance of combination therapies. If vertical rhytides are approached by direct injection of fillers alone, the results are generally unsatisfactory. Overcorrection of the rhytides results in patients complaining of lumps in the upper and lower cutaneous lip, exaggerating the problem instead of correcting it. The use of lip augmentation and vertical rhytide correction produce a more cosmetically enhanced perioral region, with the placement of the fillers in the white roll further enhancing the effects of vertical rhytide improvement. The addition of BTX-A completes the effect. If the sole concern is superficial vertical rhytides, we prefer BTX-A as the sole modality, as even the most superficial filler placement is difficult and may result in a worse cosmetic

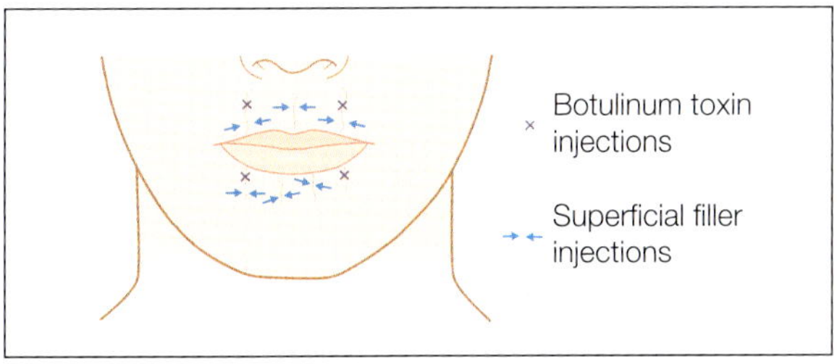

Fig. 8.6 Technique for vertical lip rhytides

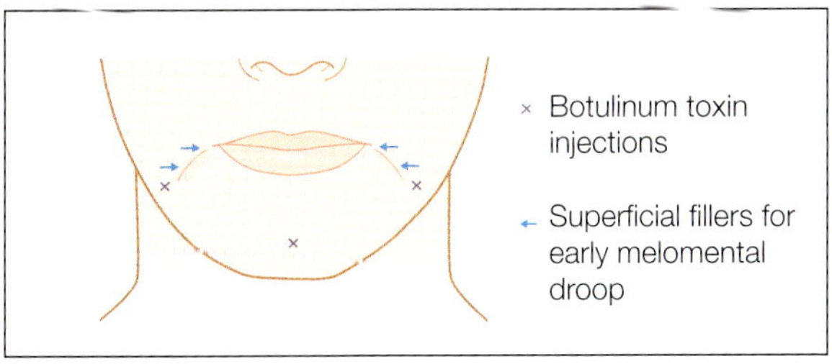

Fig. 8.7 Technique for superficial melomental folds and chin droop

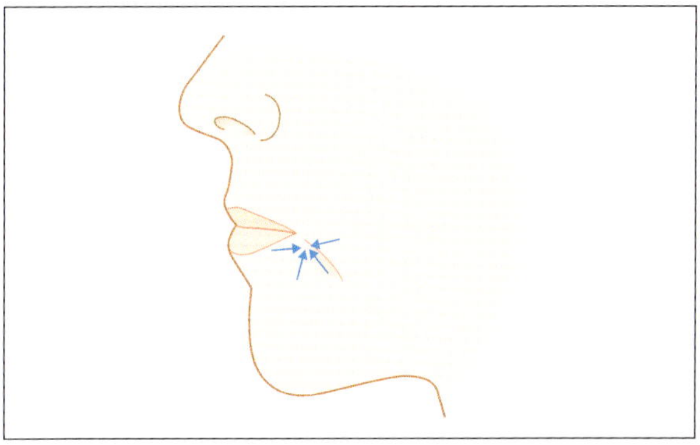

Fig. 8.8 Fanning technique for corners of mouth

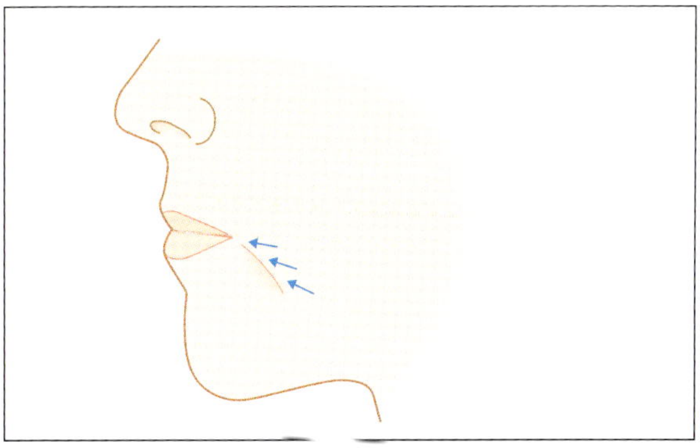

Fig. 8.9 Serial threading technique for melomental folds. Medial injection of filler towards melomental folds serial threading

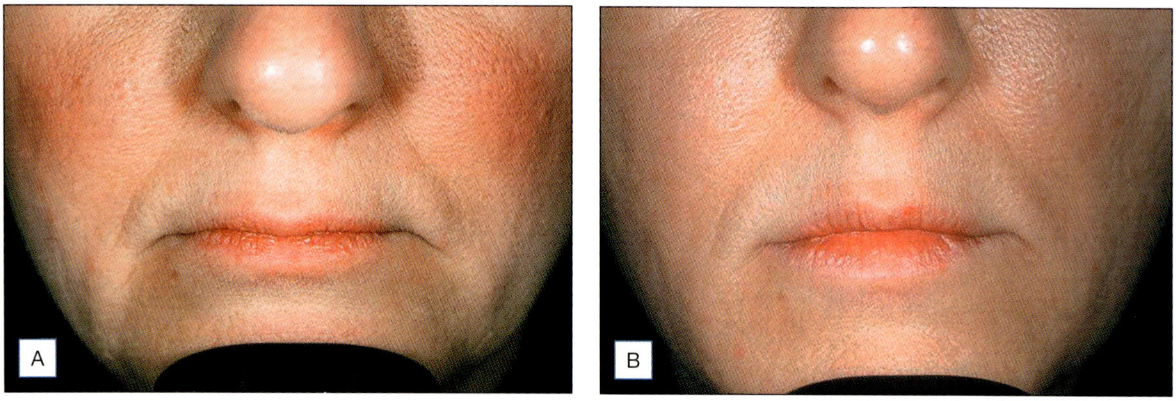

Fig. 8.10 Before (**A**) and after (**B**) photographs of Glogau type 2 photoaging patient for perioral rejuvenation

outcome. Treatment of melolabial folds and corner of the mouth droops have limited complications. Placement and correction of the filler are critical as many materials may migrate. Medially directed injections directly to the rhytide avoids lateral migration of the filler and gentle massage with a Q-tip to position the filler assures adequate placement. Inadvertent vascular injection of filler can be avoided with proper technique and is particularly critical in the lower melolabial folds to avoid intra-arteriolar injection. Use of small volumes, withdrawal prior to injection, and monitoring for tissue blanching prevents these outcomes. As placement is more superficial, inadvertent vascular injury is exceedingly uncommon in this region. Nonablative laser and pulsed light treatment of this region as a single modality is generally unsatisfactory. Typically, if photorejuvenation is being performed on the entire face, the perioral region can be treated on the same day with fillers. If longer wavelength lasers which may compromise the epidermis, such as the 1320 nm and 1540 nm lasers, are being used, we do not recommend same day treatment with fillers, as the potential for epidermal compromise with these lasers may result in undesirable outcomes with improper filler positioning, filler extrusion, and exaggerated healing sequences. We typically recommend waiting 1 week after these procedures to perform fillers in this region.

Glogau photoaging 3

These patients are ideal candidates for perioral rejuvenation with combination therapies. The chief concern in these patients is moderate vertical lip rhytides, significant vermilion atrophy, corner of mouth drooping, and prominent lower melolabial folds. It is critical to inform these patients that a multimodal approach is essential for complete correction and that adequate amounts of filler materials are necessary. These patients often have moderate photodamage and will also benefit from full face nonablative photorejuvenation.

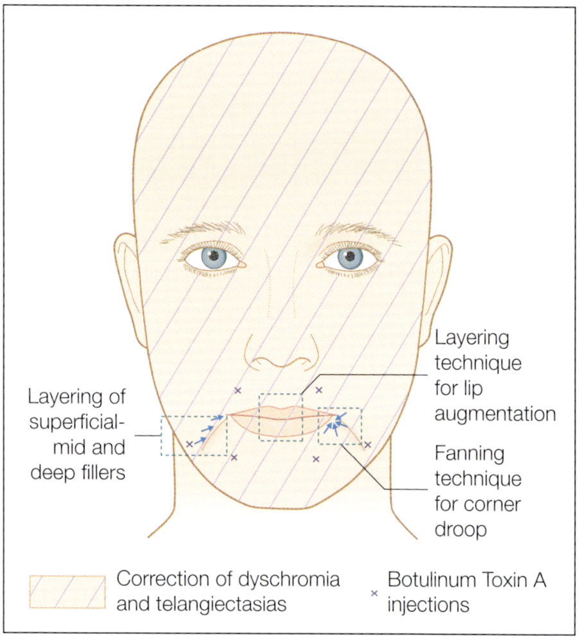

Fig. 8.11 Technique for perioral rejuvenation in more advanced Glogau photoaging type 3 stepwise approach

A stepwise approach to perioral rejuvenation in these patients (Fig. 8.11) is photorejuvenation to

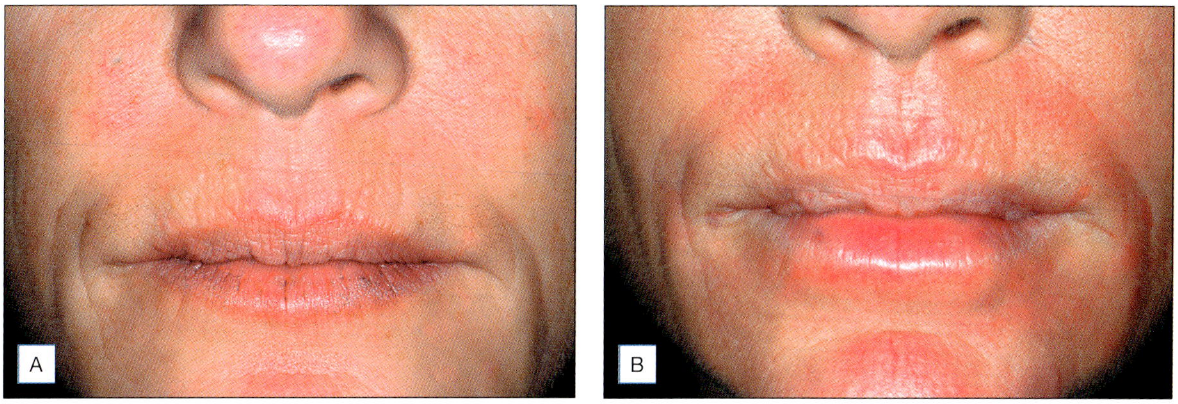

Fig. 8.12 Before (**A**) and after (**B**) photographs of Glogau type 3 photoaging for perioral rejuvenation

correct dyschromia and telangiectasias, BTX-A injections for hyperdynamic perioral rhytides, lip and lip rhytide augmentation with medium depth and superficial fillers, and lower melolabial folds and corner of mouth drooping with deep and medium depth fillers. We usually separate the photorejuvenation component and BTX-A injections from fillers, as these multiple procedures may be too time and cost prohibitive in a single session. At times, photorejuvenation is not indicated, as the primary focus is the perioral region where fillers and BTX-A may suffice alone. The interval between photorejuvenation and fillers is typically one week (Fig. 8.12).

In addition to the treatments for Glogau photoaging types 1 and 2, these patients have more exaggerated lip rhytides, further lip atrophy, very prominent lower meloabial folds, and chin drooping. Topical anesthetic and regional anesthesia are first administered followed by ice pack application. The BTX-A injections are performed first for the lip rhytides (4–6 units) and the chin (2–4 units). The melolabial folds are then addressed. Placement of the deeper filler such as Perlane is performed with a 27 gauge bent needle aimed medially, followed by layering with a superficial or medium depth filler. Typically two syringes of filler material are the absolute minimum requirement in these patients. The corner of the mouth is then treated with the identical fanning technique using a medium depth filler such as Restylane. The lip rhytides and lip augmentation is performed last, allowing the regional anesthetic to take its maximum effect. Some patients may not desire multiple regions within the perioral area to be treated at the same time. For these patients, we treat the areas that are most visible to them, typically the lower meloabial folds and chin drooping during the first visit, and then treat the lip rhytides and vermilion on a subsequent visit. This is particularly evident in new patients who have never been treated with any fillers. A conservative approach is best in these patients to familiarize them with fillers but it is critical to address all of their concerns.

While this category of patients is the ideal group for perioral rejuvenation, it is often the group of patients where undertreatment can result in patient dissatisfaction. The degree of rhytides is significant and therefore it is important to educate the patient on the synergistic approach of combination therapy. Often undercorrection is a pitfall in these patients, resulting in a high incidence of dissatisfaction. We often compare this with BTX-A injections in the male glabella where inadequate dosing results in an incomplete result. However, if the patient is focused on one particular concern (e.g. vertical lip rhytides), it is not unreasonable to address that defect initially and schedule a return appointment to assess the esthetic outcome and then address additional areas. The patient's expectations and the physician's expectations need to be synchronized.

The complications in these patients, in addition to those already discussed in the previous photoaging group, primarily deal with placement of the filler material. Layering of fillers is most critical in these patients, as the lower melolabial folds are quite deep and require the placement of a deep and superficial filler for complete correction. In addition, if the entire face shows photodamage and dynamic rhytides and the only area addressed is the perioral region, the results are generally unsatisfactory.

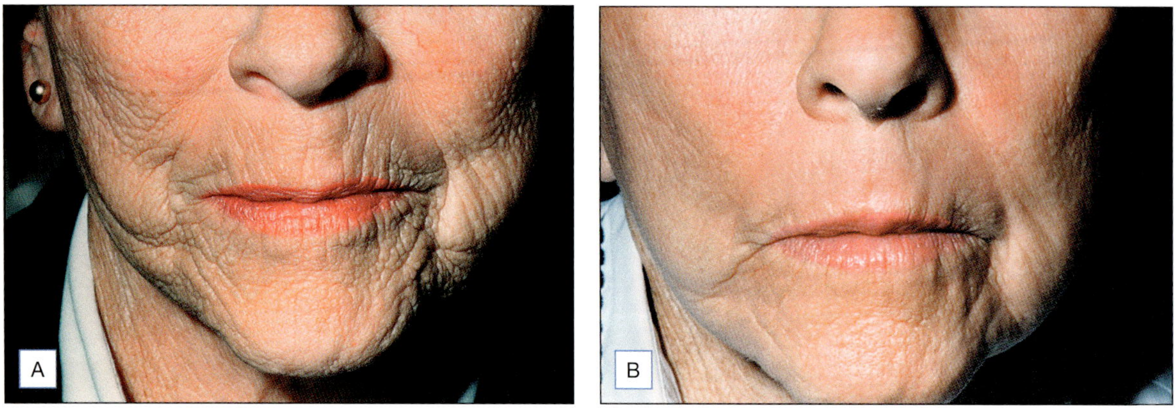

Fig. 8.13 Before (**A**) and after (**B**) photographs of Glogau type 4 photoaging of perioral areas for ablative resurfacing

These patients are ideally suited for a series of photorejuvenation procedures and BTX-A injections for the upper third of the face. Timing of perioral rejuvenation depends on patient expectations. Fillers can be performed after the first photorejuvenation as their duration is compatible with the duration of the series of photorejuvenation procedures, which usually consists of five treatments spaced 4–6 weeks apart. A more conservative approach is to introduce fillers after the final photorejuvenation procedure. This enables the patient to appreciate the dramatic effects of photorejuvenation, and establishes a relationship between the physician and patient to address the introduction of semipermanent biologic fillers as part of global esthetic enhancement.

Glogau photoaging 4

These patients are the least favorable candidates for noninvasive perioral rejuvenation as a single modality. They are best approached after definitive surgical and/or ablative procedures. However, they will often present for perioral rejuvenation as they have been misinformed about the outcomes. Thorough consultation and setting realistic expectations are particularly critical here, with the emphasis on fillers and BTX-A as adjunctive procedures. The approach to perioral rejuvenation is almost identical to those patients with Glogau photoaging 3, with the exception being that the minimally invasive procedures should be performed after definitive surgical and/or ablative procedures. The surgical approach is beyond the nature of this chapter and is discussed elsewhere. A subset of these patients benefits from ablative resurfacing prior to minimally invasive perioral rejuvenation.

Severe photodamage is best addressed with ablative resurfacing, of which pulsed erbium and pulsed carbon dioxide laser resurfacing are the most effective and precise modalities. Medium depth and deep chemical peels and dermabrasion are also effective by experienced physicians. The postoperative recovery of these procedures typically varies from 1 to 6 months and the final effects are evident after 1 year. Despite ablative resurfacing, the perioral region may still manifest significant areas that can be addressed with BTX-A and fillers. These include lip atrophy, persistent vertical lip rhytides, and lower melolabial folds and drooping (Fig. 8.13). We typically wait 6 weeks after ablative resurfacing to address perioral rejuvenation with fillers and BTX-A injections. A more conservative approach is to wait 6 months to 1 year, as that is when the complete collagen remodeling is evident, particularly with lip rhytide results. The addition of BTX-A injections and fillers augment the effects of ablative laser resurfacing (Fig. 8.14).

The main pitfall in this patient group is appropriate treatment. While fillers and BTX-A injections may have some benefit, the extent of damage is too severe for these to be the sole modality of treatment. As with Glogau type 3 patients, adequate correction and use of fillers is critical. For optimal results, these patients are best treated after surgery and/or ablative procedures and the ideal time for biologic fillers is 6 months after the resurfacing.

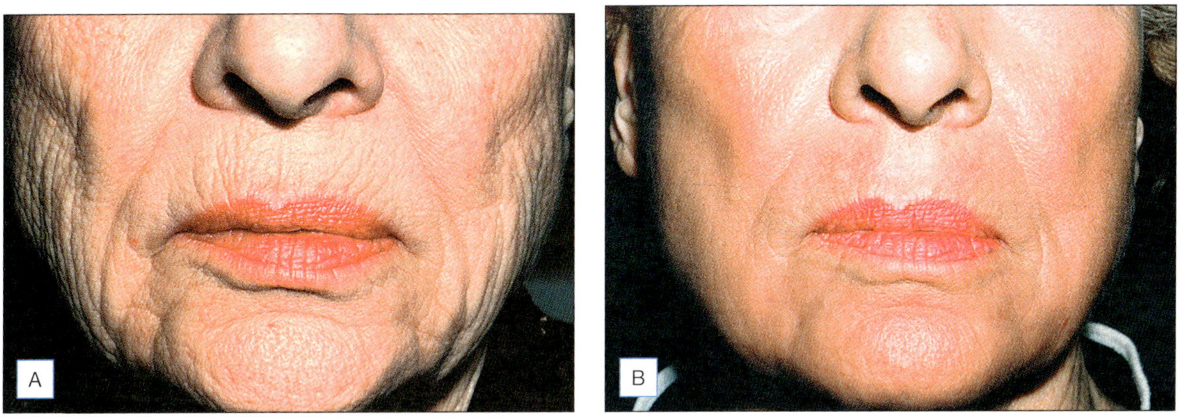

Fig. 8.14 Before (**A**) and after (**B**) photographs of Glogau type 4 photoaging with combination of ablative resurfacing, BTX-A and fillers

Conclusions

Perioral rejuvenation is approached by multiple minimally invasive procedures. Guidelines using Glogau photoaging classifications can provide a reasonable algorithm for appropriate procedures. Glogau photoaging 1 patients are primarily treated with structural fillers for lip augmentation and superficial fillers for treatment of fine lines. Glogau photoaging 2 patients are primarily treated for vertical lip rhytides, superficial melolabial rhytides, and early vermilion atrophy. BTX-A addresses isolated superficial vertical rhytides. Superficial direct placement of fillers and concurrent vermilion augmentation are indicated for vertical rhytides and lip atrophy. Superficial fillers address early melolabial folds and corner of mouth drooping. Nonablative lasers and pulsed light have a limited role as an isolated modality and produce better results when combined with BTX-A and fillers. Glogau photoaging 3 patients are ideally suited for complete perioral rejuvenation and benefit from higher volumes of correction and approaching the perioral area as an entire cosmetic unit. Deeper placement of fillers and layering techniques with superficial fillers produce a complete result in these patients. Glogau photoaging 4 patients should be first addressed surgically and/or with ablative procedures prior to minimally invasive treatments.

Further Reading

Baker TJ, Gordon HL 1979 Chemical peeling as a practical method for removing rhytides of the upper lip. Annals of Plastic Surgery 2: 209–212

Bjerring P, Clement M, Heickendorff L, Egevist H, Kiernan M 2000 Selective non-ablative wrinkle reduction by laser. Journal of Cutaneous Laser Therapy 2:9–15

Elson ML 1988 Clinical assessment of Zyplast Implant: a year of experience for soft tissue contour correction. Journal of the American Academy of Dermatology 18: 707–713

Friedman PM, Mafong EA, Kauvar AN, Geronemus RG 2002 Safety data of injectable nonanimal stabilized hyaluronic acid gel for soft tissue augmentation. Dermatologic Surgery 28: 491–494

Fulton JE Jr, Rahimi AD, Helton P, Watson T, Dahlberg K 2000 Lip rejuvenation. Dermatologic Surgery 26: 470–474

Gonzalez UM 1992 The sensuous lip. Aesthetic Plastic Surgery 16:231–236

Holmkvist KA, Rogers GS 2000 Treatment of perioral rhytides: a comparison of dermabrasion and superpulsed carbon dioxide laser. Archives of Dermatology 136: 725–731

Kesselring UK 1986 Rejuvenation of the lips. Annals of Plastic Surgery 16: 480–486

Lemperle G, Gauthier-Hazan N, Lemperle M 1998 PMMA-microspheres (Artecoll) for long lasting correction of wrinkles: refinements and statistical results. Aesthetic Plastic Surgery 22:356–365

Lowe NJ, Maxwell CA, Lowe P, Duick MG, Shah K 2001 Hyaluronic acid skin fillers: adverse reactions and skin testing. Journal of the American Academy of Dermatology 4:930–933

Sadick NS 2003 Update on non-ablative light therapy for rejuvenation. A review. Lasers in Surgery and Medicine 32:46–49

Semchyshyn N, Sengelmann RD 2003 Botulinum toxin A treatment of perioral rhytides. Dermatologic Surgery 29:490–495

Wall SJ, Adamson PA 2002 Augmentation, enhancement, and implantation procedures for the lips. Otolaryngologic Clinics of North America 35:87–102

9 Management of Nasolabial Folds

Gary D. Monheit, Betty A. Hinderks Davis

Introduction

The nasolabial fold (NLF) is the crease from the nose to the side of the oral commissure separating the cheek from the upper lip. Anatomically, the folds are the peripheral margin of the orbicularis oris muscle at the fusion of levator labii superioris medially and the zygomaticus major muscle laterally. The three branches of the levator labii superioris begin at the base of the nose, bottom edge of the orbit and zygomatic arch inserting into the skin of the upper lip. The zygomaticus major originates on the zygomatic arch inserting on the lateral mouth corner (Fig. 9.1). The repetitive action of these muscles over time contributes to the delineated NLF. As the zygomaticus major contracts and the lateral oral commissure rises to the cheekbone, a depression forms along the fold due to the bulging of the overlying cheek tissues. The NLF wrinkle gradually evolves from dynamic to static over time; as with any other rhytide, its axis always runs perpendicular to the direction of muscular pull.

In addition to the dynamic factor of the lip elevators muscles, other factors contribute to the evolution of the nasolabial wrinkle fold. This includes soft tissue atrophy including loss of skeletal muscle and fat. Loss of suspension of the pad along with skin redundancy expands the fold to a deeper groove. In addition, the loss of dermal elasticity and collagen support increases the development of photoaging wrinkles along the nasolabial area. Because the skin loses elasticity with age, gravity's pull is most effective along the lower face from the nasolabial groove over marionette lines and including the jowls along the mandibular margin. These are the major factors of the aging process – loss of soft tissue volume, repetitive muscle contraction, cutaneous ptosis from loss of support and photoaging changes of elasticity (Fig. 9.2).

The prominence of the nasolabial fold is a major change revealing mid-face aging. The fold has a dynamic stage in earlier life and a static appearance with aging. This is shown with the newborn face, which has no fold, as well as the paretic face in which the fold disappears.

Treatment efforts are directed to correct these problems as follows: volume ptosis, repetitive

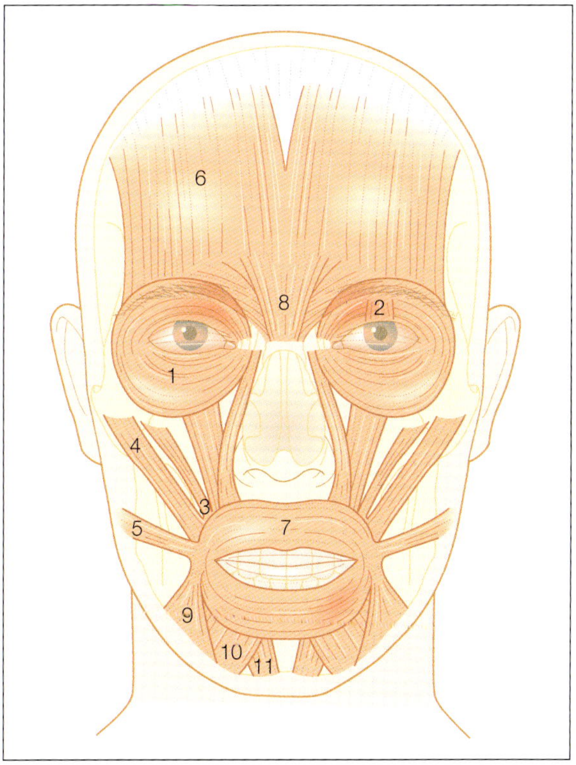

Fig. 9.1 Muscles of oral expression contribute to the fold. 1-orbicularis pars orbitalis, 2-orbicularis pars orbitalis, 3-zygomaticus minor, 4-zygomaticus major, 5-risorius, 6-frontalis, 7-orbicularis oris, 8-procerus, 9-depressor anguli oris, 10-depressor labii inferioris, 11-mentalis

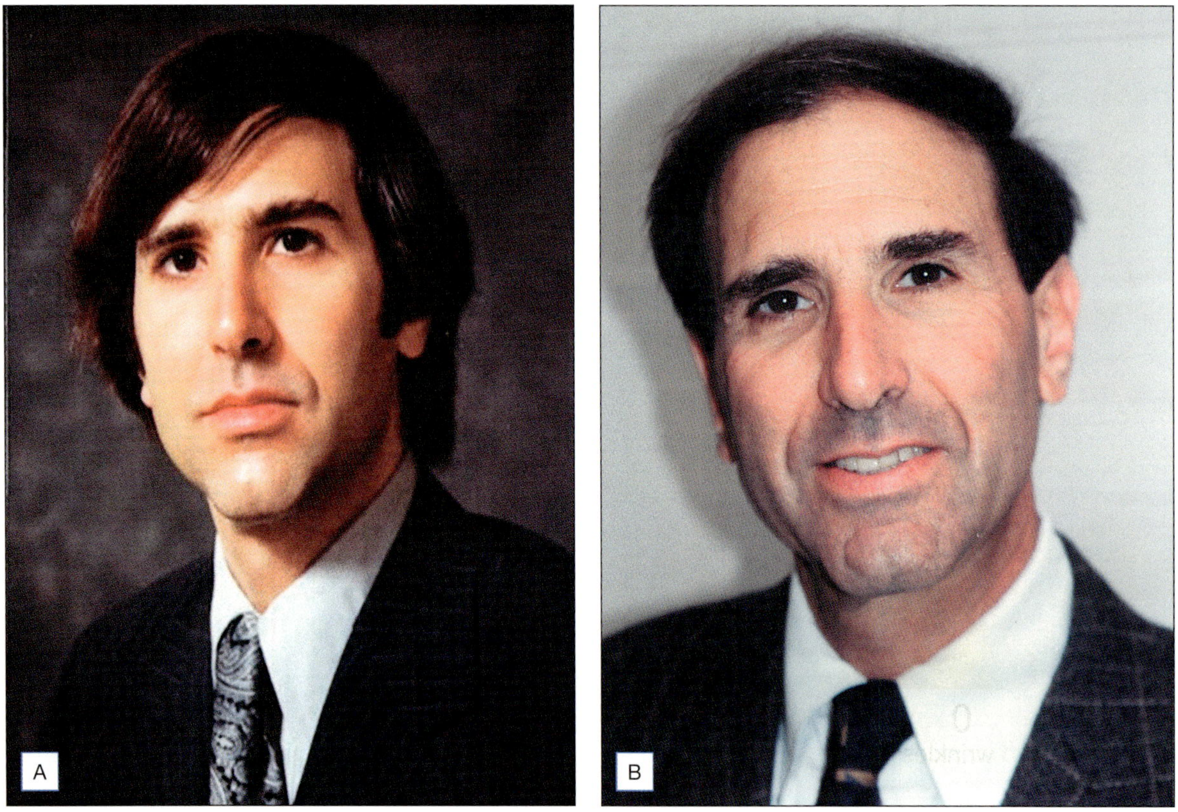

Fig. 9.2 (**A**, **B**) Changes in the NLF from dynamic expression to static ptosis: loss of soft tissue volume, repetitive muscle contraction, loss of support ptosis, and photoaging skin changes, elastolysis

muscle action and photoaging skin. Treatments are individualized in each patient relating to the degree of change within the fold and associated factors. This chapter will concentrate on volume correction with injectable fillers as this is the most common such treatment–correction. The other techniques will also be mentioned such as surgical corrections, resurfacing, and muscle relaxation with botulinum toxin (Botox), which can be a help as an adjunctive factor.

The gradual evolution of the NLF wrinkle from absence in the 20s, though mild and moderate grooves in the 30s and 40s to final severe grooves parallels the aging process. Quantitative scales of NLF prominence have been used to demonstrate the full evolution and guide the physician to proper therapy. The Genzyme 6-point scale is an example of a measuring stick to determine groove level on a 0–5 severity level (Fig. 9.3). Early changes – 0 to 1 – are mainly dynamic as the fold is only exhibited with movement (Fig. 9.4). Moderate fold prominence exhibits malar fat pad depression at rest and is present because of early fat atrophy (Fig. 9.5). These individuals will get full correction with volume filling (Fig. 9.6). The more severe forms involve ptosis as well as volume loss and may not obtain the same degree of correction with injectable filling alone (Fig. 9.7). These subjects may require face-lifting procedures.

Patient Selection

When a patient seeks cosmetic treatment, it is important that they have realistic expectations. First of all, the physician needs to understand what the patient perceives as their chief esthetic concern. After this is accomplished, the physician should begin educating the patient as to the etiology and available treatment options. Changes in the skin due to inherent aging, actinic damage, and loss of subcutaneous tissue are variables different in each patient. This review is best done while a patient is looking into a mirror and subsequently reviewing the photographs.

Different treatment is required for each separate issue – rhytids caused by recurrent movement versus

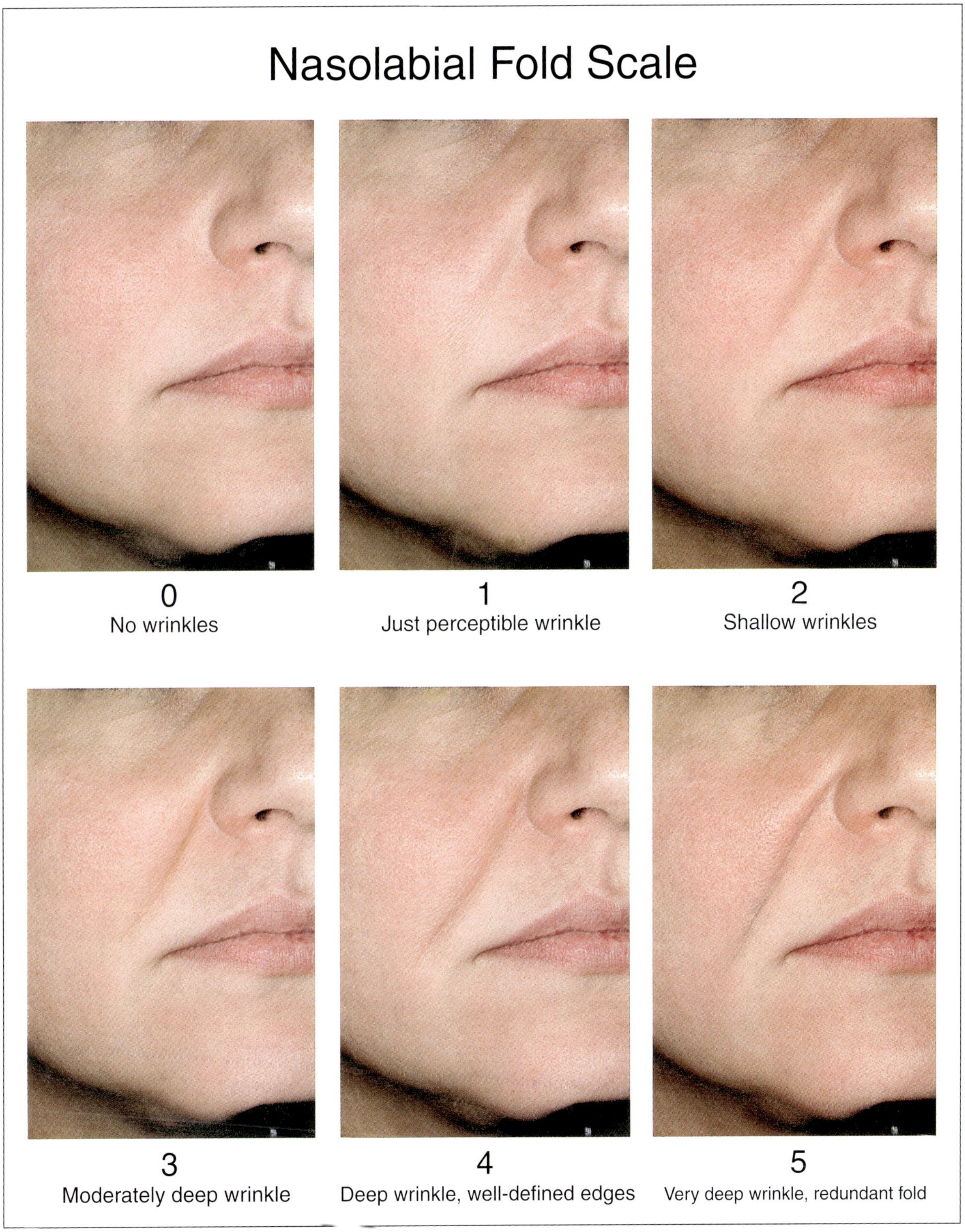

Fig. 9.3 Levels of NLF prominence: The Genzyme 6-point scale. With permission of Genzyme Corporation

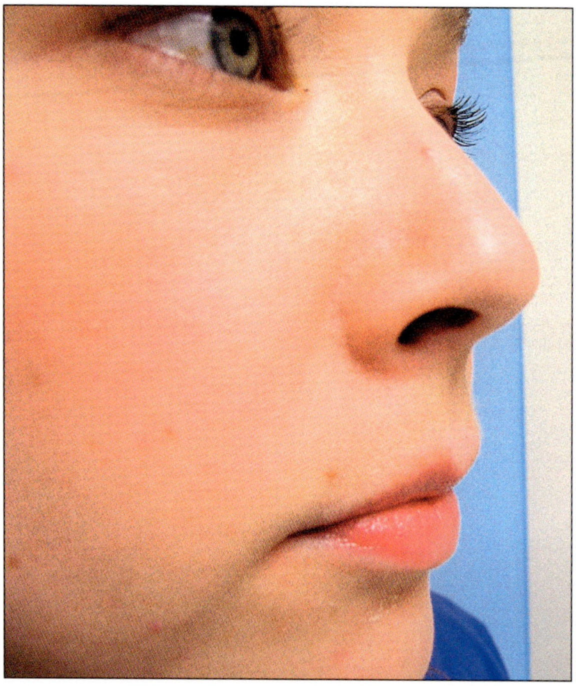

Fig. 9.4 Dynamic phase of the NLF

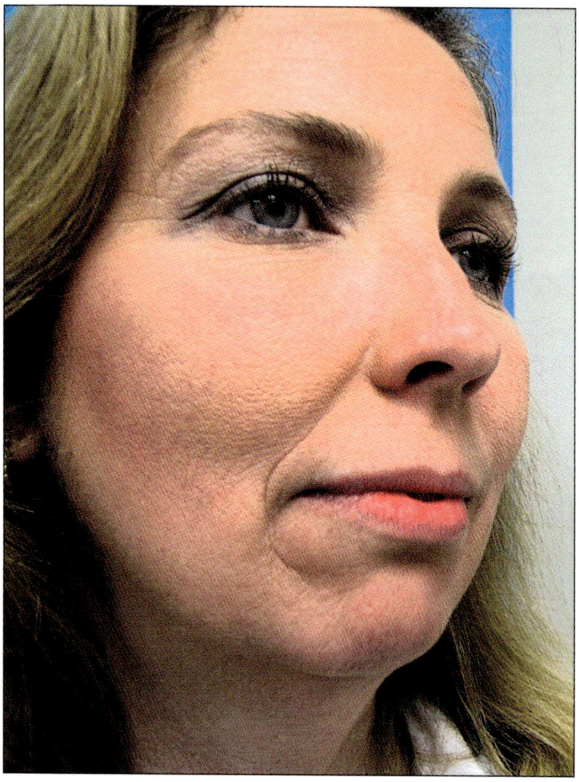

Fig. 9.6 Moderate to severe NLF with wrinkles from photoaging skin

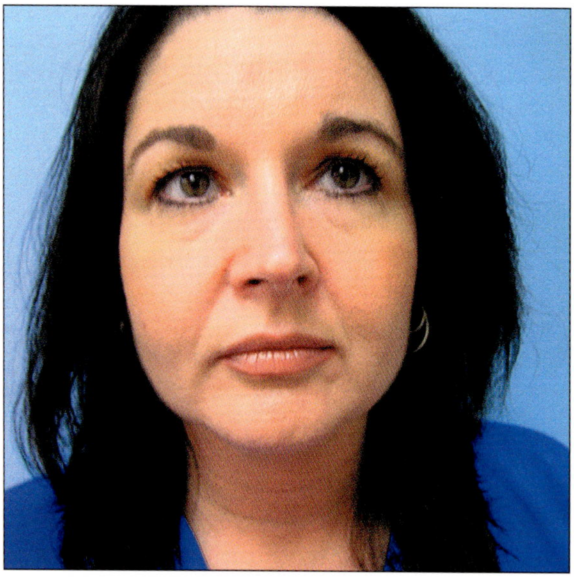

Fig. 9.5 Moderate fold at rest

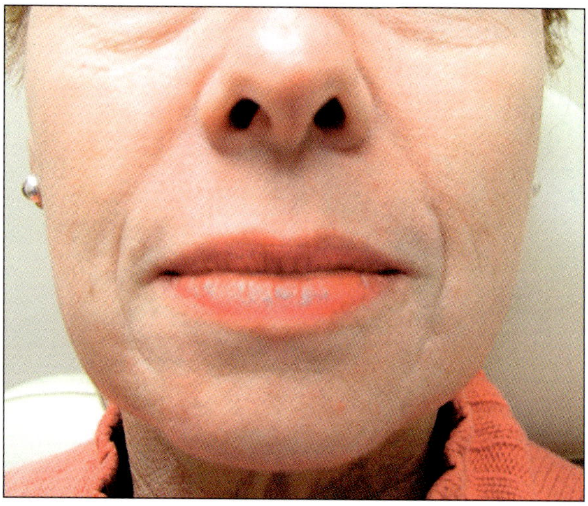

Fig. 9.7 Severe NLF with malar fat pad ptosis

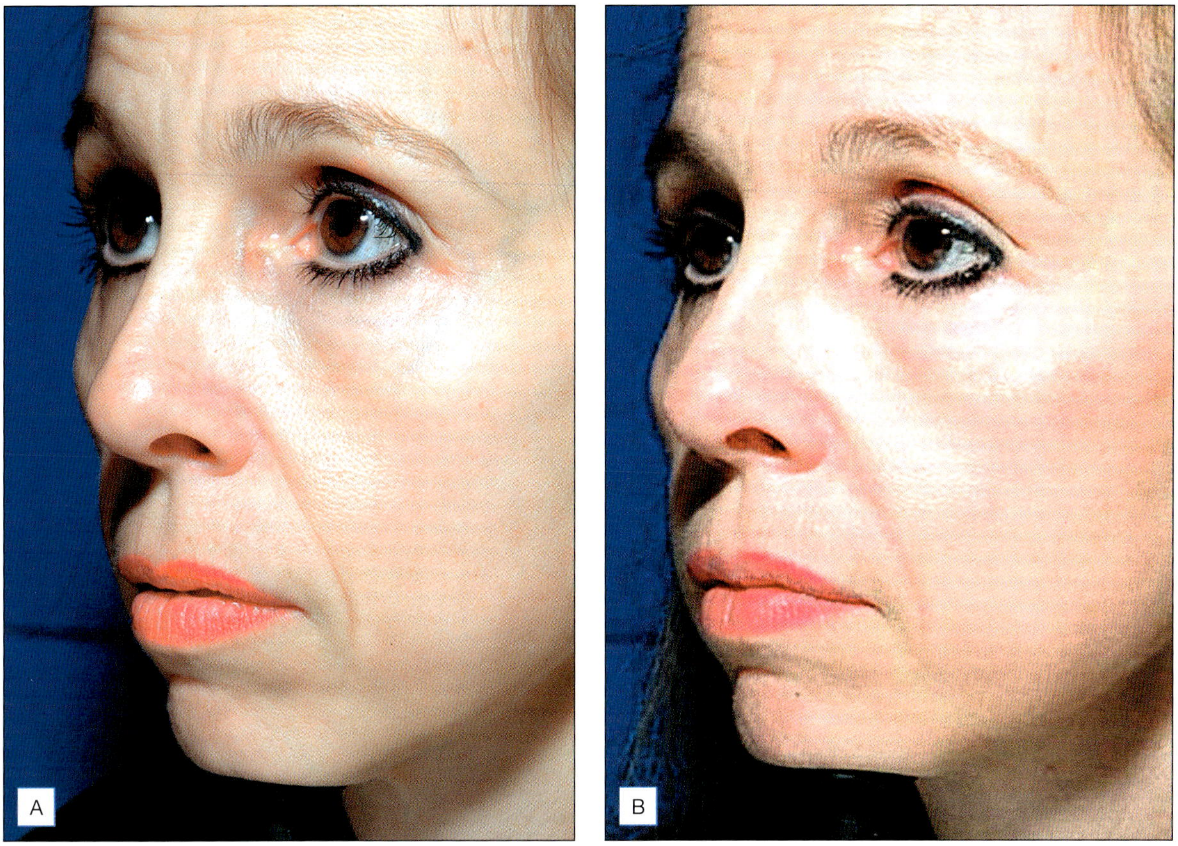

Fig. 9.8 Severe NLF with malar fat pad ptosis treated with Restylane filler and featherlift cheek suspension. (**A**) Before. (**B**) After

changes in the skin caused by increased laxity and gravity. When patients focus on prominent NLFs, it is best to begin with simple procedures that have little risk or down time. Progression to more invasive procedures that require time for recovery is usual.

The ideal patient for soft tissue augmentation of NLFs is a patient with moderate to moderately severe NLFs who wants smoothing of the contour of the mid-face, who understands the risks and benefits of the procedure, and who has realistic expectations. If a patient wants improvement more than soft tissue augmentation can offer or has a prominent cheek overhanging the NLF, a better option may be a facelift or a feather lift (Fig. 9.8). On the other hand, a patient who has almost no perceivable signs of skin aging and wants augmentation may better be treated with a good skin care regimen and possibly a noninvasive laser or microdermabrasion procedure.

Procedures for correction of the nasolabial groove concentrate on the four major causes. The dynamic phase of wrinkles in many areas is corrected with Botox. The use of Botox in the perioral area in inexperienced hands may result in severe side effects by interfering with both function and expression. Inexperienced treatment may create an asymmetric paretic appearance and thus should be used with care around the zygomaticus, levator labii or orbicularis oris muscles. Botulinum toxin A (BTX-A) can be used in the depressor anguli oris to elevate the lateral commissure as an adjunct to the insertion of filling material in the lower NLF and marionette lines. Two to five units of Botox (Botox Cosmetic, Allergan) are injected into the section of the depressor muscle just above the mandible. This procedure will give moderate enhancement of the filler esthetic (Fig. 9.9). Volume depletion may be corrected with injectable and surgically implanted filling materials. These may be temporary or permanent injectables including autologous fat, and solid implants. These procedures will be reviewed in detail for use in the NLF as volume replacement is the primary method of NLF correction.

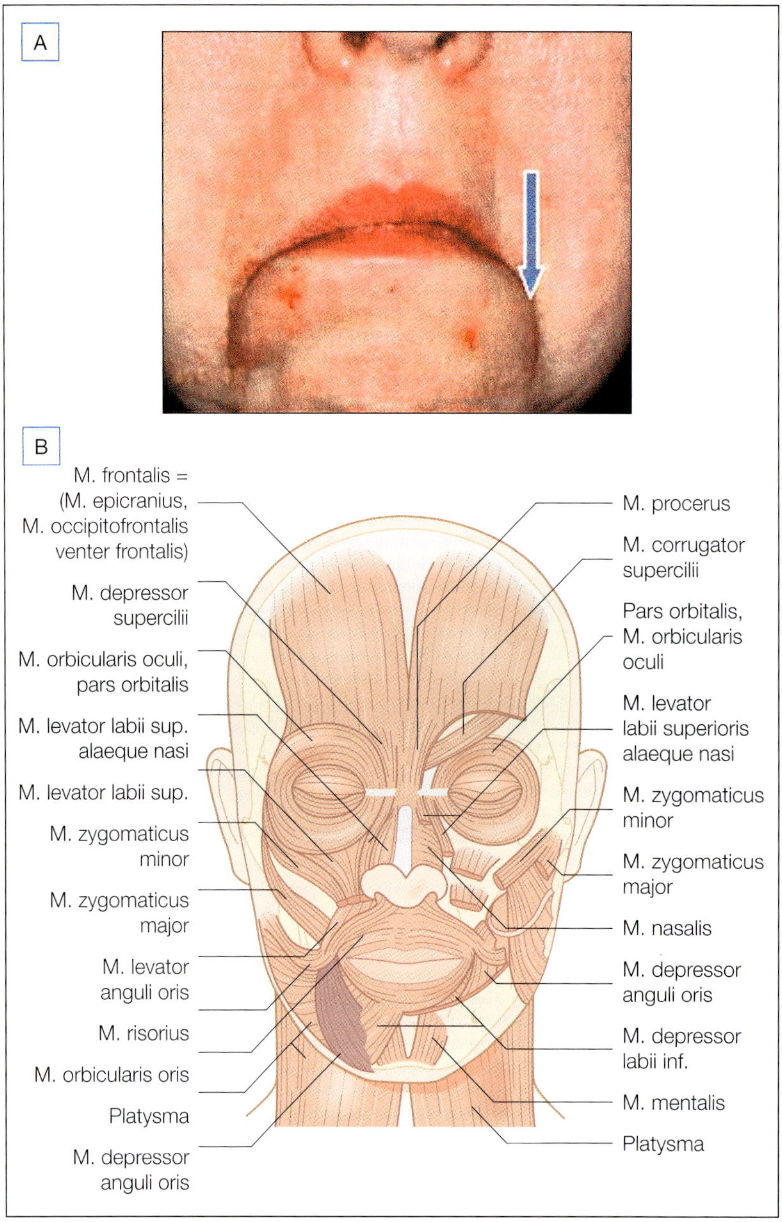

Fig. 9.9 Botox as an adjunctive procedure for the NLF and lateral lip groove

Ptosis of the medial cheek is the most difficult factor to correct and may require a surgical approach. These include mid-face lifting procedures such as subperiosteal mid-facelifts, endoscopic malar fat pad elevation, cable-suture fat pad elevations and short incision or traditional incision facelift. The technique of Sulamanidze – Aptos Threads – offers a novel nonsurgical approach to malar fat pad lifting to further correct severe NLFs. It is most commonly used in combination with injectable fillers (Fig. 9.10).

Lasers can be used to correct photoaging skin along the NLF. CO_2 or Erbium Laser Resurfacing are adjunctive techniques which can be used in combination with volume filling. Resurfacing techniques also include nonablative lasers and most recently radiofrequency devices. All of these procedures can be used to correct skin defects around the fold and may be used in combination with volume filling.

The improvement achievable with soft tissue augmentation of NLFs depends on the amount of implant used, type of implant, frequency of implantation,

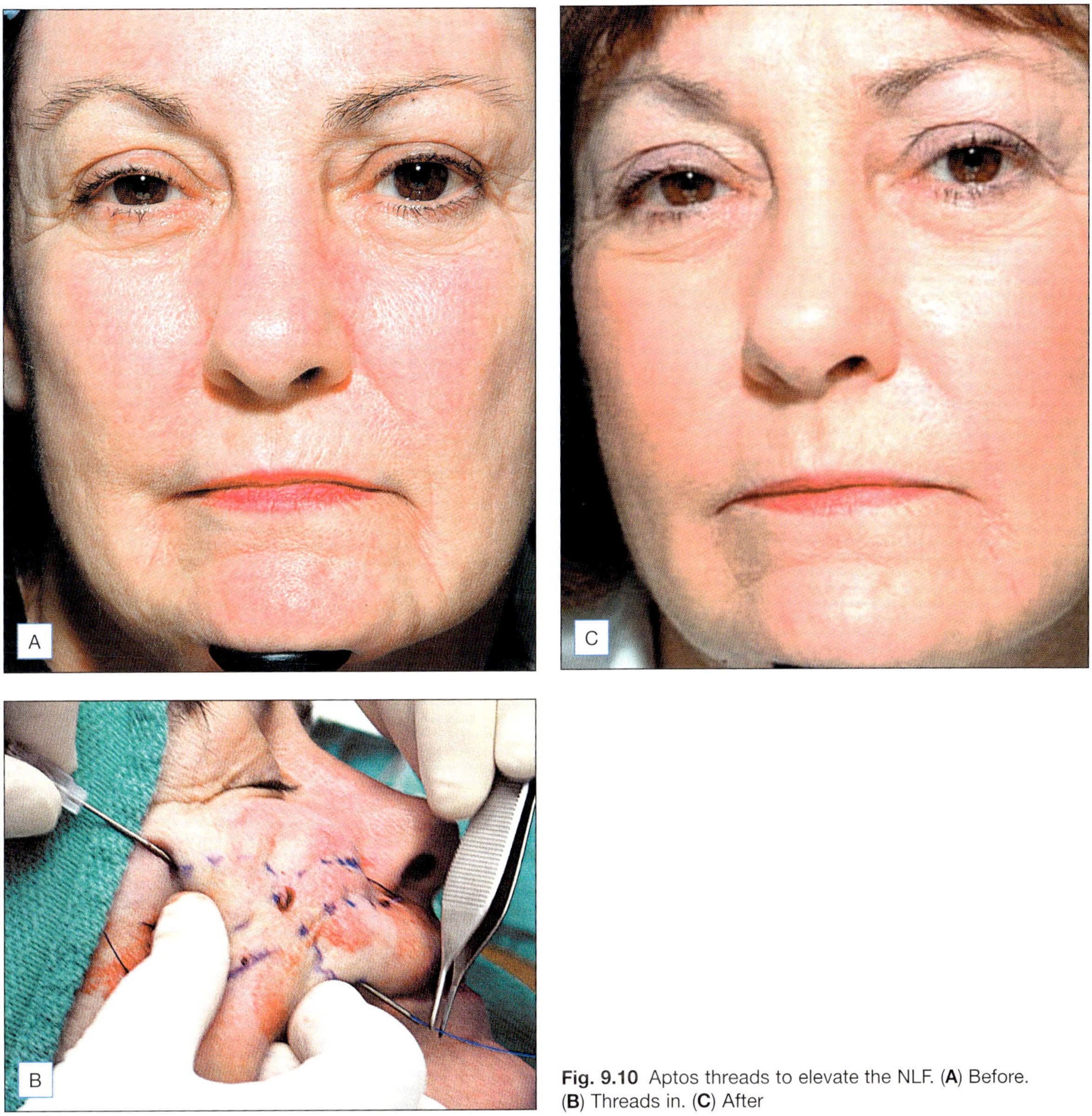

Fig. 9.10 Aptos threads to elevate the NLF. (**A**) Before. (**B**) Threads in. (**C**) After

and the intrinsic qualities of the NLF including the texture and quality of the fabric of the skin. The benefits of filler substances include softening NLFs by elevating the areas with the deficit of soft tissue. A lightening of the shadows created due to the aging face is seen in Table 9.1. A single implant or multiple implants can be used to attain the desired effect. If a patient presents with fine lines radiating from NLFs, the best treatment would be to utilize an injectable filler specific for fine lines plus filling the NLFs with a heavier volume filler for deeper furrows.

Injectable soft tissue fillers are the primary choice for treatment of the NLF from minimal to severe. This chapter will briefly review the agents most commonly used and emphasize the techniques that work best on the NLF. Soft tissue augmentation is technique sensitive so the individual procedure for each implant must be mastered (Table 9.2).

Injectable implants can be as effective as the product packaging claims as long as the implant is injected as directed on the package insert. Variables in efficacy can be noted if the material is injected into the subcutaneous tissue, causing much less aug-

NLF prominence			
None to mild	**Mild to moderate**	**Moderate**	**Severe**
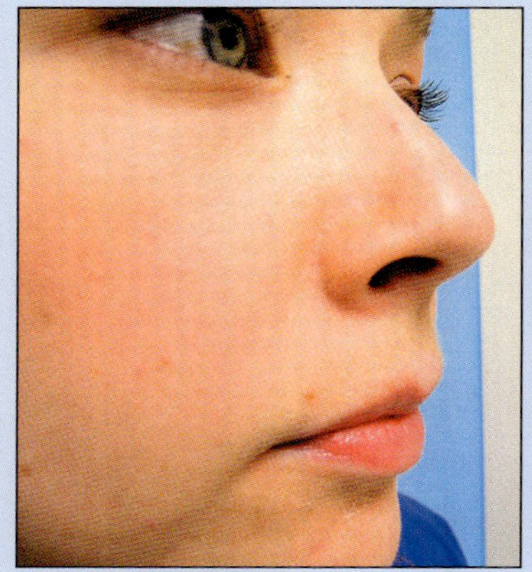	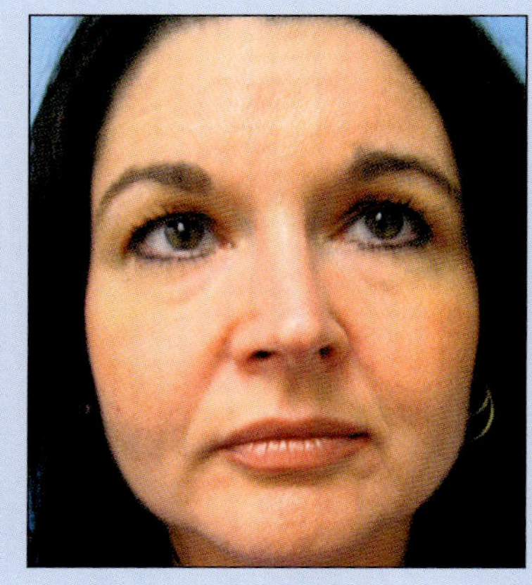	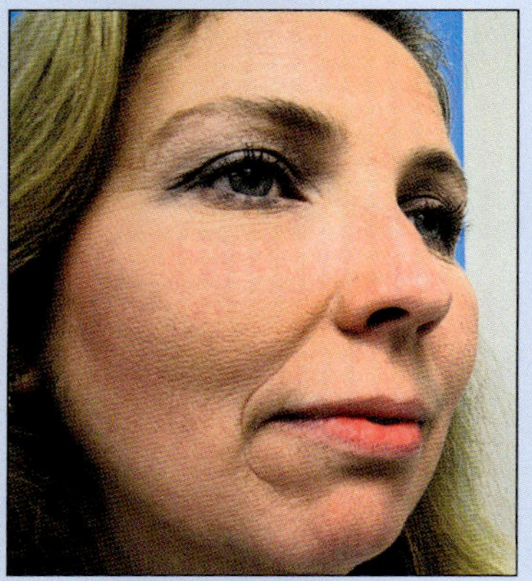	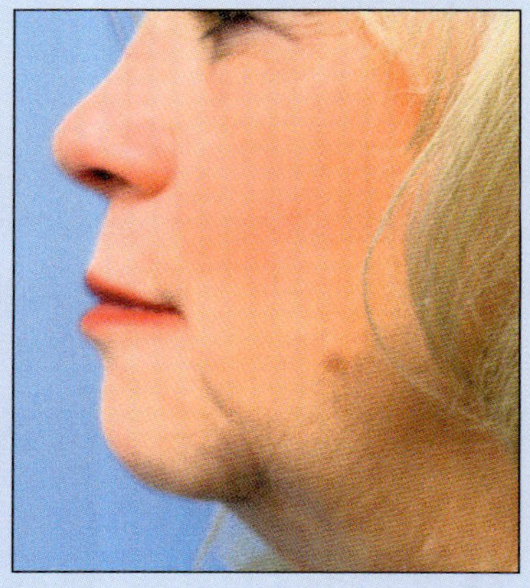
Muscular phase	Volume loss and photoaging skin	Moderate volume loss	Volume loss and ptosis

Table 9.1 NLF prominence

Fillers for the NLF	
Biodegradable	**Nonbiodegradable**
Zyderm/Zyplast	Silicone
Cosmoderm/Cosmoplast	Artecoll
Isolagen	Profill
Fascian	Gortex
Hylaform	SoftForm
Restylane	
Juvéderm	
Newfill/Sculptra	
Dermal/fascial grafts	
Fat	

Table 9.2 Fillers for the NLF

mentation compared to when it is injected correctly into the dermis. If the injectable implants are injected too superficially, beading or nodulation can occur. The beading will eventually decrease with time, decreasing fastest in areas with the most movement. When injecting into the dermis and inserting the needle in a forward fashion, the injectable material can be extruded into an area of the dermis that is not the ideal site. Firm massage of the injected sites can help to smooth the contour of the injectable filler and guide the filler to a more optimal location.

Injecting material into NLFs can cause considerable discomfort in some patients, with maximal discomfort occurring at the superior aspect of the NLFs. Some injectables contain an anesthetic, which helps with discomfort of the injection (Box 9.1). Countermeasures to avoid pain include topical anesthetics, ice, infraorbital nerve block, or simultaneous stimulation with a massaging apparatus. While it may be tempting to inject an anesthetic into the area to be treated, this can distort normal contours and should be avoided. Topical anesthetics help to decrease the pain of the needle puncture, but help minimally with the injection itself or the forward motion of the needle through the dermis. Infraorbital nerve blocks or counter nerve stimulation have mixed results, but do help to lessen the pain (Box 9.2, Fig. 9.11).

Patient Interview

A thorough medical history, family history, and physical exam should be completed for each patient. Any history of collagen vascular diseases (CVDs) should be noted, as well as hypersensitivity to ingredients of the filler substance. Skin tests should be performed when indicated. Bleeding disorders or anticoagulation medications should be noted. Bruising occurs more frequently when an anticoagulant is used and the patients should be

Anesthesia guidelines for injecting fillers

Implants with lidocaine
- Zyderm/Zyplast
- Cosmoderm/Cosmoplast

Topical anesthesia
- Elamax
- Betacaine

Nerve blocks
- Infraorbital
- Mental

Counter nerve stimulation
- Vibrator

Box 9.1 Anesthesia guidelines for injecting fillers

Commonly used topical anesthetic agents

- Betacaine enhanced gel, BetaCaine Plus
- L.M. x 4 and L.M. x 5
- EMLA (lidocaine pritocaine) cream
- Ice of other cryoesthetic agents
- Vibratory counterstimulation

Box 9.2 Commonly used topical anesthetic agents

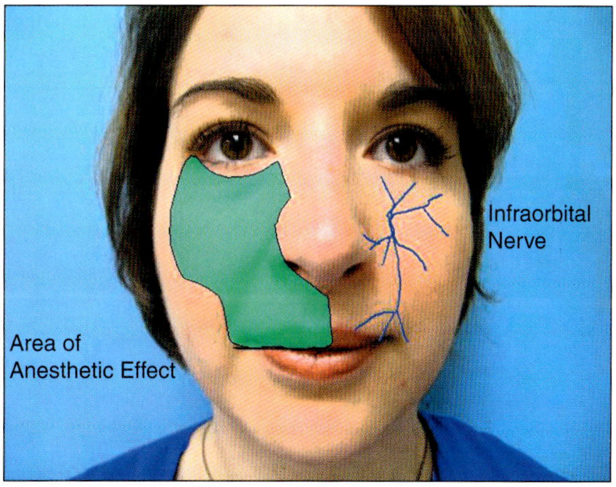

Fig. 9.11 Anesthetic distribution of infraorbital nerve block

aware of this possibility. The patient should be asked to smile and sneer to evaluate dynamics and symmetry. Any asymmetries in the patient's appearance should be noted and brought to the attention of the patient and documented with pre-treatment photographs in the chart.

The cosmetic patient is questioned as to what bothers them most about their appearance. They are asked to make a 'wish list' including up to five aspects of their appearance they would like to have improved with the most important feature to be first on the list. The list is reviewed with the patient, having them demonstrate in the mirror exactly what is meant by each topic on their list. Treatment options are then reviewed with the patient, beginning with simple procedures and combined simple procedures with little down time and ending with more long-lasting procedures requiring significant down time. If the patient has not had augmentation procedures before, the current authors typically recommend beginning with a product that lasts the least amount of time so that the patient can decide if augmentation is right for them. Although permanent fillers have the advantage of fewer injection sessions to maintain a desired effect, there is less of a margin of error when injected and the products can shift over time and with muscular movement. As the face ages, the site first injected may not be the ideal site for injection 5 or 10 years later in life. Subjects should be aware of the possibility that the aging process may result in a later unnatural appearance from the permanent implant to the area. The cost of each procedure is reviewed with the patient and written information is given to the patient, who can either proceed with treatment or can schedule a future appointment after considering their treatment options.

Treatment Technique

Every patient who is to be treated cosmetically reviews the treatment plan, and reviews the risks, benefits, and alternatives to the procedure as discussed. The patient must express understanding and sign an informed consent. Any last-minute questions are answered at this time. The patient's make-up is removed and the areas to be injected are cleansed with isopropanol and allowed to air dry. Photographs both distant and close-up are taken at this time, including a frontal view, a 45° angle view from the right and left, and a side view. It is important when comparing photographs that each picture is taken in a similar fashion under similar lighting. Make-up should be removed in all pictures and a similar background should be used.

Biodegradable Collagen

Zyderm/Zyplast

Bovine collagen is the first dermal filler approved for usage in the USA. It has a 20-year record of safety as a dermal filler and is most commonly used on the NLF. Three types of bovine collagen are presently available: (1) Zyderm I (ZI) is a 3.5% by weight bovine collagen (35 mg/mL), (2) Zyderm II (ZII which is 6.5% mg/mL), and (3) Zyplast. Zyplast 1.5 cross-linked bovine collagen, which constitutes an injectable latticework of bovine collagen, is more resistant to degradation with less immunogenicity. All of these products require skin tests to rule out allergy. Two intradermal injection tests should be performed at day 0, 2 weeks, and both evaluated in 6 weeks. The collagen is suspended in saline with 1% lidocaine. The products have different indications.

Zyderm I is primarily indicated for superficial defects while Zyderm II and Zyplast are used for deeper depressions and grooves. Zyderm I is placed in the papillary and upper reticular dermis. Overcorrection of 150–200% is required and the endpoint of injection is a 'peau d'orange' or blanching of the skin. Zyderm I is best used in combination with Zyplast or another heavier filler to correct the remaining fine wrinkles after the nasolabial groove is volume corrected (Fig. 9.12). This is a layering technique which will give a full correction to the dermal defect (Fig. 9.13).

Zyplast is a denser substance with greater longevity. It must be injected into the mid-reticular to deep dermis and is especially useful for treatment of the NLF. Zyplast is placed at a mid- to deep dermal level with a 30 gauge needle at a 10–20° angle to the skin surface. The material is deposited using a serial puncture technique.

There are variable techniques developed for NLF injections which are also applicable to other injectable fillers.

The three injection techniques most commonly used in the NLF are: serial puncture, threading and fanning (Fig. 9.14). The current authors find all three are useful for most injections. Serial puncture indicates the use of multiple injections into the

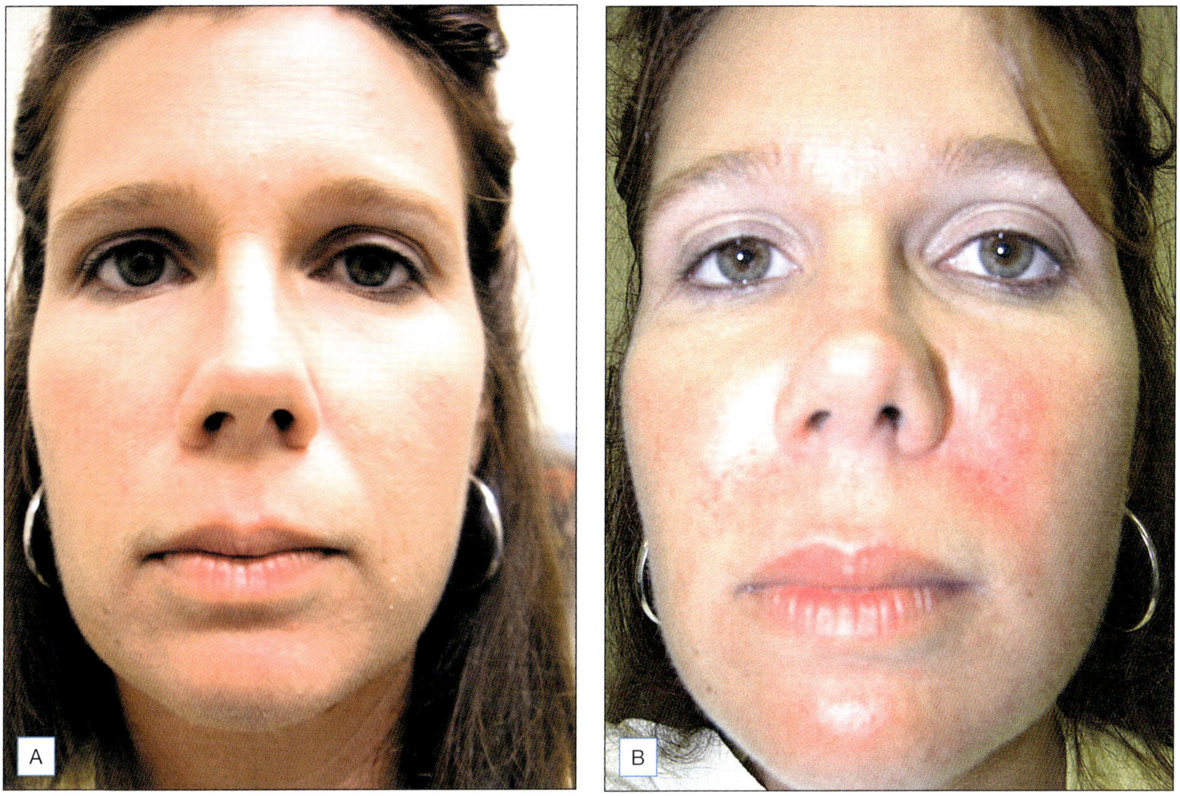

Fig. 9.12 Zyderm 1 + Zyplast layered in a NLF. (**A**) Before. (**B**) After

mid-dermis going up to the NLF, injected medial to the line/fold at a 30° angle. The injected implants are then massaged for even distribution. Threading technique uses a 1 in 30 gauge needle, which is advanced at a 30° angle below the depth of the NLF.

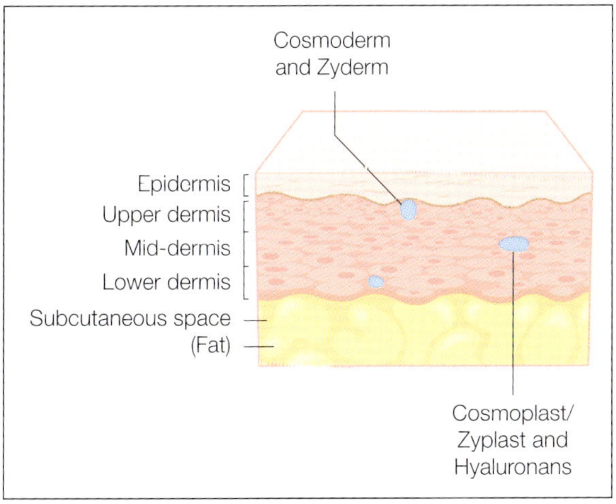

Fig. 9.13 Tissue compartment and choice of fillers

The filler is then injected as the needle is slowly withdrawn. This fills the depth of the fold through the trough evenly. The fanning technique is used for diffuse volume filling and useful for the triangle at the superior aspect of the NLF as it approaches the alar rim. Multiple 30° mid-dermal pathways are formed out and from the groove to elevate the superior angle evenly. It is also useful for volume filling at the lateral lip commissure to elevate the corner of the NLF and marionette line. Zyplast injections should never be overcorrected and always within a mid- to deep-dermal level, avoiding the peau d'orange appearance seen with superficial dermal injections.

Two or more implant sessions at intervals no less than 2 weeks apart may be needed for maximal correction. Enhancement implants are performed at 4–12-month intervals to maintain full correction (Fig. 9.15).

Best results are obtained by combining Zyplast with Zyderm I for correction of all levels of dermis within the fold. The two materials are layered with Zyplast injected first to 100% correction of the deeper groove. The authors' choice of techniques

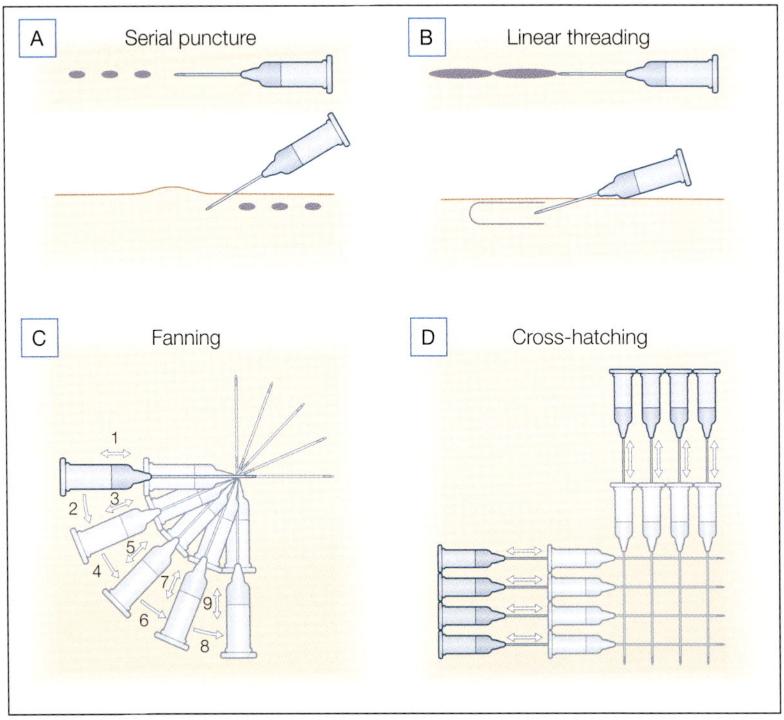

Fig. 9.14 Serial puncture, threading and fanning are all useful techniques for injecting collagen within the NLF

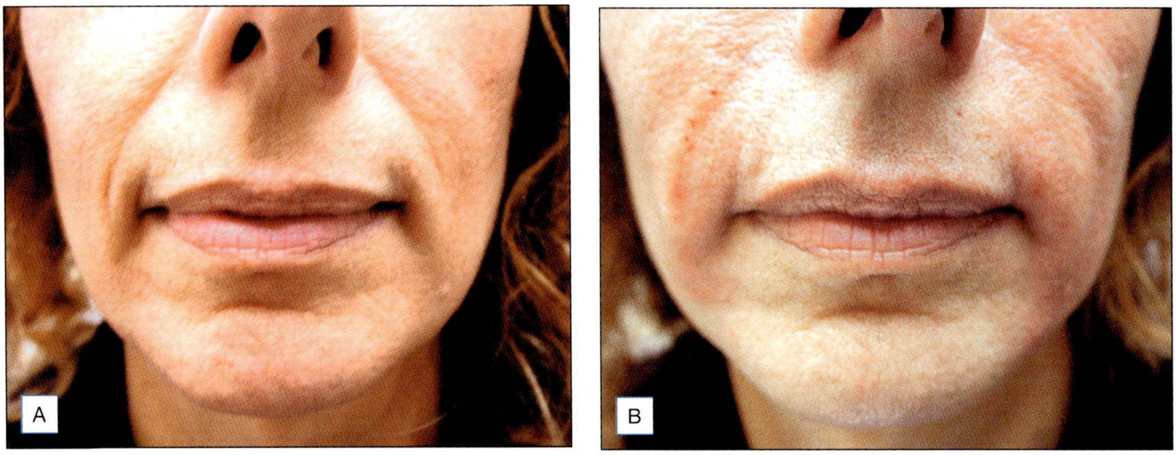

Fig. 9.15 Nasolabial lines and furrows

is to use the threading method first for volume filling and the deeper aspects of the groove. The serial puncture technique is then applied to areas of depression after full threading of the fold. Further volume filling is performed at the superior sulcus. It usually takes 1–2 cc of Zyplast to correct most NLF volume deficiencies. Then, Zyderm I is placed above the Zyplast for the remaining wrinkle within the fold and any accessory wrinkles. Massage is necessary after each injection to avoid nodulation and assure a smooth, natural implant.

Variation in longevity of augmentation is due to dynamic motion and mechanical stress along the NLF.

Though Zyderm/Zyplast is historically a reliable, forgiving product, disadvantages include the potential for allergy and need for skin tests prior to

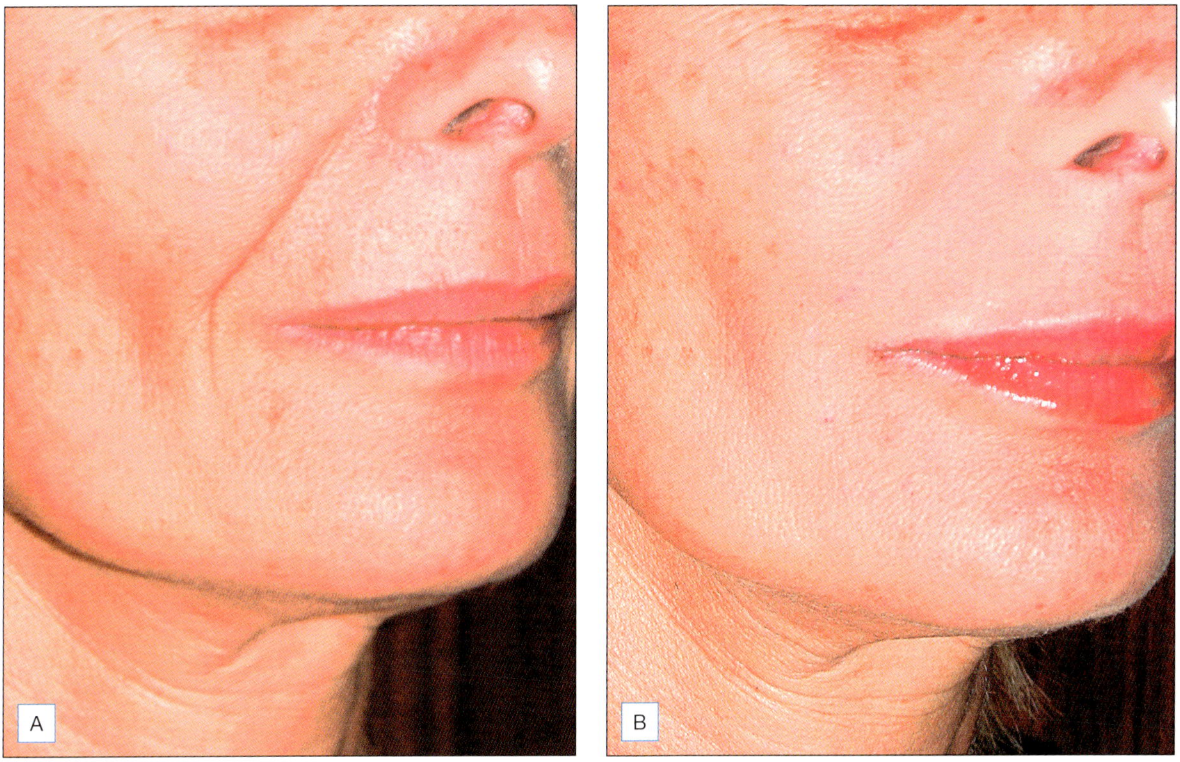

Fig. 9.16 Cosmoplast/CosmoDerm (photos courtesy of Dr Leslie Baumann). (A) Before. (B) 30 minutes after

injection, the relative short duration and potential adverse events including nodulation, allergic potential, vascular infarction with deepest injection and the rare event of cystic formation.

CosmoDerm/CosmoPlast (Inamed Corporation) is a second-generation collagen filling agent produced as a human bioengineered collagen. It is derived from dermal fibroblast cells seeded and incubated in a bioreactor to produce a human collagen product. The type I collagen is isolated from the dermal tissue, purified and mixed with lidocaine and phosphate-buffered saline. CosmoDerm I, II and CosmoPlast are used as injectable fillers in NLFs similar to the methods of Zyderm I, II and Zyplast. No skin test is required though and some clinicians believe the product may last slightly longer than Zyderm/Zyplast products. It also can be used in combination with other products including hyaluronic acid fillers. It has an excellent record of safety. It produces little swelling or bruising with the least amount of down time of any filler presently available (Fig. 9.16).

Hyaluronic Acid: Restylane (Medicis Esthetics), Hylaform (Inamed/Genzyme), Juvéderm (Inamed)

The hyaluronic acid products are the most recently approved family of injectable fillers for contour defects. These are especially applicable for the NLF, in which the unique viscoelastic properties and high water retention capacity fill the groove in a very natural manner. Hyaluronic acid is chemically, physically and biologically identical in the tissues of all species. It is biocompatible with little or no allergenicity. The body rapidly clears the noncross-linked hyaluronic acid molecule in 24–48 hours so that the product needs stabilization to be effective as a dermal implant. Restylane is a bacterial-based product while Hylaform is derived from chicken combs. Both products are purified and stabilized by cross-linking, producing a hydroscopic gel that is gradually eliminated. Both Restylane and Hylaform have been approved by the FDA for intradermal injection to correct NLFs. This is especially applicable since the NLF was the area chosen for the paired double-blind studies used for efficacy and safety of the products. Both studies used Zyplast as a control. The Restylane study compared products on either side of the face in a double-blind paired comparison. It was to demonstrate efficacy and longevity. The Hylaform study was a 'noninferiority' study with outcomes for efficacy at 4 months. Both products were successful with the following outcomes:

1. Both products achieved correction equal to or better than Zyplast at 4 months
2. Both products were declared safe with no need for skin testing
3. Both were declared safe and effective treatments for correction of NLFs.

Neither product has lidocaine, thus pretreatment topical anesthesia and/or local blocks are needed for patient comfort. The current authors prefer using topical betacaine or lidocaine infraorbital nerve block.

The products are packaged as a gel within a syringe with 0.7 ml product and a 30 gauge 0.5 in needle. They should be injected into the mid-dermis with only 100% correction (no overcorrection).

Restylane and Hylaform can be injected into the NLF by all three defined techniques: serial puncture, threading and fanning. The viscoelastic properties of the gel make it malleable for massage in the fold, resulting in a very natural correction (Fig. 9.17). The implant should not be placed superficially as it results in nodularity with a visibly bluish discoloration to the skin.

The hyaluronic acids are relatively free of side effects and carry a very small risk of allergic or inflammatory reactions. Rare granulomas have been reported from both products. This filler, like all the biodegradable products, is forgiving because it will be resorbed and side effects disappear with time (Fig. 9.18).

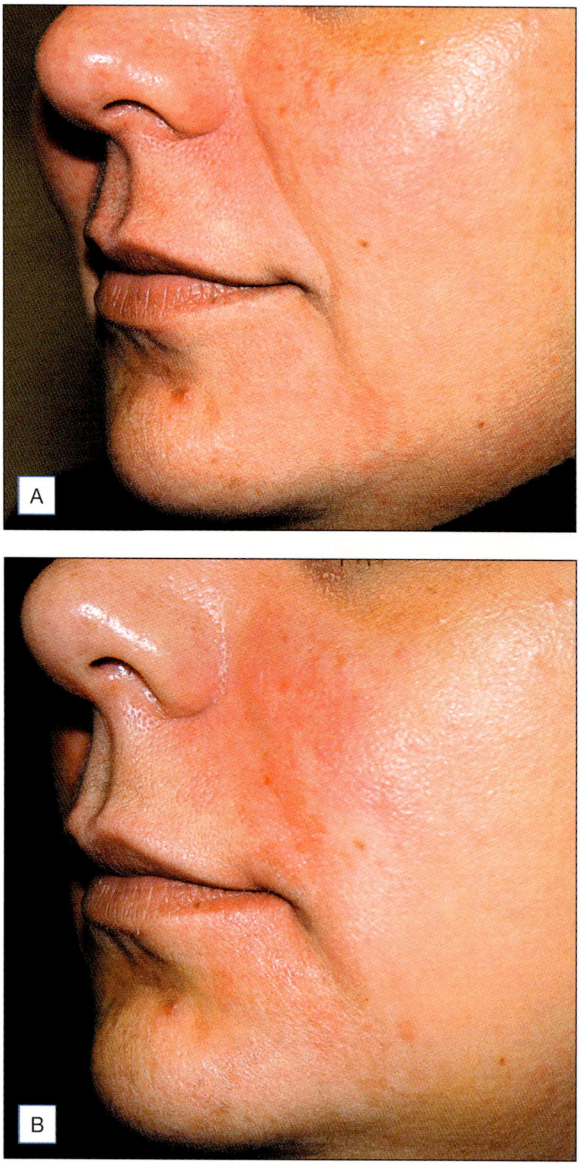

Fig. 9.17 Mid-dermal injection of Hylaform to correct NLFs. (**A**) Before. (**B**) After

Calcium Hydroxylapatite (Radiance: Bioform)

Calcium hydroxylapatite (CaHA) is an inorganic substance that mimics the structure of bone. In the USA, it is marketed as Radiance. Radiance is currently FDA approved for use in oral maxillofacial defects and for soft tissue vocal fold augmentation and as a radiographic tissue marker. CaHA is currently widely used in Europe as a soft tissue filler. Radiance is not approved in the USA by the FDA for cosmetic applications and use for soft tissue augmentation is classed as off-label use.

In its soft tissue injectable form, CaHA microspheres are suspended in a sodium carboxymethyl cellulose absorbable gel, and it is injected into the dermis or subcutaneous tissue. As the gel is absorbed, collagen deposition into and around the microspheres causes collagen formation and enhances augmentation. It is expected to last between 2 and 5 years with breakdown products of calcium and phosphorus.

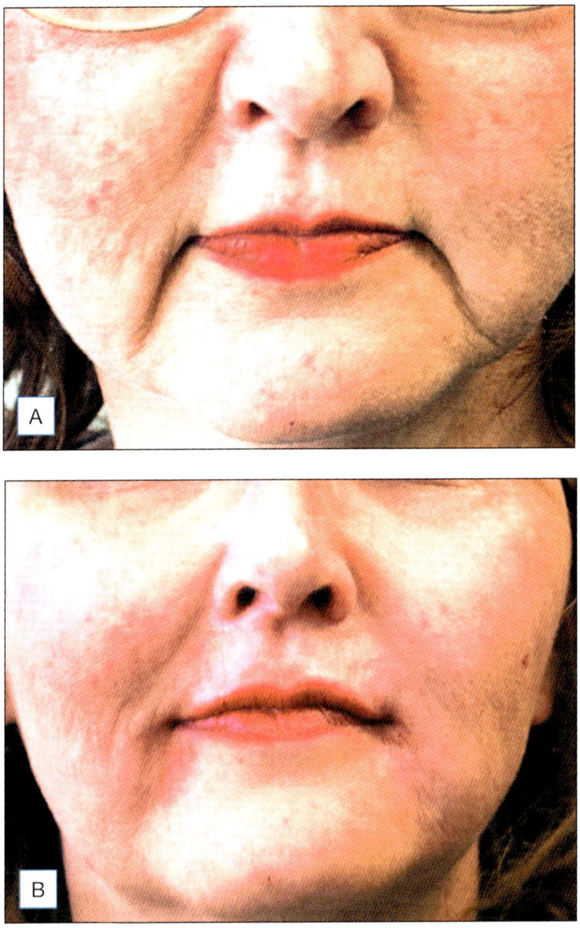

Fig. 9.18 Deep marionette lines treated with Restylane 0.7 cc within each fold. (**A**) Before. (**B**) After

Radiance has been used effectively for correction of NLF defects by deep dermal injection. A local nerve block is needed for its comfortable usage. The gel is injected through a 25 or 27 gauge needle and the correction is usually 1:1. It is advisable to undercorrect the fold as lumpiness and medial overcorrection can produce a deformity. Conservative correction with follow-up correction in 2–4 weeks is advisable. The pliability of the substances allows postinjection massage, minimizing irregularities or lumpiness which can occur. It is expected to last longer than 2 years (Fig. 9.19).

Poly-L-lactic Acid: Sculptra (New-Fill): Dermik

Poly-L-lactic acid (PLLA) received conditional approval from an FDA advisory panel for treatment of HIV-related lipoatrophy under the trade name Sculptra in March 2004. However, the FDA itself has not yet approved Sculptra for use in the USA. Studies of this product are currently underway to gain FDA approval. PLLA has been marketed as New-Fill in Europe since November 1999.

PLLA is a synthetic polymer which is resorbable, biocompatible, and biodegradable. It has been used for several years in multiple medical devices and is a component of vicryl sutures. PLLA can be injected into the deep dermal tissue or subcutaneous tissue. The area to be filled should be undercorrected. After injection, gradual degradation takes place by hydrolysis while gradual deposition of collagen occurs.

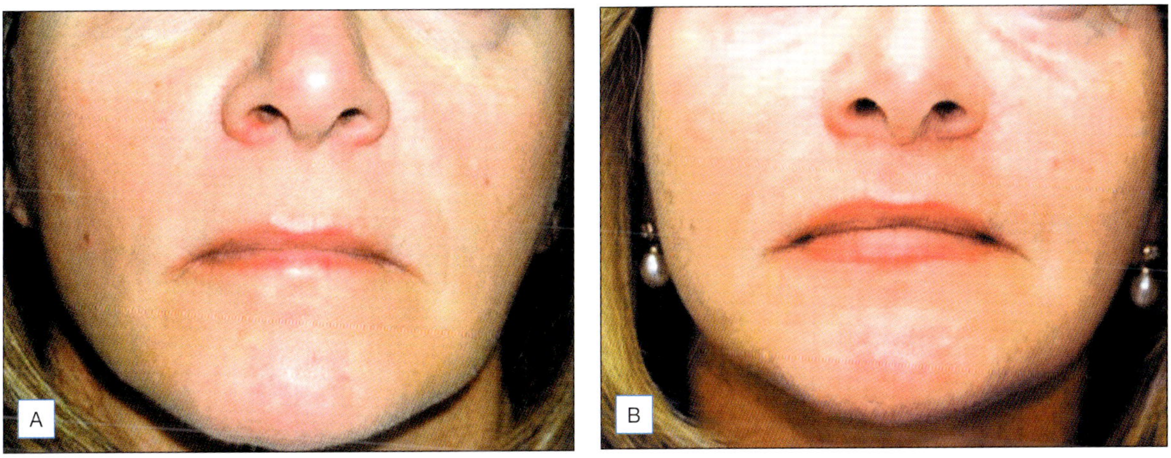

Fig. 9.19 Deep NLFs treated with Radiance. (**A**) Before. (**B**) After

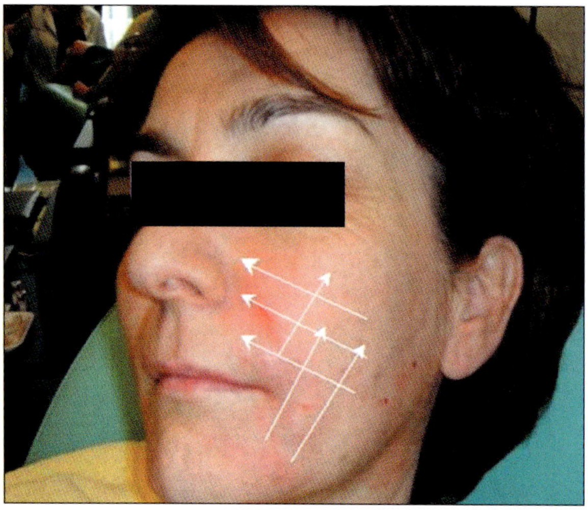

Fig. 9.20 Sculptra is a deep volume filler injected in a criss-cross pattern

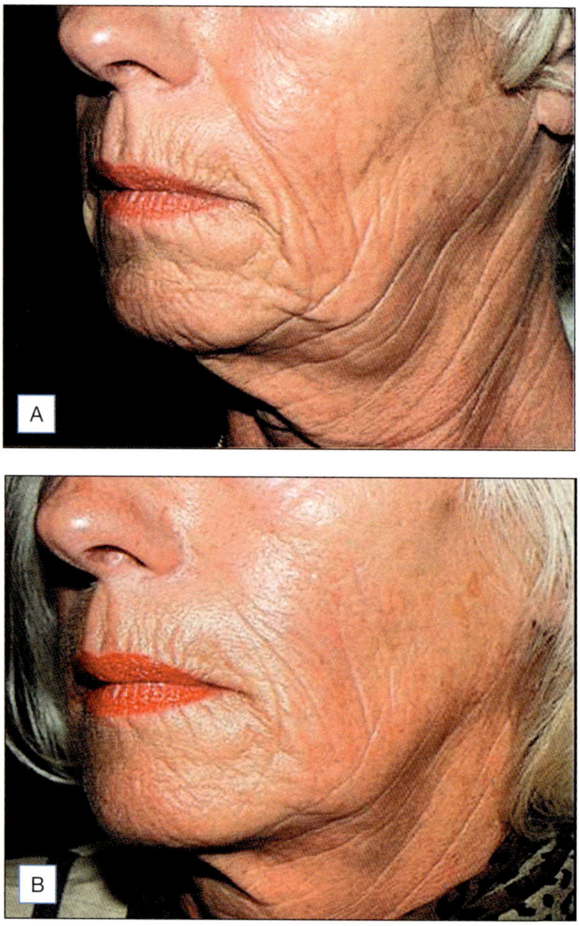

Fig. 9.21 Volume filling redefines facial features as well as fills wrinkle folds. (**A**) Before. (**B**) 10 months after treatment

The initial correction due to implantation of the PLLA decreases over the next few days as the diluent is resorbed. The area treated with PLLA will then slowly refill as the tissue reacts to the implant. A gradual increase in the volume will continue to occur over the next few months.

The side effects of this material are similar to those of other injectables and include erythema, edema, and bruising at the injection site. Palpable but nonvisible subcutaneous nodules have been noted in some patients, which can resolve spontaneously. These nodules on the lip may be due to over-correction. Massaging the treated area after injection may reduce the incidence of this side effect. Rare cases of sterile abscess, late granuloma formation and hypersensitivity reactions have been reported.

Sculptra is injected with a different technique than the other wrinkle fillers. It is layered as a deep dermal and subcutaneous soft tissue filler that is used mainly to correct volume deficits rather than wrinkle correction alone. The technique of Vleggar demonstrates injection with a criss-cross pattern to lay down a uniform matrix for new collagen to be deposited in the deep dermis (Fig. 9.20). To correct NLFs, the entire lower facial area should be blended to augment tissue and provide a volume-enhancing effect. That not only corrects the furrow but also redefines the lost volume in surrounding skin and soft tissues (Fig. 9.21). A 27 gauge needle is used to implant the gel into deep dermis and subcutaneous tissue in a criss-cross pattern. No more than 1–2 ml is injected with undercorrection. The area is then massaged and iced to decrease inflammation. Two or three repeat procedures are performed for full correction. The product has been found to last 2–4 years.

Nonbiodegradable Fillers

Nonbiodegradable fillers include both injectables and solid products (Table 9.3). Over a period of time, the current authors' patients do request longer lasting fillers and discuss permanence. There are both advantages and disadvantages of these products. Most importantly, the physician must understand that errors and complications are not forgiving and in some cases, not correctable.

Nonbiodegradable synthetic fillers	
Injectables	**Solids**
Silicone Artecoll Bioplastique	Gortex SoftForm

Table 9.3 Nonbiodegradable synthetic fillers

Silicone

Silicone is the oldest filling material in the USA, first used in 1930 and used for NLF augmentation since 1965 by Orentreich and associates. The Dow Corning material had a viscosity of 360 cs, ideal for microdroplet deep dermal injection. The fine droplets are deposited as an undercorrection with only minimal change in the NLF. Collagen is laid down around the droplets and the process is repeated at 6-month intervals until the desired correction is obtained. Optimal correction has been followed for over 30 years by Orentreich and Barnett with good cosmetic correction. The patient though must be alerted to the fact that aging changes facial contour and the silicone may 'bead up' or change position as wrinkles and features fall. The most common complications seen are implant migration and nodulation. These are usually technique related (Fig. 9.22).

Dow Corning silicone is not approved by the FDA. Other forms of silicone, though, are presently approved for ophthalmic usage. These are: Adato-Sil (5000 cs) and Silikon (1000 cs). They are presently being used as a dermal filler in off-label usage.

Artecoll/Artefill

Artecoll is a permanent injectable filler used to correct the NLF since 1994. Polymethyl-methacrylate (PMMA) microspheres are suspended in bovine

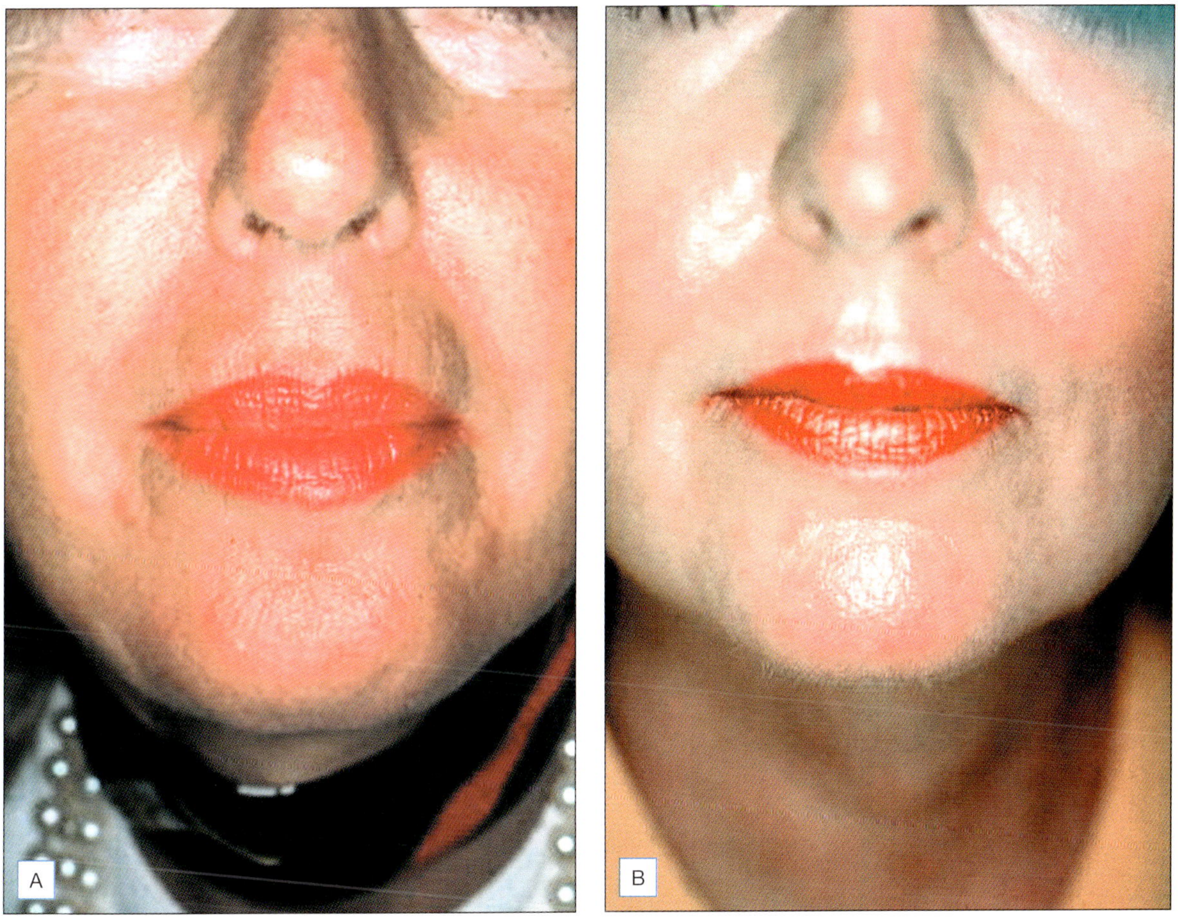

Fig. 9.22 Long-term nodulation – silicone (**A** & **B**)

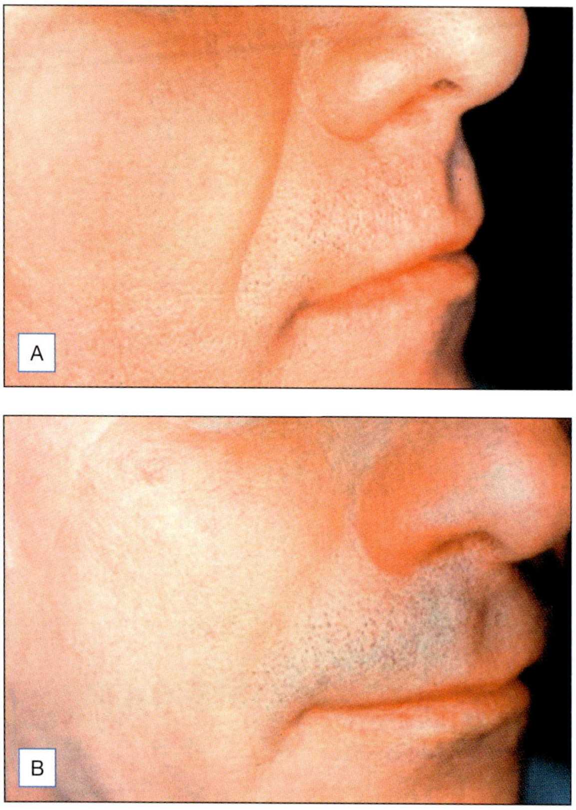

Fig. 9.23 Artecol injection within the NLFs. (**A**) Before. (**B**) 3 years after

collagen for intradermal injection. The product is manufactured by Rofil Medical International but presently is not FDA approved. The product has had clinical trials in the USA under the name of Artefill (Fig. 9.23).

The suspension of bovine collagen and PMMA microspheres is injected into the deep dermis and subdermal plane with 100% correction of the fold, yet not overcorrection. Within 3–4 months, the collagen is degraded as new collagen is formed around the microspheres. The product is well indicated for deep NLFs for long-term correction.

Artefill is designed for implantation into the deep reticular dermis. Implanting Artefill is more technique sensitive than injecting collagen due to its viscosity and permanence. The viscosity of Artefill is three times higher than that of Zyplast and therefore a greater and a constant pressure should be applied to the plunger of the syringe throughout the injection procedure. Also due to the increased viscosity, more pain occurs during injection compared to collagen. Before injecting, one should exert a firm and steady push on the plunger of the syringe to ensure that there is no blockage of the needle and that the material is moved to the tip of the needle and is ready for injection. The needle should be inserted into the deep reticular dermis tunneled just beneath the area to be filled while maintaining constant pressure on the plunger of the syringe.

The material should only be injected while withdrawing the needle since if injection on entering the tissue is as if injecting into a wall of tissue; material injected can move in any direction away from the needle tip, taking the path of least resistance. When injecting into the reticular dermis, a firm resistance is felt and a lifting of the skin is noticed. If the needle is in the subcutaneous tissue, the resistance will be much less and a much greater amount of product will be needed to achieve a lifting of the skin. If while injecting Artefill a blanching occurs, the needle is placed too superficially. If this occurs, it is important to stop the injection immediately and massage the area with firm pressure, helping to deepen the injected material. At the end of implantation, massage all areas gently. If lumpiness is noted, massage more firmly. Patients should limit movement of the injected site for the next 3 days as Artefill can be pushed deeper into the skin with pronounced movement during this time. The implant site can be taped for approximately 3 days, serving more as a reminder to try to keep the area still than as a dressing. The patients should be instructed that they may develop edema and erythema over the next few days.

The area should be allowed to settle for several weeks and the patient should then be re-evaluated to see if any further augmentation is needed. If further augmentation is needed, Artefill should be injected in a layered fashion with care taken not to inject the material too superficially.

When correcting NLFs with Artefill, two to three strands are implanted in a parallel fashion 1–2 mm medial to the NLF. This is because NLFs are involved in many facial expressions. For the first 3 days after injection, Artefill is more easily dislodged and due to muscular movement of this area can be moved laterally with facial expression during this time.

Side effects/complications

The tolerability and acceptability of side effects due to Artefill is low due to the longevity of the implant

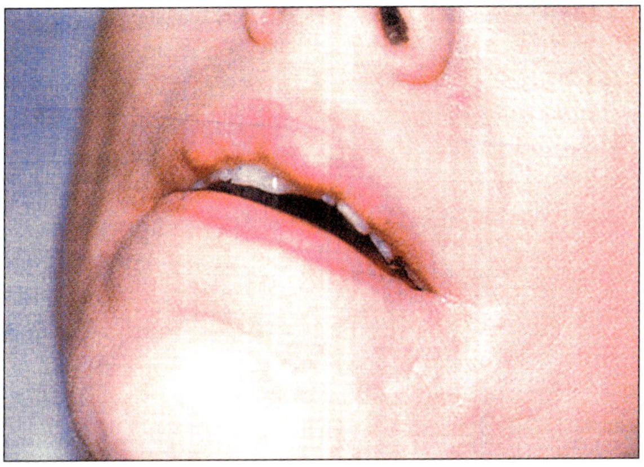

Fig. 9.24 Artefill – granuloma formation on lip injection

and therefore the potential for nonresolving side effects. Although the PMMA microspheres are nonallergenic, allergic reaction can occur with Artefill as it can with any injectable collagen preparation. Even with a test site, allergic reaction can occur.

True granuloma formation is a rare occurrence, occurring in less than 0.01% of patients and occurring 6–24 months after Artefill treatment. This side effect may not be reversible. In summary, Artefill is a permanent product with permanent results and permanent complications. Care must be taken to avoid the latter (Fig. 9.24).

Autologous Fat

As opposed to these injectable products, long-term correction can also be attained with fat injections. This is a more complicated surgical procedure involving fat harvesting, centrifuging and then injecting. There is down time with significant swelling, inflammation and bruising; thus it is not a procedure to be taken lightly. In fact, the current authors like to try a simpler temporary filler first prior to fat injection procedures. This will show the patient the type of correction that can be obtained before this longer lasting procedure is performed. The following concepts have made fat injection a reliable and long-lasting procedure:

1. Fat is harvested atraumatically and handled in vitro carefully to preserve the live fat cells
2. Small aliquots of fat are injected into tissue using a layering technique – microlipoinjection

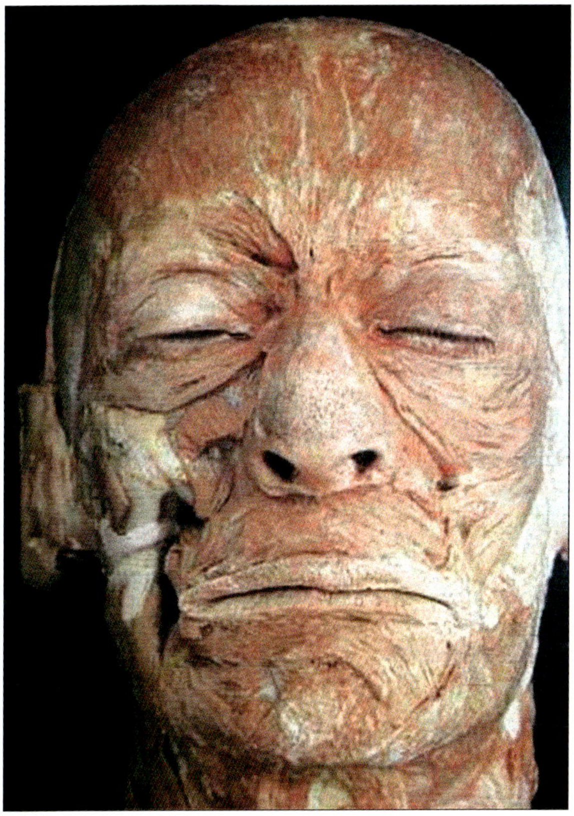

Fig. 9.25 Facial muscles

3. Fat is injected deeply into muscle and deep subcutaneous tissue for best survival.

The fat autograft muscle injection (FAMI) technique developed by Roger Amar is a reliable method of deep fat injection to correct the lower face and NLF. It involves a careful analysis of muscle and fat loss around the NLF with correction of fat into those areas of loss. For example, deep NLFs are corrected by microlipoinjection into the following muscles: levator labii, zygomaticus major, orbicularis oris. This is performed through the use of a specially designed cannula through which the fat is injected longitudinally through the muscle mass and fat above (Fig. 9.25).

The thin patient with severe folds and a skeletonized lower face responds well to this operative procedure. The fat is injected through definitive incision sites for volume replacement of the lower face. Volume replacement will give long-lasting (1–5 years) correction of folds and a new contouring of the lower face (Fig. 9.26).

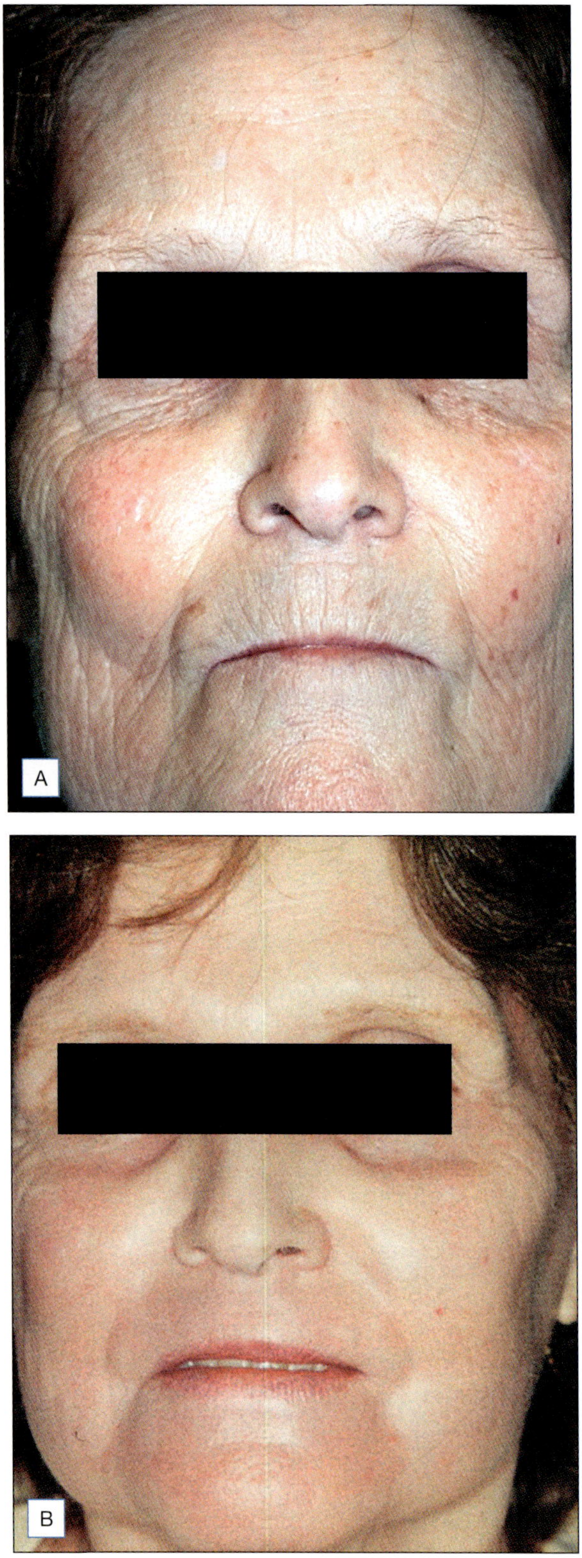

Fig. 9.26 FAMI injection – lips and folds. (**A**) Before. (**B**) 2 years post-injection

Conclusion

This chapter has explored the available techniques to correct the NLFs with emphasis on individualizing correction to meet each patient's needs.

Further Reading

Allevato MA, Pastorale E, Zamboni M, Kerdel F, Woscoss A 1996 Complications following industrial liquid silicone injection. International Journal of Dermatology 20:267–276

Anderson RD, Lo MW 1998 Endoscopic malar/midface suspension procedure. Plastic and Reconstructive Surgery 102(6):2196–2208

Atamoros FP 2003 Botulinum toxin in the lower one third of the face. Clinical Dermatology 21(6):505–512

Barton FE Jr, Kenkel JM 1997 Direct fixation of the malar pad. Clinical Plastic Surgery 24(2):329–335

Berry J 2002 New-Fill for an old face. Positively Aware. 13(3):34–35

Butterwick KJ, Lack EA 2003 Facial volume restoration with the fat autograft muscle injection technique. Dermatologic Surgery 29(10):1019–1026

Carruthers J, Carruthers A 2003 Aesthetic botulinum A toxin in the mid and lower face and neck. Dermatologic Surgery 29(5):468–476

Charriere G, Bejot M, Schnitzler L, Ville G, Hartmann DJ 1989 Reactions to a bovine collagen implant. Clinical and immunologic study in 705 patients. Journal of the American Academy of Dermatology 21(6):1203–1208

Cheonis N 2002 New-Fill to treat facial wasting. Bulletin of Experimental Treatments for AIDS 15(2):10–15

Clark DP, Hanke CW, Swanson NA 1989 Dermal implants: safety of products injected for soft tissue augmentation. Journal of the American Academy of Dermatology 21(5 Pt 1):992–998 (Review)

de Maio M 2003 Challenges in the mid and the lower face. Journal of Cosmetic Laser Therapy 5(3–4):213–215

Donofrio L 2000 Structural autologous lipoaugmentation: a pan-facial technique. Dermatologic Surgery 26:1129–1134

Duffy DM 1998 Injectable liquid silicone: new perspectives. In: Klein AW (ed.) Tissue Augmentation in Clinical Practice: Procedures and Techniques. Marcel Dekker, New York, pp 237–267

Duranti F, Salti G, Bovani B, Calandra M, Rosati ML 1998 Injectable hyaluronic acid gel for soft tissue augmentation: A clinical and histological study. Dermatol Surg 24(12):1317–1325

Eremia S, Newman N 2000 Long-term follow-up after autologous fat grafting. Dermatologic Surgery 26:1150–1158

Faigin G 1990 The Artist's Complete Guide to Facial Expression, Watson-Guptill Publications, New York

Fernandez-Acenero MJ, Zamora E, Borbujo J 2003 Granulomatous foreign body reaction against hyaluronic acid: report of a case after lip augmentation. Dermatologic Surgery 29(12):1225–1226

Friedman PM, Mafong EA, Kauvar AN, Geronemus RG 2002 Safety data of injectable nonanimal stabilized hyaluronic acid gel for soft tissue augmentation. Dermatologic Surgery 28(6):491–494

Hanke CW 1998 Adverse reactions to bovine collagen. In: Klein AW (ed.) Tissue Augmentation in Clinical Practice. Procedures and Techniques. Marcel Dekker, New York, pp 145–154

Homicz MR, Watson D 2004 Review of injectable materials for soft tissue augmentation. Facial Plastic Surgery 20(1):21–29

Jacobson LG, Alexiades-Armenakas M, Bernstein L, Geronemus RG 2003 Treatment of nasolabial folds and jowls with a noninvasive radiofrequency device. Archives of Dermatology 139(10):1371–1372

Klein AW 2001 Skin filling. Collagen and other injectables of the skin. Dermatology Clinics 19(3):491–508, ix (Review)

Lemperle G, Romano J, Busso M 2003 Soft tissue augmentation with Artecoll: 10-year history, indications, techniques, and complications. Dermatologic Surgery 29:573–578

Lombardi T, Samson J, Plantier F, Husson C, Kuffer R 2004 Orofacial granulomas after injection of cosmetic fillers. Histopathologic and clinical study of 11 cases. Journal of Oral Pathology and Medicine 33(2):115–120

Lowe NJ 2003 Arterial embolization caused by injection of hyaluronic acid (Restylane). British Journal of Dermatology 148(2):379 (author reply 379–380)
Markey A, Glogau R 2000 Autologous fat grafting: Comparison of techniques. Dermatological Surgery 26:1135–1139
Narins RS, Brandt F, Leyden J, Lorenc ZP, Rubin M, Smith S 2003 A randomized, double-blind, multicenter comparison of the efficacy and tolerability of Restylane versus Zyplast for the correction of nasolabial folds. Dermatologic Surgery 29(6):588–595
Orentreich NO 1983 Soft tissue augmentation with medical grade fluid silicone. In: Rubin LR (ed.) Biomaterials in Reconstructive Surgery. CV Mosby, St Louis 859–881
Rudkin F, Miller TA 1999 Aging nasolabial fold and treatment by direct excision. Plastic and Reconstructive Surgery 104(5): 1502–1505
Sommer B, Sattler G 2000 Current concepts in fat graft survival: histology of aspirated adipose tissue and review of the literature. Dermatologic Surgery 26;1159–1166

10 NewFill: A New Material in Subdermal Sculpting

Nicholas J. Lowe, Kenneth R. Beer

Introduction

Of the numerous filling agents presently used in Europe, only a few are available in the USA. One recent addition to the wide range of dermal correction procedures for creases, lines and scars is the polymerized lactic acid (PLA) product known as NewFill in Europe and Sculptra in the USA. PLA was first introduced in Europe for the treatment of AIDS-related facial lipoatrophy. Subsequently, experience over the last 2 years has confirmed its value as a dermal correcting injection in the non-HIV-infected population.

It is probably best not to refer to this as simply a dermal filler, as unpublished data shows that this agent stimulates increased dermal connective tissue regeneration. Although the mechanism of the regeneration is presently unclear, it probably involves the induction of dermal fibroblast activity. For a comparison of NewFill with other fillers, see Tables 10.1 and 10.2.

What is NewFill?

NewFill is polymerized lactic acid (PLA) in a powdered lyophilized form. This is similar to the material used for skin sutures (Vicryl).

The powdered material is reconstituted with sterile water into a suspension, which is then injected into the area of dermis to be elevated or corrected.

Early history of polymerized lactic acid

The earliest clinical use for soft tissue augmentation was for the treatment of AIDS-related facial lipoatrophy. The initial successes from this treatment led to the use of PLA for cosmetic correction.

One possible mechanism of action is the stimulation of dermal and subcutaneous macrophage and fibroblast activity with subsequent neovascularized fibrosis and increased collagen deposition.

Problems That Can Be Treated with Polymerized Lactic Acid and Treatment Techniques

Facial lines and hollows

Over the last 2 years, one of the authors (NJL) has had experience with over 130 polymerized lactic acid treatments in London, UK. He has successfully treated lower facial lines, hollows, and atrophic scars with PLA injection. Areas that respond safely and adequately include nasolabial folds (Fig. 10.1), hollows of the cheek (particularly where there is fat atrophy from age-related thinning of the face or pathologic fat atrophy such as post-traumatic fat atrophy). PLA is also helpful in augmenting the malar and zygomatic arch areas for the correction of age-related midface descent, as well as cheek bone 'sculpting' for better definition. Other indications for PLA may include the correction of atrophic scars, including those resulting from acne, trauma, and skin cancer surgery.

There is presently a paucity of data regarding the use of PLA for the following indications: the neck, dorsal hands, lips, periorbital area, and forehead. The authors believe that well controlled studies are needed to demonstrate the safety and efficacy of the product for several of these areas, as there have been case reports and personal communications suggesting that using PLA in the lips may result in post-treatment nodules. This may be a result of the action of the orbicularis oris muscle moving the material into clumps during the course of normal mouth activities.

Comparison of fillers				
	Location of injection	**Duration of correction**	**Mechanism of correction**	**Composition of correcting substance**
NewFill (Sculptra)	Deep dermal–subcutaneous junction	1–2 years (may be longer)	Stimulation of collagen and other connective tissue synthesis	Innate collagen and connective tissue stimulated by polylactic acid injection
Restylane Thin	Superficial dermal	4–6 months	Direct tissue filling	Nonanimal stabilized hyaluronic acid (NASHA)
Restylane	Mid dermal	6–8 months	Direct tissue filling augmentation with volume	NASHA
Perlane	Deep dermal	9–18 months	Direct tissue augmentation with material injected	NASHA
CosmoPlast and Zyplast	Mid to deep dermal	3–5 months	Direct tissue augmentation with material injected	Crosslinked collagen (bovine for Zyplast, human for CosmoPlast)
CosmoDerm and Zyderm	Upper dermal	3–5 months	Direct tissue augmentation with material injected	Collagen (bovine for Zyderm and human for Cosmoderm)
Radiance	Deep dermal–subcutaneous junction	Months to years (trials still pending)	Stimulation of innate connective tissue using hydroxylapatite injection that will form scaffolding	Calcium hydroxylapatite in an aqueous carrier
Silicone	Deep dermis	Years to possibly permananent	Replacement with volume injected as well as encapsulation of material by ingrowth of native connective tissue	Silicone
Artecoll/Artefill	Deep dermis	Years	Encapsulation of polymethylmethacrylate (PMMA) spheres	PMMA microspheres, suspended in a solution of collagen

Table 10.1 Comparison of fillers

Technical considerations for various fillers		
	Anesthesia required	**Degree of correction required**
NewFill (Sculptra)	No—if mixed with lidocaine (lignociane) when reconstituted	Undercorrection
Restylane	Anesthesia (usually injected) required in most cases	Correction but not overcorrection
Perlane	Anesthesia (usually injected) required in most cases	Correction but not overcorrection
CosmoPlast and Zyplast	Product contains lidocaine	Overcorrection by 125–150%
CosmoDerm and Zyderm	Product contains lidocaine	Overcorrection by 150%
Radiance	Nerve blocks or local infiltration of anesthesia required	Correction
Silicone	Nerve blocks or local infiltration of anesthesia required	Gradual correction—no overcorrection
Artecoll/Artefill	Anesthesia (local or regional) required	Correction

Table 10.2 Technical considerations for various fillers

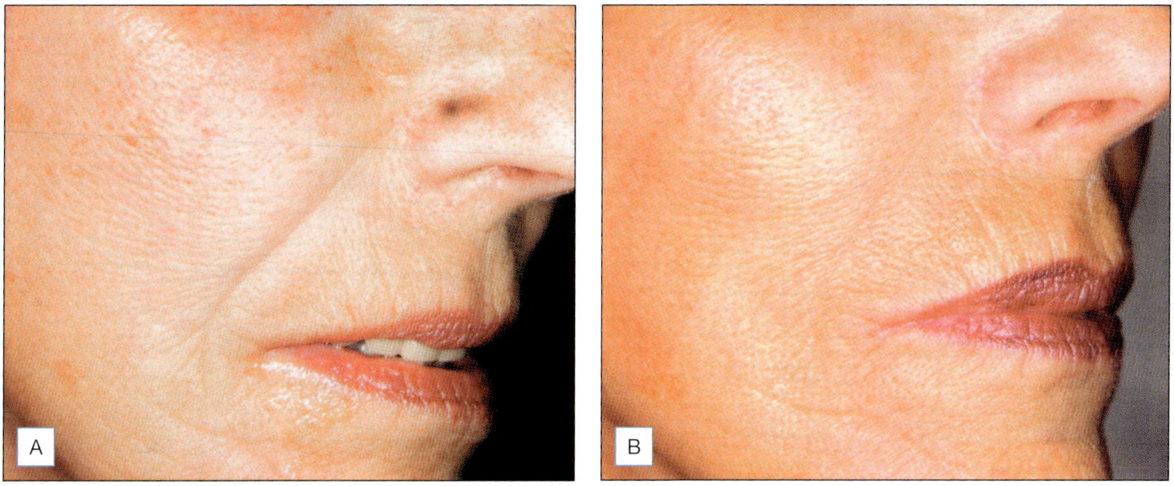

Fig. 10.1 A patient with deep nasolabial and melolabial lines before (**A**) and after (**B**) NewFill—three treatment sessions, 4 weeks apart. (**B**) was taken 2 months after the last injection session

Dilution technique

The current dilution technique used (by NJL) involves dilution of each vial (containing 350 µg of polymerized lactic acid) with 4 mL of sterile water. This is then allowed to form a suspension that should be left at room temperature for at least 2–4 hours before injection. Immediately before injection, a further 1 mL of 1% Xylocaine (lidocaine (lignocaine)) is added to this suspension for a total dilution of 5 mL per vial.

The suspension is vigorously shaken and is drawn up into 1 mL Luer–Lok syringes using an 18 gauge needle. The PLA suspension is injected using a half-inch 26 gauge needle. The syringes are shaken and rotated before injection to ensure as uniform a suspension as possible.

Injection technique

The injection is into a high subcutaneous deep dermal plane. The concept is to lay down a smooth layer of the polymerized lactic acid that will stimulate dermal fibroblasts from the deep dermis to produce dermal connective tissues including collagen.

Usually, the best technique is a retrograde injection. In this technique the needle is placed in the subcutaneous–dermal junction. The plunger is then withdrawn to minimize the risk of intravascular injection. Multiple injections utilizing 0.01–0.02 mL amounts of the suspension are then injected into multiple areas of the high subcutaneous–deep dermal plane.

It is important not to overcorrect, as there will be a delayed fibroblastic response to the injection. This may result in overcorrection if too large a volume is administered. In addition, overcorrection will increase the risk of delayed lumping of the material. In the event that lumps are noted following injection of PLA, the affected areas should be gently massaged for the following week.

Potential problems

Early problems include the risks of bruising and initial swelling. If a patient has a history of possible lidocaine (lignocaine) sensitivity, then the dilution should be with 5 mL of water without Xylocaine to avoid the risk of an allergic reaction to lidocaine.

Usually sufficient local anesthesia is obtained using LMX cream without occlusion.

Early technique problems

Problems that have been noted with PLA include the occurrence of reactive nodules. The authors have found these to be largely absent since using the dilution guidance as above, i.e. 5 mL of volume dilution. In 132 patient treatments we noted only five transient subcutaneous nodules which dispersed over several weeks.

One earlier technique utilizing a 2 mL dilution produced a much more viscous and less smooth suspension. Some patients that were injected with this viscous suspension developed nodules. Most of these resolved over several weeks after treatment with dilute intralesional corticosteroid injections and massage of the affected areas. There have been anecdotal reports of nodule formation, but little accurate information on these cases is available.

Duration of effect

Reports from the European literature suggest a duration of benefit of between 2 and 4 years. It is the experience of one of the authors (NJL) that patients still show signs of benefits 2 years after injection of PLA.

Detailed photographic facial studies are needed to accurately assess duration. Also further long term studies including histopathologic or ultrasound image analysis are required to judge the duration of correction for PLA.

It is our impression that PLA will last longer in areas that are less mobile (i.e. scarred areas, the malar eminence, the lateral cheeks) than in mobile areas such as the nasolabial folds. Adjunctive use of Botox (particularly around the mouth) to decrease the mobility of areas treated with PLA is an area that will require further study.

Summary

In summary, polymerized lactic acid represents a dermal stimulating correcting injection that may be of help in a number of situations. These include deep nasolabial folds and hollow cheeks where other temporary fillers give a more transient effect. In addition, PLA has the potential to lift cheeks and define bony prominences in order to accomplish a truly nonsurgical facelift.

Further experience is recommended before some of the other areas for future injection (e.g. hips, neck, hands, forehead, and periorbital areas) are investigated in large numbers of patients.

Advanced Techniques

Advanced techniques using PLA include the use of other soft tissue augmentation products as well as Botox.

It has been our experience that because PLA does not lead to immediate correction it may be safely combined with hyaluronic acid fillers such as Restylane and Perlane. Frequently we inject nasolabial folds and/or lips with Restylane and/or Perlane to get an immediate effect, followed by PLA injections. The Restylane and Perlane fillers produce immediate correction while the PLA programme of injections then produces a more prolonged, but delayed improvement by stimulating new dermal connective tissue.

As a final note, it is appropriate to say that our favorite immediate volume fillers remain Restylane—Thin, Restylane, and Perlane—and these fillers will probably retain their 'most favored filler' status for lips, forehead, and periorbital skin. However, we think that PLA will have a role in the long term correction of some facial problems.

Further Reading

Day JN, Raobe A, Shiner AM, et al 2002 Intradermal polylactic acid (NewFill) for treatment of severe HIV-associated facial lipoatrophy. HIV Medicine 3:162

Gogolewski S 1993 Tissue response and in vivo degradation of selected polyhydroxyacids: polylactide (PLA), poly (3-hydroxybutyrate) PHB, and poly (3-hydroxybutyrate-co-3-hydroxysolerate) (PHB/VA). Journal of Biomedical Materials Research 27:1335–1348

Lemperle G, Morhenn V, Charrier U 2003 Human histology and persistence of various injectable filler substances for soft tissue augmentation. Aesthetic Plastic Surgery 27:354–366

Lowe NJ 2002 Temporary dermal fillers—European experiences. in: Lowe NJ (ed) Textbook of facial rejuvenation. Martin Dunitz/Taylor & Francis, London, pp 177–188

Valantin MA, Aubron-Oliver C, Ghon J, et al 2003 Polylactic acid implants (NewFill) to correct facial lipoatrophy in HIV infected patients: results of an open-label study VEGA. AIDS 17:2471–2477

11 Pain Control in Cosmetic Facial Surgery

Joseph Niamtu, Jean Carruthers

Introduction

In cosmetic facial surgery practices, the majority of patients require regional anesthesia, topical or injected. The aesthetic physician and surgeon can do a better job on a pain free patient. The reputation for excellence in amelioration of pain and discomfort serves as an extraordinary internal marketing enhancer. Conversely, even the most talented cosmetic surgeon can produce negative marketing effects if they have the reputation of hurting their patients.

This chapter is designed to teach basic methods of pain control for cosmetic facial surgical procedures. It is impossible within the scope of this text to provide full details on each technique, but after reading this chapter the doctor should be able to understand the most basic techniques of local anesthesia as well as the neuroanatomy involved in anesthetizing specific dermatomes related to the injection of fillers in the face.

Patient selection

Patient selection for any aesthetic procedure includes an assessment of aesthetic needs and expectations within the traditional medical framework of an assessment of general health, allergy, and previous response to analgesic medications. It is often helpful to inquire about previous dental work and the response to injected anesthetic.

Expected benefits

The expected benefits for local anesthetic techniques are primarily focused on the subjective comfort of the patient.The physician will be able to more completely address the aesthetic concerns in a subject who is relaxed. The safety profile of these techniques is high and the complication rate is low.

Complications are related to individual patient susceptibility and to physician technique. The former can include allergic reaction, vasoconstrictor overdose, ineffective block, and extended anesthesia. Technique related complications are largely avoidable and include hematoma, nerve damage, bruising, and intravascular injection.

Sensory Dermatomes of the Head and Neck

The main sensory innervation of the face is derived from cranial nerve V (trigeminal nerve) and the upper cervical nerves (Fig. 11.1).

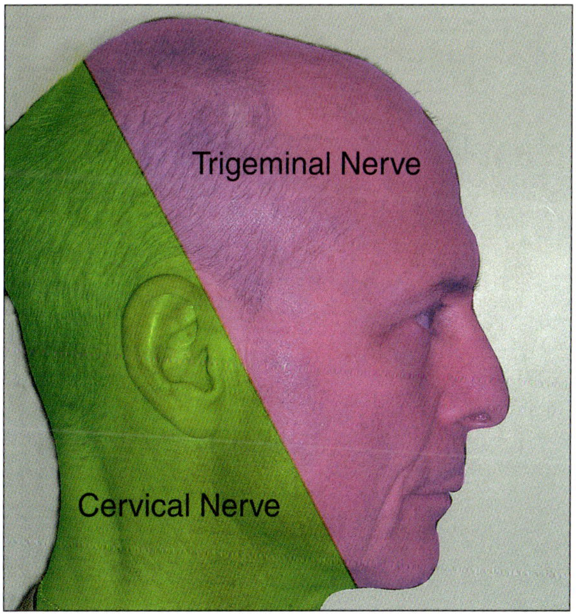

Fig. 11.1 The entire head and neck is supplied by the trigeminal and cervical nerves

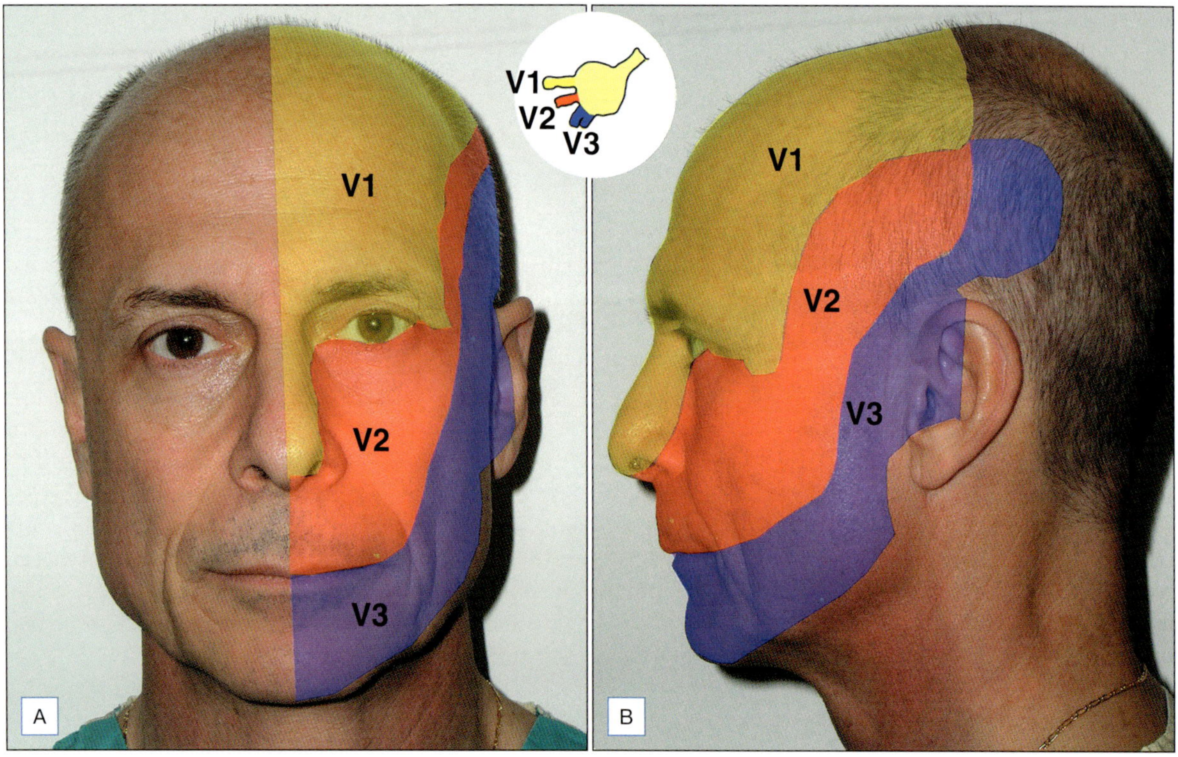

Fig. 11.2 (**A,B**) The main branches of the trigeminal nerve supplying sensation to the respective facial areas. The inset shows the trigeminal ganglion with the three main nerve branches

Trigeminal nerve

The trigeminal nerve is the fifth of the 12 cranial nerves. Its branches originate at the semilunar ganglion (gasserian ganglion) located in the temporal bone. Three large nerves, the ophthalmic, maxillary, and mandibular, proceed from the ganglion to supply sensory innervation to the face (Fig. 11.2).

Often referred to as 'the great sensory nerve of the head and neck', the trigeminal nerve is named for its three major sensory branches. The ophthalmic nerve (V1), maxillary nerve (V2), and mandibular nerve (V3) are literally 'three twins' (trigeminal) carrying sensory information of light touch, temperature, pain, and proprioception from the face and scalp to the brainstem. The main branches of the trigeminal nerve supply sensation to the well defined and consistent facial areas (Fig. 11.2). The inset in Figure 11.2 shows the trigeminal ganglion with the three main nerve branches.

Ophthalmic nerve (V1)

The ophthalmic nerve, or first division of the trigeminal, is a sensory nerve only. It supplies branches to the cornea, ciliary body, and iris; to the lacrimal gland and conjunctiva; to part of the mucous membrane of the nasal cavity; and to the skin of the eyelids, eyebrow, forehead, and upper lateral nose (see V1 on Fig. 11.2). It divides into three branches, the frontal, nasociliary, and lacrimal. The frontal nerve divides into the supraorbital and supratrochlear nerves providing sensation to the forehead and anterior scalp.

Anesthetizing branches of V1 has clinical significance for procedures in the forehead, brow regions, and glabella.

The maxillary nerve (V2)

The maxillary nerve or second division of the trigeminal is a sensory nerve that appears upon the face at the infraorbital foramen as the infraorbital nerve. At its termination, the nerve divides into branches which spread out upon the side of the nose, the lower eyelid, and the upper lip (see V2 on Fig. 11.2). Additional branches include the zygomaticotemporal which supplies sensation to the skin on the side of the forehead and zygomaticofacial nerve which supplies sensation to the skin on the prominence of the cheek (see V2 on Fig. 11.2). Anesthetizing branches of V2 has clinical significance for procedures in the temporal area, midface, nasolabial folds, and the upper lip.

The mandibular nerve (V3)

The mandibular nerve supplies the teeth and gums of the mandible, the skin of the temporal region, part of the auricle, the lower lip, and the lower part of the face (see V3 on Fig. 11.2). Sensory branches of the mandibular nerve include the auriculotemporal nerve which supplies sensation to the skin covering the front of the helix and tragus (Fig. 11.2). The inferior alveolar nerve is the largest branch of the mandibular nerve. It exits the ramus of the mandible at the mandibular foramen. It then passes forward in the mandibular canal, beneath the teeth, as far as the mental foramen, where it divides into two terminal branches, the incisive and mental nerves. The mental nerve emerges at the mental foramen, and divides into three branches of which one descends to the skin of the chin, and two ascend to the skin and mucous membrane of the lower lip. The buccal nerve is a branch of V3 which supplies sensation to the skin over the buccinator muscle. Anesthetizing branches of V3 has clinical significance for procedures in the lower lip and perioral areas of the lower face.

Topical Anesthesia

Despite the effectiveness of injectable anesthetics, the injection itself is often as painful as the procedure for which the anesthetic is used. This is especially true for minor procedures such as botulinum exotoxin injection and nonablative lasers. In these cases, topical anesthetics are useful to alleviate mild to moderate discomfort.

There are several commonly used topical anesthetics. Eutectic Mixture of Local Anesthetics (EMLA) is a 5% eutectic mixture of lidocaine (lignocaine) and prilocaine. One of the most widely used topical agents, it was briefly removed from the market recently due to a faulty child resistant cap, but is now available once again with a redesigned child resistant closure. EMLA provides suboptimal analgesia when applied for 30 minutes or less, but gives adequate dermal analgesia when applied under occlusive dressing for 60 minutes. Dermal analgesia continues for 15–30 minutes after its removal.

ELA-Max, which recently has been renamed LMX-5, is a 5% lidocaine (lignocaine) cream which uses a liposomal encapsulation system. Liposomes enhance the penetration into the skin, provide sustained release, and protect the drug from metabolic degradation. It appears superior to EMLA in providing analgesia when applied for 30 minutes.

Betacaine is also a combination of lidocaine (lignocaine) and prilocaine with an added vasoconstrictor, although the manufacturer has not revealed the exact proportion. The vasoconstrictive agent and the proprietary microemulsion delivery system speed the onset of the analgesia, and the petrolatum base makes the gel self occlusive. The manufacturer recommends an application time of 30–45 minutes without occlusive dressing. This product is not approved by the FDA and must be purchased from the manufacturer.

Tetracaine gel, previously known as amethocaine in the UK, is a compounded, proprietary ester anesthetic with a recommended application time of 30–45 minutes under occlusion. Its advantage is the long duration of analgesia, up to 4–6 hours. A comparison study shows that tetracaine is more efficacious than lidocaine-prilocaine mixture when both anesthetics are applied for the same amount of time. However, unlike the amide anesthetics, allergic contact reactions to ester anesthetics are quite common.

The average time of application of topical anesthetics ranges from 30–60 minutes, which can be a frustrating rate limiting step in clinical practice. S-Caine peel is a new development that may have a quicker onset. S-Caine peel is a eutectic lidocaine (lignocaine) and tetracaine (amethocaine) cream mixture that dries to a flexible film that easily peels off. This property precludes the need for extra time-consuming steps such as application of occlusive dressing and removal of the creams. Furthermore, adequate anesthesia is achieved in as little as 20 minutes of application. A recent double blinded study concluded that S-Caine peel is superior to EMLA cream under occlusion for 30 minutes.

Vibratory Anesthesia

Vibration has been used for many years to reduce pain in disciplines such as dentistry and physiotherapy, and is now becoming recognized as a simple, safe, and effective form of anesthesia in dermatology. Vibration anesthesia can be explained by the 'gate theory of pain control' popularized by Melzack and Wall in the 1960s. Noxious nerve impulses evoked by injuries are influenced in the spinal cord by other nerve cells that act like gates, either preventing the impulses from getting through, or facilitating their passage. Without vibratory modulation, noxious impulses are carried through small C fibers uninhibited through a 'gate' in the spinal cord that ultimately sends the signal to the brain. When applied simultaneously, vibratory stimulation excites large A fibers, which activates inhibitory interneurons at the gate and mitigates the perception of pain in the brain.

Any vibratory massager can be used to produce the vibratory stimulation. A study has shown that pain sensitivity gradually declines as vibration amplitude increases, but no specific frequency is more effective in interference with nociception. The vibratory massager should be applied approximately 2–3 seconds prior to the injection or laser application and 1–2 cm from the site, and continue throughout the procedure.

Infiltrative Peripheral Anesthesia versus Regional Nerve Block Anesthesia

Local anesthesia can be effectively obtained both by infiltrations and nerve blocks. Infiltrative local anesthesia applies to the injection of the local anesthesia solution in the area of the peripheral innervation distant from the site of the main nerve. An advantage of infiltrative anesthesia is that no specific skill is necessary, only the selected area of innervation is involved and vasoconstrictors can improve local hemostasis. A drawback of infiltrative local anesthesia is the distortion of the tissue at or around the site of injection which may obscure the tissue detail required in cosmetic procedures such as filler injection.

Nerve blocks

A nerve block involves placing the local anesthetic solution in a specific location at or around the main nerve trunk that will effectively depolarize that nerve and obtund sensation in the area of sensory distribution of that particular nerve. Advantages of nerve blocks include the fact that a single accurately placed injection can obtund large areas of sensation without tissue distortion at the operative site. Disadvantages of peripheral nerve block include the sensation of numbness in areas other than the operative site and the lack of hemostasis at the operative site from the vasoconstrictor component of the local anesthetic injection.

Individual anatomic variation is responsible for the sometimes unpredictable effect of peripheral nerve block. Nerves that innervate areas close to the midline may receive innervation from the contralateral side and require bilateral blocks. Some nerve blocks may also require infiltrative local anesthesia to obtain adequate pain control.

Since many nerves are accompanied by corresponding veins and arteries, preinjection aspiration should always be performed to prevent intravascular injection. Using local anesthetics with vasoconstrictors will prolong anesthesia which may be undesirable for most patients who want to return to normal activities after filler injection. Prolonged anesthesia makes speaking and normal lip posture difficult, so most doctors only prefer to use shorter acting anesthetics so that the anesthetic effect persists through the injection sequence.

Anatomic arrangement of the facial foramina

Successful nerve block anesthesia is largely dependent upon knowing the positions of the nerve foramina. The surgeon can take advantage of the alignment of the major facial foramina as they relate to a vertical line through the midpupillary line with the eye in the primary position of natural forward gaze (Fig. 11.3).

Blocking the scalp and forehead

The use of fillers has recently expanded beyond the lips. Multiple areas of all sensory dermatomes may be sites for the use of dermal fillers. Using filler agents in the glabellar area and frontalis lines may require local anesthesia of the frontal nerve to anesthetize the forehead.

Supraorbital nerve

The supraorbital nerve exits through a notch (in some cases a foramen) on the superior orbital rim approximately 27 mm lateral to the glabellar midline (Fig. 11.4). This supraorbital notch is readily palpable in most patients. After exiting the notch or foramen, the nerve traverses the corrugator supercilii muscles and branches into a medial and lateral portion. The lateral branches supply the lateral forehead and the medial branches supply the scalp.

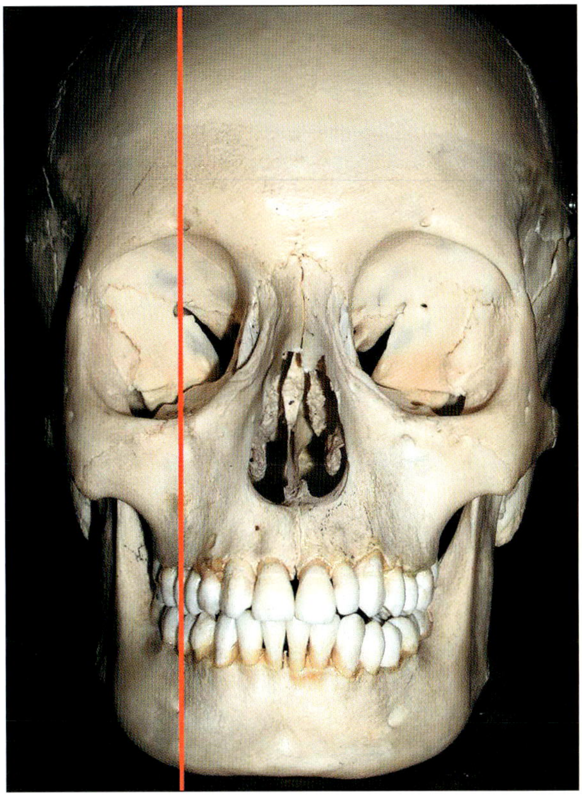

Fig. 11.3 The supraorbital, infraorbital and mental foramina are all in line with an imaginary vertical line passing through the mid pupil

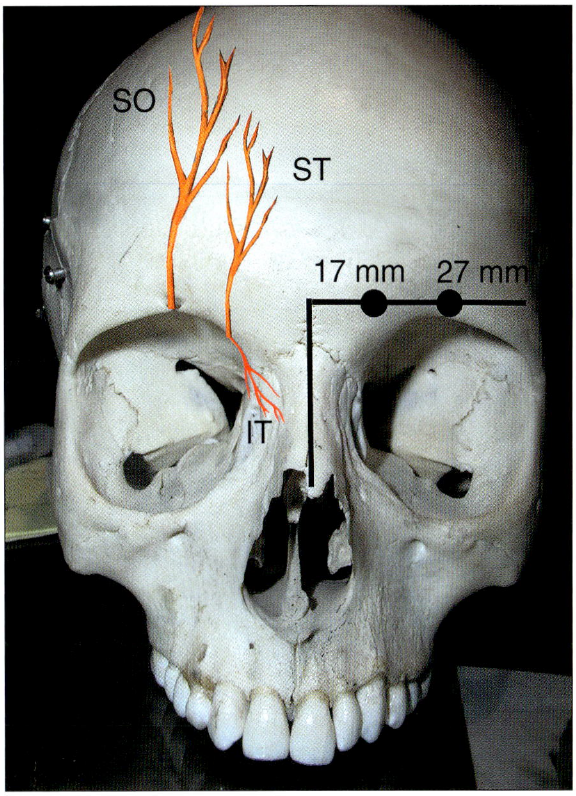

Fig. 11.4 The supraorbital nerve (SO) exits about 27 mm from the glabellar midline and the supratrochlear nerve (ST) is located approximately 17 mm from the glabellar midline. The infratrochlear nerve (IT) exits below the trochlea

Supratrochlear nerve

The supratrochlear nerve exits a foramen approximately 17 mm from the glabellar midline (Fig. 11.4) and supplies sensation to the middle portion of the forehead. The infratrochlear nerve exits a foramen below the trochlea and provides sensation to the medial upper eyelid, canthus, medial nasal skin, conjunctiva, and lacrimal apparatus (Fig. 11.4).

When injecting this area it is prudent to always use the nondominant hand to palpate the orbital rim to ensure that the needle tip is exterior to the bony orbital margin. To anesthetize this area, the supratrochlear nerve is measured 17 mm from the glabellar midline and 1–2 mL of local anesthetic are injected (Fig. 11.5A). The supraorbital nerve is blocked by palpating the notch (and/or measuring 27 mm from the glabellar midline) and injecting 1–2 mL of local anesthetic solution (Fig. 11.5B). The infratrochlear nerve is blocked by injecting 1–2 mL of local anesthetic solution at the junction of the orbit and the nasal bones (Fig. 11.5C; Fig. 11.6 shows the regions anesthetized from the above blocks).

Infraorbital nerve block

This block is one of the most commonly utilized facial blocks in order to anesthetize the upper lip and upper nasolabial fold for injection of fillers. Obviously, a bilateral block must be performed to achieve anesthesia on both sides of the lip.

The infaorbital nerve exits the infraorbital foramen 4–7 mm below the orbital rim in an imaginary line dropped from the midpupillary midline. The anterior superior alveolar nerve branches from the infraorbital nerve before it exits the foramen, and thus some patients will manifest anesthesia of the anterior teeth and gingiva if the branching is close to the foramen. Areas anesthetized include the lateral nose, anterior cheek, lower eyelid, and upper

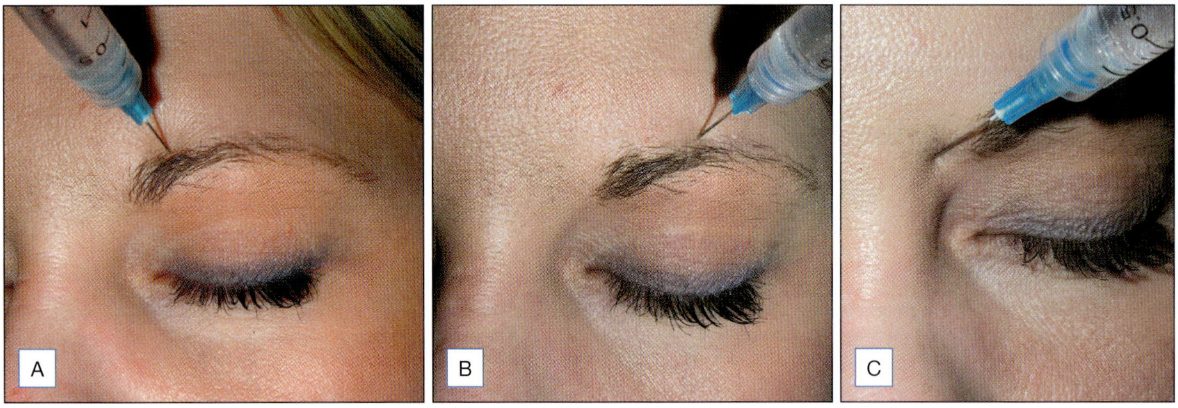

Fig. 11.5 (A–C) The forehead and scalp is blocked by a series of injections from the central to the medial brow

lip on the injected side. This nerve can be blocked by intraoral or extraoral routes. To perform an infraorbital nerve block from an intraoral approach, topical anesthesia is placed on the oral mucosa at the vestibular sulcus just under the canine fossa (between the canine and first premolar tooth) and left for several minutes. The lip is then elevated and a ½ inch 30 gauge needle is inserted in the sulcus and directed superiorly toward the infraorbital foramen (Fig. 11.7). Bending the needle at a 45 degree angle upward can facilitate the needle insertion (Fig. 11.8). The needle needs only to approach the vast branching around the foramen to be effective. It is important to use the other hand to palpate the inferior orbital rim to avoid injecting superiorly the orbit. 2–4 mL of 2% lidocaine (lignocaine) are injected in this area for the infraorbital block and the palpating finger can feel the local anesthetic bolus below the infraorbital rim, confirming the correct area of placement.

We find it important to ask the patient to open the eyes and look straight ahead when performing the infraorbital block. This way, the injector can see the pupil and better appreciate the position of the infraorbital foramen which is 4–7 mm below the infraorbital rim in the midpupillary line.

The infraorbital nerve can also be very easily blocked by the transcutaneous facial approach and may be the preferred route in dental phobic patients. A 32 gauge ½ inch needle is used and is placed through the skin and aimed at the foramen in a perpendicular direction. Between 2 and 4 mL of local anesthetic solution is injected at or close to the foramen (Fig. 11.9). Again, the other hand must constantly palpate the inferior orbital rim to prevent inadvertent injection into the orbit. Care must be used in this approach to avoid superficial vessels that may cause noticeable bruising.

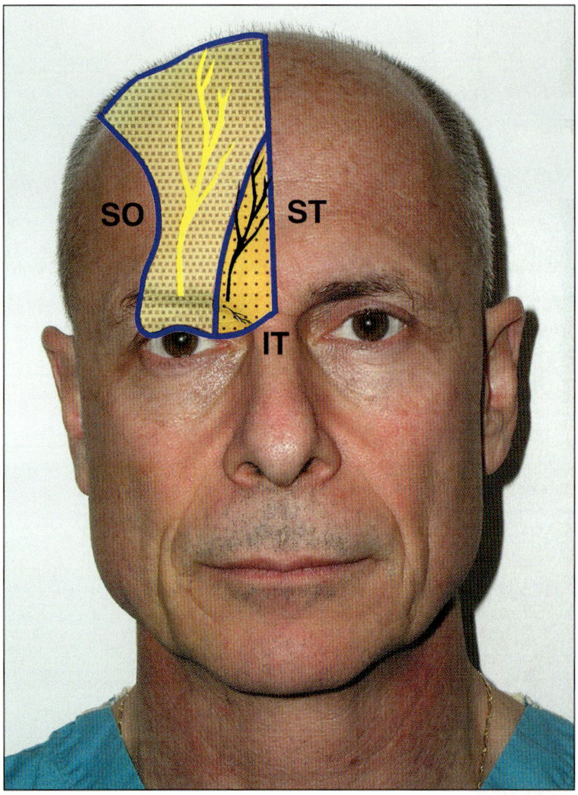

Fig. 11.6 The shaded areas indicate the anesthetized areas from supraorbital nerve (SO) and supratrochlear nerve (ST) and infratrochlear nerve (IT) blocks

A successful infraorbital nerve block will anesthetize the infraorbital cheek, the lower palpebral

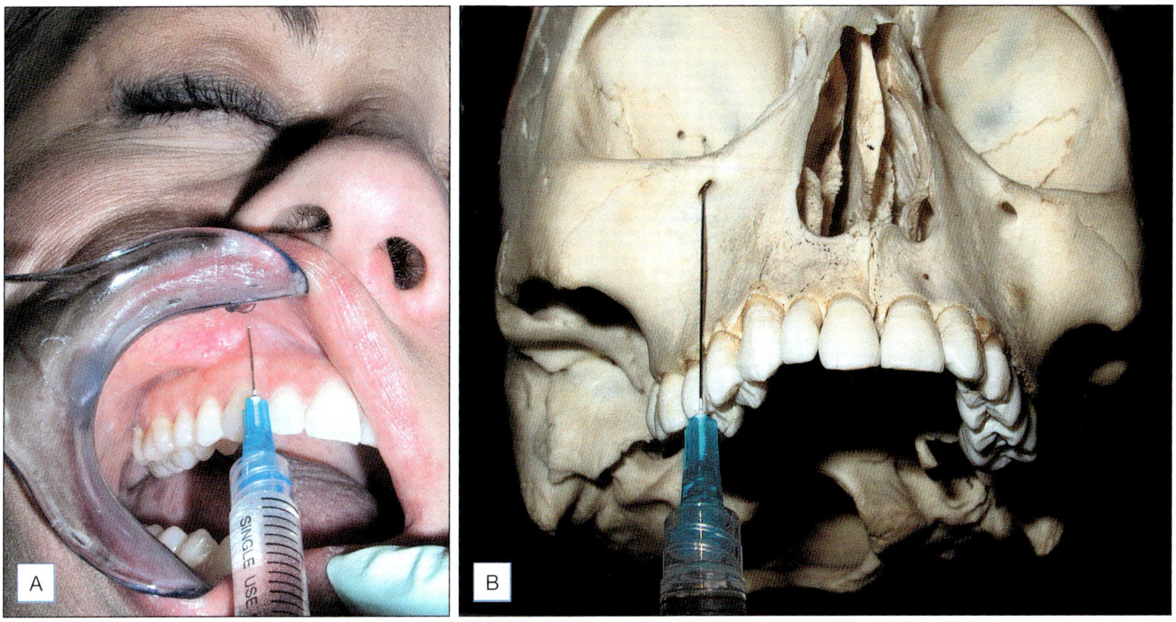

Fig. 11.7 (**A,B**) The intraoral approach for local anesthetic block of the infraorbital nerve

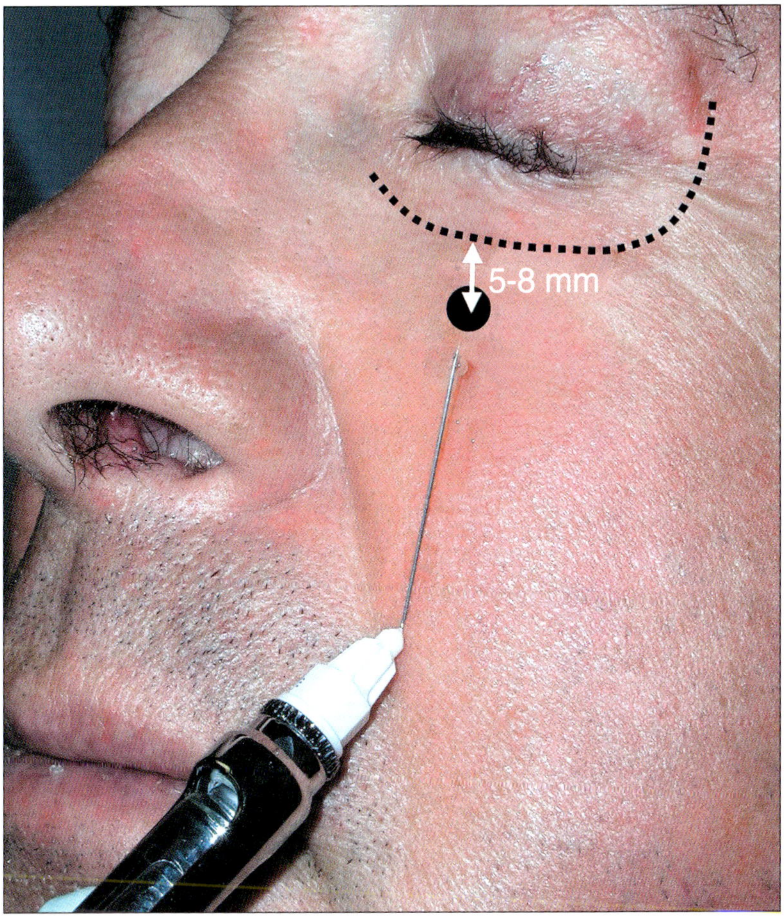

Fig. 11.8 Bending the 1½ inch 28 gauge needle at a 45 degree angle can facilitate the injection technique of the infraorbital nerve. Note the needle is shown outside the mouth for illustrative purposes only. The actual injection is intraoral

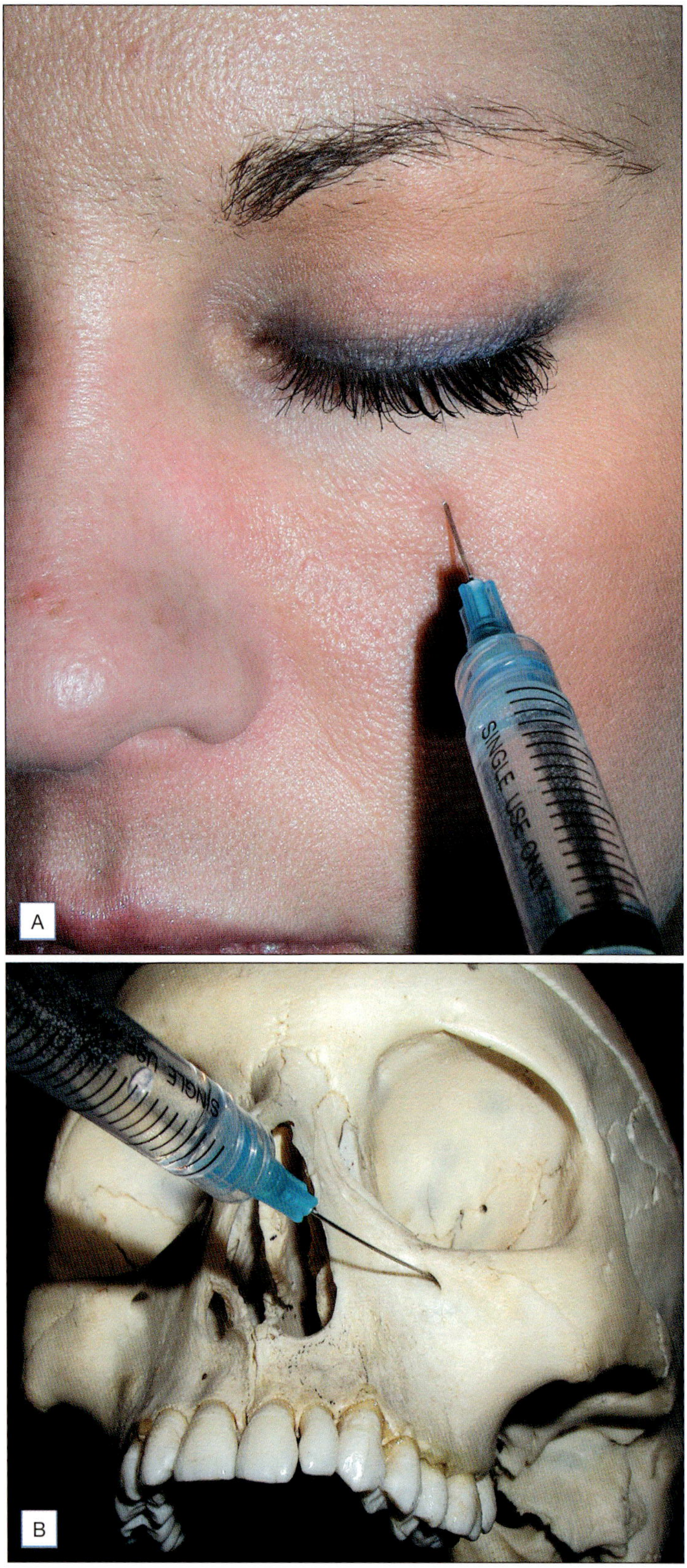

Fig. 11.9 (**A,B**) The facial approach for local anesthetic block of the infraorbital nerve

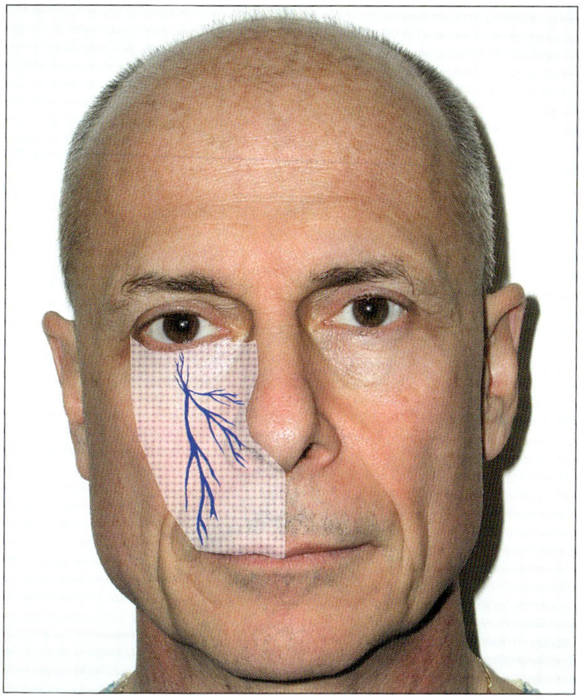

Fig. 11.10 Area of anesthesia from unilateral infraorbital nerve block

area, the lateral nasal area, and superior labial regions as shown in Figure 11.10.

Anesthesia for aesthetic lip augmentation

Although in theory a bilateral infraorbital block should anesthetize the entire upper lip, some patients may still perceive pain for various anatomic (or sometimes psychological) reasons detailed earlier in this article. The author recommends the injection of 1.0mL of local anesthetic solution in the maxillary labial frenum (Fig. 11.11). Whether for psychological or physiological reasons, this seems to provide additional anesthesia. This can also be performed in the lower lip labial frenum area to augment bilateral mental blocks, as will be discussed later in this chapter. The combination of bilateral infraorbital and mental blocks and the just described infiltrative augmentation (when necessary) is an ideal technique for anesthetizing the lips for filler injection or lip implant placement.

Zygomaticofacial nerve

Two often overlooked nerves in facial local anesthetic blocks are the zygomaticotemporal and zygo-

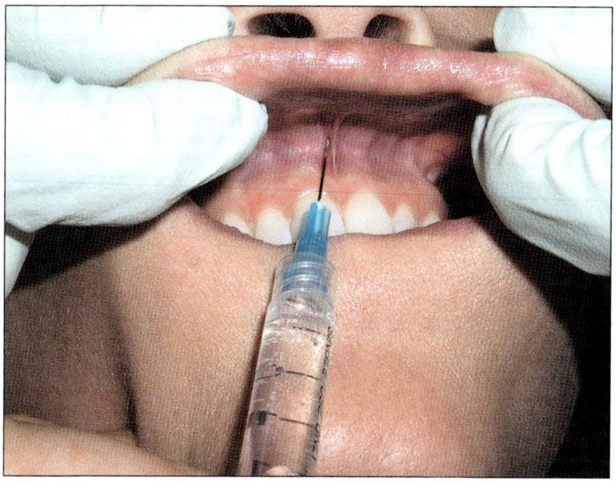

Fig. 11.11 An augmentative injection of local anesthesia in the maxillary frenum can assist subtotal anesthesia from infraorbital blocks when the upper lip is anesthetized

maticofacial nerves. This may assist the injection of fillers in facial rhytides on the lateral temporal and lateral canthal areas or in the malar areas. These nerves represent terminal branches of the zygomatic nerve. The zygomaticotemporal nerve emerges through a foramen located on the anterior wall of the temporal fossa. This foramen is actually behind the lateral orbital rim posterior to the zygoma at the approximate level of the lateral canthus (Fig. 11.12).

The injection technique involves sliding a 1½ inch 27 gauge needle behind the concave portion of the lateral orbital rim. It is suggested that this area should be closely examined on a model skull prior to attempting this injection as it will facilitate understanding of the anatomy and make the technique simpler. To orient for this injection it is necessary to palpate the lateral orbital rim at the level of the frontozygomatic suture (which is frequently palpable). With the index finger in the depression of the posterior lateral aspect of the lateral orbital rim (inferior and posterior to the frontozygomatic suture), the operator places the needle just behind the palpating finger (which is about 1 cm posterior to the frontozygomatic suture (Fig. 11.12)). The needle is then 'walked' down the concave posterior wall of the lateral orbital rim to the approximate level of the lateral canthus. After aspirating, 1–2mL of 2% lidocaine (lignocaine) is injected in this area with a slight pumping action to ensure deposition of the local anesthetic solution at or about the foramen. Again, it is important to hug the back

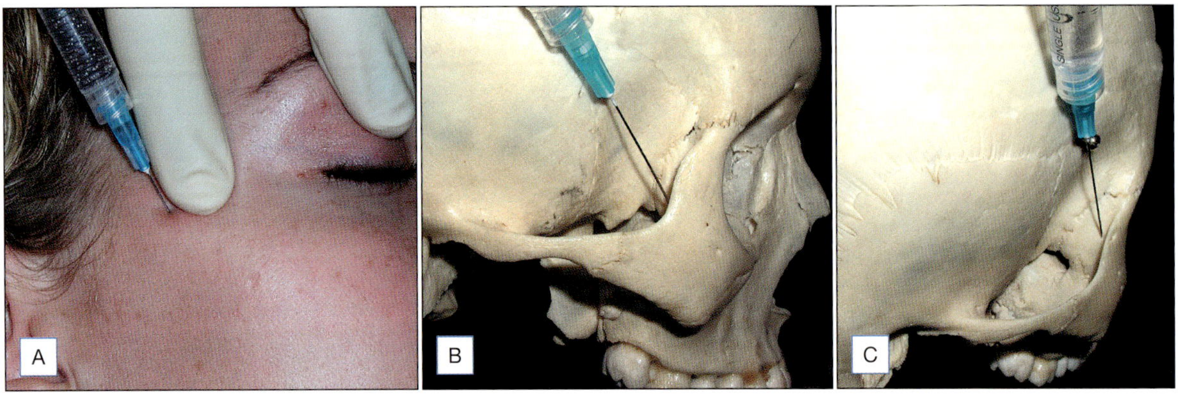

Fig. 11.12 (A–C) The zygomaticotemporal nerve is blocked by placing the needle on the concave surface of the posterior lateral orbital rim

concave wall of the lateral orbital rim with the needle when injecting.

Blocking the zygomaticotemporal nerve causes anesthesia in the area superior to the nerve, including the lateral orbital rim and the skin of the temple from above the zygomatic arch to the temporal fusion line (see ZT on Fig. 11.13).

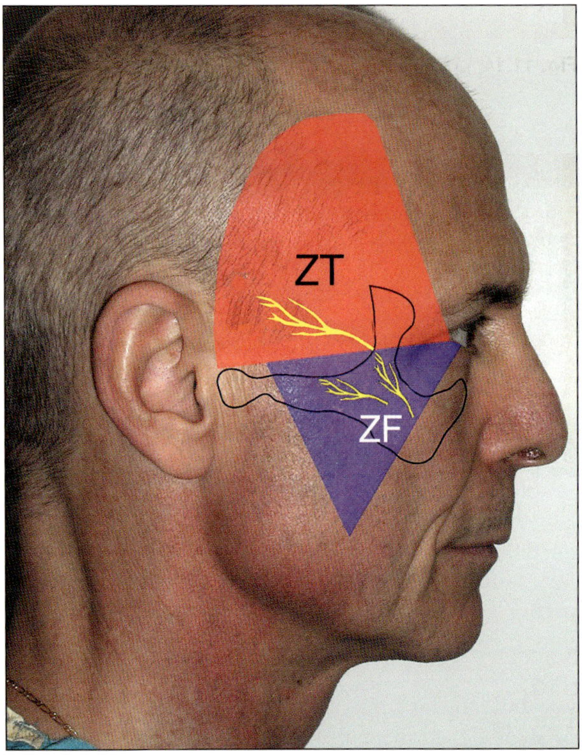

Fig. 11.13 The anesthetized areas form the zygomaticotemporal (ZT) and the zygomaticofacial (ZF) nerves

Zygomaticofacial nerve

The zygomaticofacial nerve exits through a foramen (or foramina in some patients) in the inferior lateral portion of the orbital rim at the zygoma. If the surgeon palpates the junction of the inferior lateral portion of the lateral orbital rim, the nerve emerges several millimeters lateral to this point. By palpating this area and injecting just lateral to the finger, this nerve is successfully blocked with 1–2 mL of local anesthetic (Fig. 11.14). Blocking this nerve will result in anesthesia of a triangular area from the lateral canthus and the malar region along the zygomatic arch and some skin inferior to this area (see ZF on Fig. 11.13).

Mental nerve block

The mental nerve exits the mental foramen on the hemimandible at the base of the root of the second premolar (many patients may be missing a premolar due to orthodontic extractions). The mental foramen is on average 11 mm inferior to the gum line (Fig. 11.15). There is variability with this foramen (like all foramina), but by injecting 2–4 mL of local anesthetic solution about 10 mm inferior to the gum line or 15 mm inferior to the top of the crown of the second premolar tooth the block is usually successful. In a patient without teeth, the foramen is often times located much higher on the jaw and can sometimes be palpated. This block is performed more superiorly in the denture patient. As stated earlier, the foramen does not need to be entered as a sufficient volume of local anesthetic solution in the general area will be effective. By placing traction on

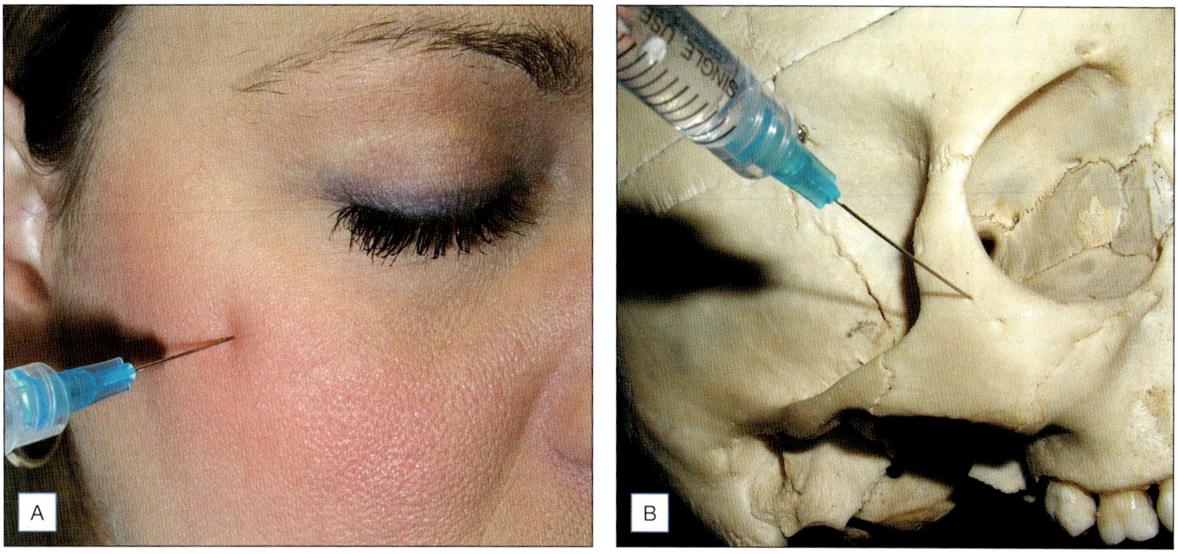

Fig. 11.14 (**A,B**) The zygomaticofacial nerve(s) are blocked by injecting the inferior lateral portion of the orbital rim

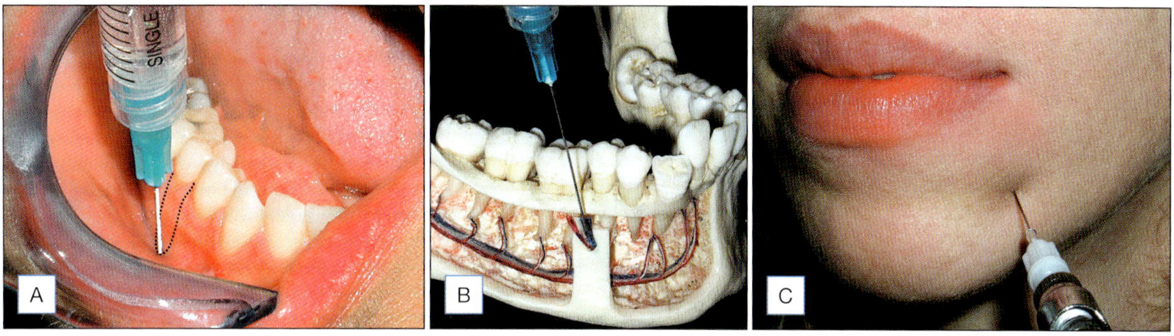

Fig. 11.15 The mental foramen is approached intraorally below the root tip of the lower second premolar (**A,B**) or from a facial approach (**C**)

the lip and pulling it away from the jaw, the labial branches of the mental nerve can sometimes be seen traversing through the thin mucosa (Fig. 11.16). The mental nerve gives off labial branches to the lip and chin (Fig. 11.17).

Alternatively, the mental nerve may be blocked through the skin of the cheek with a facial approach, aiming for the same target.

When anesthetized the distribution of numbness will be the unilateral lower lip to the midline and laterally to the mentolabial fold, and in some patients the anterior chin and cheek depending on the individual furcating anatomy of that patient's nerve (Fig. 11.18).

As mentioned earlier, sometimes patients may perceive pain despite bilateral nerve block in the upper or lower lips. When injecting fillers in the lower lip and bilateral mental nerve blocks are not totally effective, a supplemental infiltration of several milliliters of local anesthesia into the region of the mandibular labial frenulum can assist the blocks (Fig. 11.19).

The author after performing hundreds of facial blocks for filler injection now uses a simple infiltration technique. Instead of blocking the infraorbital and mental nerves, the author first places topical anesthetic on the maxillary and mandibular vestibule from the canine tooth no one side to the canine tooth on the other side. After several minutes, a 32 gauge needle is used to inject 1/4 cc of local anesthetic solution at the depth of the maxillary and/or mandibular vestibule. The vestibule is defined as the

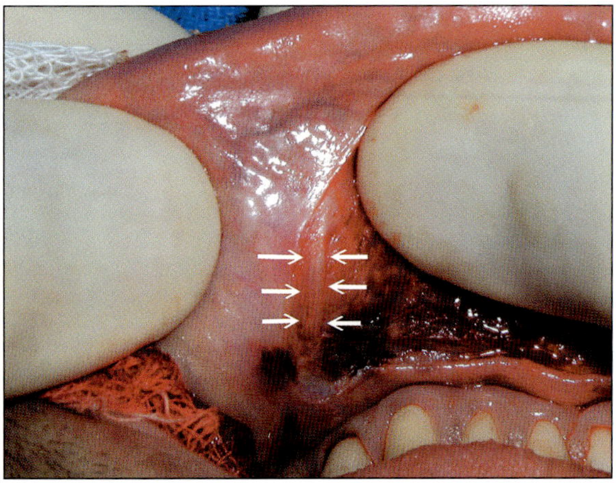

Fig. 11.16 By stretching the lower lip mucosa the underlying labial branches of the mental nerve are sometimes visible. This image shows the very superficial labial sensory nerve exposed with mucosal incision for a chin implant

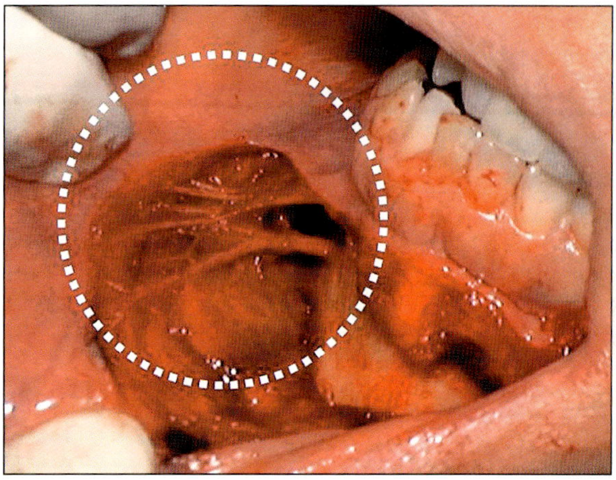

Fig. 11.17 The vast arborization of the distal branches of the mental nerve (in circle) are visualized intraoperatively in a genioplasty incision

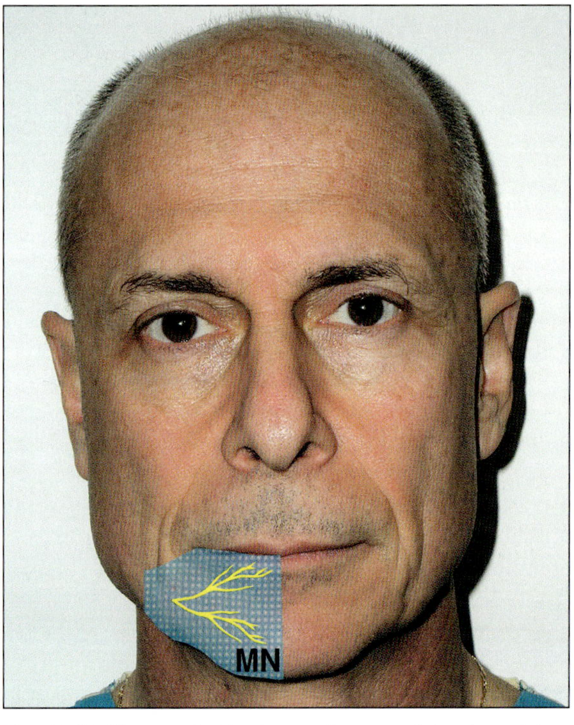

Fig. 11.18 The anesthetized areas from a unilateral mental nerve block. Due to various anatomic factors, the area below the mentolabial fold or at the midline may share other innervation

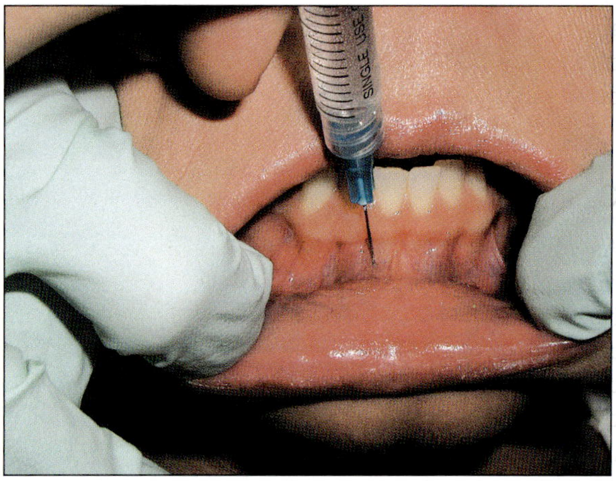

Fig. 11.19 Supplemental anesthetic infiltration of the lower labial frenum area can be used to augment bilateral mental blocks when the patient still perceives pain

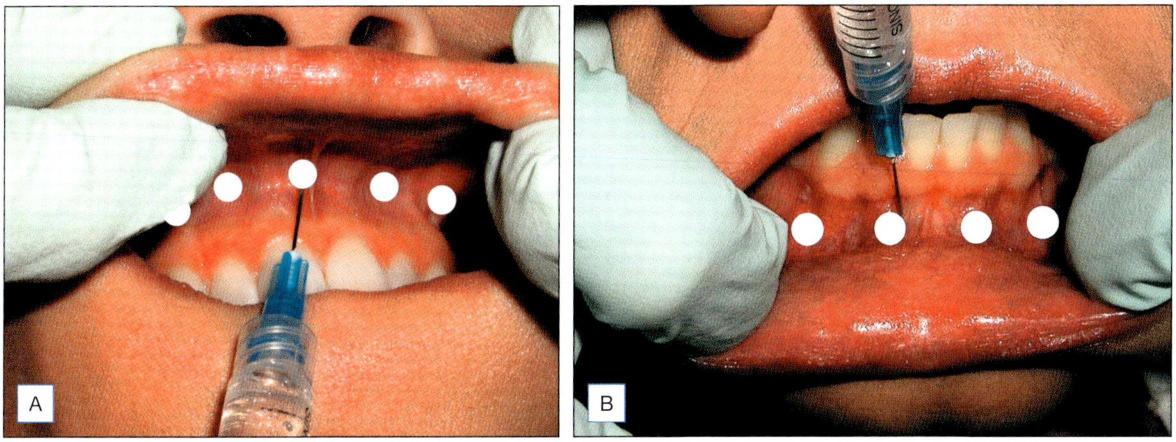

Fig. 11.20 (**A–B**) Submucosal lip infiltration can be used to augment or in place of bilateral mental nerve block to treat the lower lip. Very small volumes will create adequate anesthesia. The solution is injected across the entire lip. The same technique can be used on the upper lip as well

junction of the attached gingiva (gum) and the lip mucosa. These injections are made just above the periosteum in 4 or 5 spots between the upper or lower canine teeth. This technique provides remarkable anesthesia suitable for filler injection and is often easier for the doctor and patient than nerve blocks. This technique is shown in Figure 11.20.

Conclusion

As advances are made in the science of facial fillers more products and indications will become available for these minimally invasive, highly effective aesthetic procedures. This chapter outlines some of the more basic anatomy and techniques for anesthetizing the common areas of the face amenable to injectible fillers.

Further Reading

Aceves J, Machne X 1963 The action of calcium and of local anesthetics on nerve cells and their interaction during excitation. Journal of Pharmacology and Experimental Therapeutics 140:138–148

Alster TS, Lupton JR 2002 Evaluation of a novel topical anesthetic agent for cutaneous laser resurfacing: a randomized comparison study. Dermatologic Surgery 28:1004–1006

Bucalo BD, Mirikitani EJ, Moy RL 1998 Comparison of skin anesthetic effect of liposomal lidocaine, nonliposomal lidocaine, and EMLA using 30-minute application time. Dermatologic Surgery 24:537–541

Covino BG, Vassalo HG 1976 Chemical aspects of local anesthetic agents. In: Kitz RJ, Laver MB (eds) Local anesthetics: mechanism of action and clinical use. Grune & Stratton, New York, pp 1–11

Fink BR 1988 History of neural blockade. In: Cousins MJ, Bridenbaugh PO (eds) Neural blockade in clinical anesthesia and management of pain, 2nd edn. JB Lippincott, Philadelphia, pp 3–21

Friedman PM, Fogelman JP, Nouri K, Levine VJ, Ashinoff R 1999 Comparative study of the efficacy of four topical anesthetics. Dermatologic Surgery 25:950–954

Gray H 1918 Anatomy of the human body, 13th edn. Lea & Febiger, Philadelphia, 1158–1169

Hadda SE 1962 Procaine: Alfred Einhorn's ideal substitute for cocaine. Journal of the American Dental Association 64:841–845

Hersh EV 2000 Local anesthetics. In: Fonseca RJ (ed) Oral and maxillofacial surgery. WB Saunders, Philadelphia, pp 58–78

Hersh EV, Condouis GA 1987 Local anesthetics: a review of their pharmacology and clinical use. Compendium of Continuing Education in Dentistry 8:374–382

Hollins M, Roy EA, Crane SA 2003 Vibratory antinociception: effects of vibration amplitude and frequency. Journal of Pain 4:381–391

Jastak JT, Yagiela JA, Donaldson D 1995 Local anesthesia of the oral cavity. WB Saunders, Philadelphia

Kakigi R, Shibasaki H 1992 Mechanisms of pain relief by vibration and movement. Journal of Neurology, Neurosurgery and Psychiatry 55:282–286

Kosten TR, Hollister LE 1998 Drugs of abuse. In: Katzung BG (ed) Basic and clinical pharmacology, 7th edn. Appleton & Lange, Norwalk, CT, pp 516–531

Lathers CM, Tyau LSY, Spino MM, Agarwal I 1988 Cocaine-induced seizures, arrhythmias, and sudden death. Journal of Clinical Pharmacology 28:584–593

Lener EV, Bucalo BD, Kist DA, Moy RL 1997 Topical anesthetic agents in dermatologic surgery. A review. Dermatologic Surgery 23:673–683

Malamed SF 1997 Handbook of local anesthesia, 4th edn. Mosby, St Louis, MO

Mendel N, Puterbaugh PG 1938 Conduction, infiltration and general anesthesia in dentistry, 4th edn. Dental Items of Interest Publishing Company, p 140

Stricharatz D 1976 Molecular mechanisms of nerve block by local anesthetics. Anesthesiology 45:421–441

Yagiela JA 1991 Local anesthetics. In: Dionne RA, Phero JC (eds) Management of pain and anxiety in dental practice. Elsevier, New York, pp 109–134

Zide BM, Swift R 1998 How to block and tackle the face. Plastic and Reconstructive Surgery 101:840–851

Subject Index

Notes
Index entries in **bold** refer to information in tables or boxes: index entries in *italics* refers to figures.
vs. indicates a comparison or differential diagnosis.

G

H

M

N

ELSEVIER DVD-ROM LICENSE AGREEMENT

PLEASE READ THE FOLLOWING AGREEMENT CAREFULLY BEFORE USING THIS DVD-ROM PRODUCT. THIS DVD-ROM PRODUCT IS LICENSED UNDER THE TERMS CONTAINED IN THIS DVD-ROM LICENSE AGREEMENT ("Agreement"). BY USING THIS DVD-ROM PRODUCT, YOU, AN INDIVIDUAL OR ENTITY INCLUDING EMPLOYEES, AGENTS AND REPRESENTATIVES ("You" or "Your"), ACKNOWLEDGE THAT YOU HAVE READ THIS AGREEMENT, THAT YOU UNDERSTAND IT, AND THAT YOU AGREE TO BE BOUND BY THE TERMS AND CONDITIONS OF THIS AGREEMENT. ELSEVIER INC. ("Elsevier") EXPRESSLY DOES NOT AGREE TO LICENSE THIS DVD-ROM PRODUCT TO YOU UNLESS YOU ASSENT TO THIS AGREEMENT. IF YOU DO NOT AGREE WITH ANY OF THE FOLLOWING TERMS, YOU MAY, WITHIN THIRTY (30) DAYS AFTER YOUR RECEIPT OF THIS DVD-ROM PRODUCT RETURN THE UNUSED, PIN NUMBER PROTECTED, DVD-ROM PRODUCT, AND ALL ACCOMPANYING DOCUMENTATION TO ELSEVIER FOR A FULL REFUND.

DEFINITIONS As used in this Agreement, these terms shall have the following meanings:

"Proprietary Material" means the valuable and proprietary information content of this DVD-ROM Product including all indexes and graphic materials and software used to access, index, search and retrieve the information content from this DVD-ROM Product developed or licensed by Elsevier and/or its affiliates, suppliers and licensors.

"DVD-ROM Product" means the copy of the Proprietary Material and any other material delivered on DVD-ROM and any other human-readable or machine-readable materials enclosed with this Agreement, including without limitation documentation relating to the same.

OWNERSHIP This DVD-ROM Product has been supplied by and is proprietary to Elsevier and/or its affiliates, suppliers and licensors. The copyright in the DVD-ROM Product belongs to Elsevier and/or its affiliates, suppliers and licensors and is protected by the national and state copyright, trademark, trade secret and other intellectual property laws of the United States and international treaty provisions, including without limitation the Universal Copyright Convention and the Berne Copyright Convention. You have no ownership rights in this DVD-ROM Product. Except as expressly set forth herein, no part of this DVD-ROM Product, including without limitation the Proprietary Material, may be modified, copied or distributed in hardcopy or machine-readable form without prior written consent from Elsevier. All rights not expressly granted to You herein are expressly reserved. Any other use of this DVD-ROM Product by any person or entity is strictly prohibited and a violation of this Agreement.

SCOPE OF RIGHTS LICENSED (PERMITTED USES) Elsevier is granting to You a limited, non-exclusive, non-transferable license to use this DVD-ROM Product in accordance with the terms of this Agreement. You may use or provide access to this DVD-ROM Product on a single computer or terminal physically located at Your premises and in a secure network or move this DVD-ROM Product to and use it on another single computer or terminal at the same location for personal use only, but under no circumstances may You use or provide access to any part or parts of this DVD-ROM Product on more than one computer or terminal simultaneously.

You shall not (a) copy, download, or otherwise reproduce the DVD-ROM Product in any medium, including, without limitation, online transmissions, local area networks, wide area networks, intranets, extranets and the Internet, or in any way, in whole or in part, except for printing out or downloading nonsubstantial portions of the text and images in the DVD-ROM Product for Your own personal use; (b) alter, modify, or adapt the DVD-ROM Product, including but not limited to decompiling, disassembling, reverse engineering, or creating derivative works, without the prior written approval of Elsevier; (c) sell, license or otherwise distribute to third parties the DVD-ROM Product or any part or parts thereof; or (d) alter, remove, obscure or obstruct the display of any copyright, trademark or other proprietary notice on or in the DVD-ROM Product or on any printout or download of portions of the Proprietary Materials.

RESTRICTIONS ON TRANSFER This License is personal to You, and neither Your rights hereunder nor the tangible embodiments of this DVD-ROM Product, including without limitation the Proprietary Material, may be sold, assigned, transferred or sublicensed to any other person, including without limitation by operation of law, without the prior written consent of Elsevier. Any purported sale, assignment, transfer or sublicense without the prior written consent of Elsevier will be void and will automatically terminate the License granted hereunder.

TERM This Agreement will remain in effect until terminated pursuant to the terms of this Agreement. You may terminate this Agreement at any time by removing from Your system and destroying the DVD-ROM Product. Unauthorized copying of the DVD-ROM Product, including without limitation, the Proprietary Material and documentation, or otherwise failing to comply with the terms and conditions of this Agreement shall result in automatic termination of this license and will make available to Elsevier legal remedies. Upon termination of this Agreement, the license granted herein will terminate and You must immediately destroy the DVD-ROM Product and accompanying documentation. All provisions relating to proprietary rights shall survive termination of this Agreement.

LIMITED WARRANTY AND LIMITATION OF LIABILITY NEITHER ELSEVIER NOR ITS LICENSORS REPRESENT OR WARRANT THAT THE DVD-ROM PRODUCT WILL MEET YOUR REQUIREMENTS OR THAT ITS OPERATION WILL BE UNINTERRUPTED OR ERROR-FREE. WE EXCLUDE AND EXPRESSLY DISCLAIM ALL EXPRESS AND IMPLIED WARRANTIES NOT STATED HEREIN, INCLUDING THE IMPLIED WARRANTIES OF MERCHANTABILITY AND FITNESS FOR A PARTICULAR PURPOSE. IN ADDITION, NEITHER ELSEVIER NOR ITS LICENSORS MAKE ANY REPRESENTATIONS OR WARRANTIES, EITHER EXPRESS OR IMPLIED, REGARDING THE PERFORMANCE OF YOUR NETWORK OR COMPUTER SYSTEM WHEN USED IN CONJUNCTION WITH THE DVD-ROM PRODUCT. WE SHALL NOT BE LIABLE FOR ANY DAMAGE OR LOSS OF ANY KIND ARISING OUT OF OR RESULTING FROM YOUR POSSESSION OR USE OF THE SOFTWARE PRODUCT CAUSED BY ERRORS OR OMISSIONS, DATA LOSS OR CORRUPTION, ERRORS OR OMISSIONS IN THE PROPRIETARY MATERIAL, REGARDLESS OF WHETHER SUCH LIABILITY IS BASED IN TORT, CONTRACT OR OTHERWISE AND INCLUDING, BUT NOT LIMITED TO, ACTUAL, SPECIAL, INDIRECT, INCIDENTAL OR CONSEQUENTIAL DAMAGES. IF THE FOREGOING LIMITATION IS HELD TO BE UNENFORCEABLE, OUR MAXIMUM LIABILITY TO YOU SHALL NOT EXCEED THE AMOUNT OF THE LICENSE FEE PAID BY YOU FOR THE SOFTWARE PRODUCT. THE REMEDIES AVAILABLE TO YOU AGAINST US AND THE LICENSORS OF MATERIALS INCLUDED IN THE SOFTWARE PRODUCT ARE EXCLUSIVE.

If this DVD-ROM Product is defective, Elsevier will replace it at no charge if the defective DVD-ROM Product is returned to Elsevier within sixty (60) days (or the greatest period allowable by applicable law) from the date of shipment.

Elsevier warrants that the software embodied in this DVD-ROM Product will perform in substantial compliance with the documentation supplied in this DVD-ROM Product. If You report a significant defect in performance in writing to Elsevier, and Elsevier is not able to correct same within sixty (60) days after its receipt of Your notification, You may return this DVD-ROM Product, including all copies and documentation, to Elsevier and Elsevier will refund Your money.

YOU UNDERSTAND THAT, EXCEPT FOR THE 60-DAY LIMITED WARRANTY RECITED ABOVE, ELSEVIER, ITS AFFILIATES, LICENSORS, SUPPLIERS AND AGENTS, MAKE NO WARRANTIES, EXPRESSED OR IMPLIED, WITH RESPECT TO THE DVD-ROM PRODUCT, INCLUDING, WITHOUT LIMITATION THE PROPRIETARY MATERIAL, AND SPECIFICALLY DISCLAIM ANY WARRANTY OF MERCHANTABILITY OR FITNESS FOR A PARTICULAR PURPOSE.

If the information provided on this DVD-ROM Product contains medical or health sciences information, it is intended for professional use within the medical field. Information about medical treatment or drug dosages is intended strictly for professional use, and because of rapid advances in the medical sciences, independent verification of diagnosis and drug dosages should be made.

IN NO EVENT WILL ELSEVIER, ITS AFFILIATES, LICENSORS, SUPPLIERS OR AGENTS, BE LIABLE TO YOU FOR ANY DAMAGES, INCLUDING, WITHOUT LIMITATION, ANY LOST PROFITS, LOST SAVINGS OR OTHER INCIDENTAL OR CONSEQUENTIAL DAMAGES, ARISING OUT OF YOUR USE OR INABILITY TO USE THE DVD-ROM PRODUCT REGARDLESS OF WHETHER SUCH DAMAGES ARE FORESEEABLE OR WHETHER SUCH DAMAGES ARE DEEMED TO RESULT FROM THE FAILURE OR INADEQUACY OF ANY EXCLUSIVE OR OTHER REMEDY.

U.S. GOVERNMENT RESTRICTED RIGHTS The DVD-ROM Product and documentation are provided with restricted rights. Use, duplication or disclosure by the U.S. Government is subject to restrictions as set forth in subparagraphs (a) through (d) of the Commercial Computer Restricted Rights clause at FAR 52.22719 or in subparagraph (c)(1)(ii) of the Rights in Technical Data and Computer Software clause at DFARS 252.2277013, or at 252.2117015, as applicable. Contractor/Manufacturer is Elsevier Inc., 360 Park Avenue South, New York, NY 10010 USA.

GOVERNING LAW This Agreement shall be governed by the laws of the State of New York, USA. In any dispute arising out of this Agreement, You and Elsevier each consent to the exclusive personal jurisdiction and venue in the state and federal courts within New York County, New York, USA.